Efficiency of Health System Units
in Africa

Efficiency of Health System Units in Africa: *A Data Envelopment Analysis*

Edited by

Joses Muthuri Kirigia

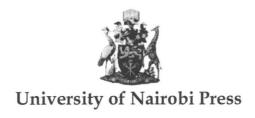

University of Nairobi Press

First Published 2013
University of Nairobi Press
University of Nairobi
P.O. Box 30197, Nairobi – 00100
Kenya

Tel: +254-20-2314316, +254-726-610570

E-mail: **nup@uonbi.ac.ke**   **http://www.uonbi.ac.ke/press**

The University of Nairobi Press supports and promotes University of Nairobi's objectives of discovery, dissemination and preservation of knowledge, and stimulation of intellectual and cultural life by publishing works of the highest quality in association with partners in different parts of the world. In doing so, it adheres to the University's tradition of excellence, innovation, and scholarship.

The moral rights of the editor have been asserted.

University of Nairobi Library CIP Data

RA	Efficiency of health system units in Africa: a data
410	envelopment analysis/ ed. by Joses Muthuri Kirigia. -
.E34	Nairobi : University of Nairobi Press, 2013.
	xxii, 567 p. : ill.

1. Medical economics -- Africa
2. Medical care – Africa – Evaluation
I. Kirigia, Joses Muthuri.   II. Title

ISBN 10-9966 792 15 5
ISBN 13-978 9966 792 15 0

Printed by
Aliki Printers, P.O. Box 9434-00300
Nairobi, Kenya

Contents

List of Figures vii

List of Tables ix

List of Appendices...ix

Preface...xv

Acknowledgements xviii

List of Contributors..xxi

Abbreviations and Acronyms..xxiv

Part I

Health Systems and Economic Theory of Health Service Decision-Making Units

1   Overview of Health Situation in Africa... 3

2   Health Challenges in Africa and the Way Forward....................................... 37

3   Lecture Notes on Efficiency Analysis of Health Systems............................. 43

4   Introduction to Health Services Production and Cost Theory 69

Part II

Application of Data Envelopment Analysis in Health Systems in Africa

5   Technical Efficiency of Public Hospitals and Health Centres in
       Ghana 139

6   Measurement of Technical Efficiency of Public Hospitals in Kenya:
       Using Data Envelopment Analysis 161

7   Using Data Envelopment Analysis to Measure the Technical
       Efficiency of Public Health Centres in Kenya................................. 171

8   Technical Efficiency of Peripheral Health Units in Pujehun District of
       Sierra Leone: *A DEA Application* 185

9   Are Public Hospitals in Kwazulu-Natal Province of South Africa
       Technically Efficient? 203

10   Technical Efficiency of Public Clinics in Kwazulu-Natal Province of South Africa 217

11   Technical Efficiency of Primary Health Units in Kailahun and Kenema Districts of Sierra Leone 239

12   Efficient Management of Health Centres Human Resources in Zambia 267

13   A Performance Assessment Method for Hospitals: *The Case of Municipal Hospitals in Angola* 291

14   A Comparative Assessment of Performance and Productivity of Health Centres in Seychelles 312

15   Productivity Changes in Benin Zone Hospitals: *A nonparametric Malmquist approach* 337

16   Assessment of Productivity of Hospitals in Botswana: *A DEA Application* 367

17   Technical Efficiency, Efficiency Change, Technical Progress, and Productivity Growth Among National Health Systems in African Continent 395

Part III
Case Studies for Developing Skills in Economic Efficiency Analysis

18   Technical Efficiency Analysis: *A Case Study of Muthuleni Health Centres* 419

19   Measurement of Total Cost Efficiency or Economic Efficiency: *A Case Study of Health Centres in the Democratic Republic of Njuri-Ncheke* 451

20   Measurement of Efficiency Change and Productivity Growth: *A Case Study of National Health Systems in the African Union* 479

Part IV
Advancing Knowledge and Skills in Efficiency Analysis using Data Envelopment Analysis

21   Advancing Knowledge and Skills in DEA 507

Glossary 516

Index 519

List of Figures

Figure 3.1   The WHO health system framework.. 44

Figure 3.2   Health promoting schools programme 50

Figure 3.3   Production process for a health institution 51

Figure 3.4   Technical, allocative, and cost efficiencies of a household health education visits programme........................ 54

Figure 3.5   Relative efficiency of health districts in Kibari State with one input and two outputs 58

Figure 4.1   Relationship between number of children immunised and number of nurses at Kathera Health Centre..................... 73

Figure 4.2   Average and marginal product curves for labour 74

Figure 4.3   Alternative combinations of two inputs needed to immunise 2,000 children 76

Figure 4.4   Fixed proportions input-output isoquants when inputs are used in fixed proportions 77

Figure 4.5   Linear isoquants when inputs are perfect substitutes of each other 78

Figure 4.6   Linear programming isoquant 79

Figure 4.7   Smooth convex isoquant 80

Figure 4.8   Isoquant map of a health centre immunisation of children.. 81

Figure 4.9   Health system factor/input intensity... 84

Figure 4.10   Technical efficiency or efficiency of production 85

Figure 4.11   Production in the Edgeworth box to illustrate efficiency in production... 89

Figure 4.12   Health service production possibilities frontier...................... 92

Figure 4.13   Fixed, variable, and total cost of Kathera Health Centre... 96

Figure 4.14   Average fixed cost for Kathera Health Centre 98

Figure 4.15   Average variable cost for Kathera Health Centre..................... 99

Figure 4.16   Average total cost of Kathera Health Centre........................... 100

Figure 4.17   Average and marginal costs of Kathera Health Centre 102

Figure 4.18   Kathera Health Centre long-run average costs as an envelop of short-run average total cost curves 103

Figure 4.19   Kathera Health Centre long-run average cost function 104

Figure 4.20   Kathera Health Centre total cost function 104

Figure 4.21   Kathera Health Centre long-run marginal cost (LMC) function 105

Figure 4.22   Technical efficiency or efficiency of production of a HIV/AIDS prevention community-based programme 107

Figure 4.23   Output-oriented technical efficiency measure of a community-based condom distribution programme 109

Figure 4.24   Community health centre output-oriented technical and allocative efficiencies 110

Figure 4.25   Efficiency frontier graph for 11 health centres in Kenya 115

Figure 4.26   Output distance functions 128

Figure 5.1   Relationship between inputs and the production process and resulting outputs 143

Figure 5.2   DEA Models 144

Figure 5.3   Production possibilities frontier graph 146

Figure 6.1   DEA models 163

Figure 7.1   DEA ratio model 175

Figure 7.2   Input-oriented DEA model 176

Figure 8.1   Relationship between inputs and the production process and resulting outputs 192

Figure 11.1   Relationship between inputs and the production process and resulting outputs outputs 249

Figure 11.2   DEA models 250

Figure 12.1   Health centre technical and allocative efficiencies 273

Figure 14.1   Technical efficiency 316

Figure 14.2   Output-based Malmquist productivity index 320

Figure 15.1   Hospital technical efficiency 341

Figure 17.1   Concept and measurement of technical efficiency 398

Figure 17.2   Frequency distribution of technical efficiency scores of national health systems in Africa (1999-2003) 404

Figure 19.1   Production process for a hospital 454

List of Tables

Table 3.1   Distribution of global health workforce across the six
             WHO regions (2006) 46

Table 3.2   Estimated critical shortages of doctors, nurses, and
             midwives by WHO region (2006) 46

Table 3.3   Relative efficiency of health districts in Kibari State with
             one input and one output 56

Table 3.4   Relative efficiency of health districts in Kibari State with
             one input and two outputs 57

Table 3.5   Technical efficiency of Kibari health districts 63

Table 4.1   Output of children immunised when various numbers of
             nurses are applied to a fixed health centre space of
             300 sq. ft 72

Table 4.2   Average and marginal product of labour (nurses) at
             Kathera Health Centre 74

Table 4.3   Alternative combinations of two inputs that yield the same
             level of total output for a representative health centre 75

Table 4.4   Production function of a health promotion programme 87

Table 4.5   Regression results 88

Table 4.6   Derivation of the production possibility curve 93

Table 4.7   Short-run costs for Kathera Health Centre in Kathera
             dollars (K$) 95

Table 4.8   Derivation of average fixed cost for Kathera Health Centre 97

Table 4.9   Derivation of average variable cost for Kathera Health
             Centre 98

Table 4.10   Derivation of average total cost of Kathera Health Centre 100

Table 4.11   Derivation of marginal cost of Kathera Health Centre 101

Table 4.12   Health centre performance 113

Table 4.13   Input and output data for selected health centres in Kenya 114

Table 4.14   Estimation of technical and scale efficiency among health
             centres with multiple inputs and multiple outputs 119

Table 4.15   Data needs for estimating cost efficiency for selected
             health centres in Zambia 122

Table 4.16   DEAP efficiency summary output 123

Table 4.17   Health systems' inputs and outputs for the Njuri-Ncheke
             Health Centre for 2000 and 2007 125

Table 4.18   Outputs and inputs in selected municipal hospitals in
             Angola 130

Table 4.19   Malmquist index summary of annual means (output oriented) 131

Table 4.20   Malmquist index summary of firm (DMU) means 132

Table 5.1   Illustration of DEA analysis using a hypothetical example of nine hospitals 145

Table 5.2   Means and standard deviations for public hospital inputs and outputs 149

Table 5.3   Technical and scale efficiency scores for district hospitals 150

Table 5.4   Means and standard deviations for public health centre inputs and outputs 151

Table 5.5   Technical and scale efficiency scores for public health centres.. 152

Table 5.6   Total output increases and/or input reductions needed to make inefficient district public hospitals efficient...................... 153

Table 5.7   Total output increases and/or input reductions needed to make inefficient public health centres efficient 154

Table 6.1   Means and standard deviations for public hospitals inputs and outputs... 164

Table 6.2   Technical and scale efficiency scores for public hospitals......... 165

Table 6.3   Total input reductions and/or output increases needed to make inefficient public hospitals efficient................................ 166

Table 6.4   Input reductions and/or output increases needed to make individual inefficient public hospitals efficient 167

Table 7.1   Means and standard deviations for efficient and inefficient health centres... 177

Table 7.2   Technical and scale efficiency scores for health centres 178

Table 7.3   Input reductions and/or output increases needed to make individual inefficient health centres efficient............................. 179

Table 8.1   Functioning PHUs and hospitals... 187

Table 8.2   Estimated number and ratio of health personnel in 2002 188

Table 8.3   Manifestations of inaccessibility to basic health services in Sierra Leone 191

Table 8.4   Means and standard deviations for public PHUs outputs and inputs 193

Table 8.5   Technical and scale efficiency scores for public PHUs.............. 193

Table 8.6   Total output increases needed to make inefficient public PHUs efficient 194

Table 8.7   Ranking of WHO African Region countries on the basis of overall health system goal attainment (out of 191 WHO Member States in 2000) 198

Table 9.1	DEA efficiency rating of general hospitals in Kwazulu-Natal Province	208
Table 9.2	Comparison of Hospital 9 with its efficiency reference set hospitals 23, 25, 26, 48, and 55	209
Table 9.3	Input reductions needed to make inefficient hospitals efficient in Kwazulu-Natal Province	210
Table 10.1	Means and standard deviations for various variables	223
Table 10.2	Distribution of clinics by their technical and scale efficiency scores	224
Table 10.3	Total increases in outputs and input reductions needed to make inefficient clinics efficient	224
Table 12.1	Descriptive statistics (mean and standard deviation) for the inputs and output	277
Table 12.2	Descriptive statistics (mean and standard deviation) of efficiency scores	277
Table 12.3	Frequency distribution of health centres efficiency by ownership	278
Table 12.4	Input reductions (or increases) needed to make individual inefficient health centres efficient	280
Table 18.1	Summary of the health centres' technical efficiency scores	425
Table 18.2	Summary of health centres' efficiency scores	425
Table 18.3	Summary of excess inputs and output deficits	425
Table 19.1	Descriptive statistics for inputs and outputs	458
Table 19.2	Efficiency scores for individual hospitals	459
Table 19.3	Descriptive statistics for efficiency scores	459
Table 19.4	Frequency distribution of hospitals' efficiency by ownership	459
Table 19.5	Output increases needed to make individual inefficient hospitals efficient	460
Table 19.6	Input reductions (or increases) needed to make individual inefficient hospitals efficient	460

List of Appendices

Appendix 1.1   Health in the Millennium Development Goals 26

Appendix 1.2.   Health-related Millennium Development Goals
indicators 27

Appendix 1.3   Global mortality and burden of disease 31

Appendix 1.4   Cause-specific mortality and morbidity 32

Appendix 1.5   Health service coverage 33

Appendix 1.6   Risk factors 34

Appendix 1.7   Health workforce and infrastructure 34

Appendix 1.8   Health expenditure 35

Appendix 10.1   Efficiency score, scale efficiency score and excess
numbers of staff 229

Appendix 10.2   Input reductions needed to make inefficient clinics
efficient 231

Appendix 10.3   Increases in outputs needed to make inefficient clinics
efficient 233

Appendix 10.4   Linear probability regression model results 236

Appendix 10.5   Logistic regression model results 237

Appendix 11.1   Descriptive statistics for community health posts,
maternal, child health and family planning centres,
and community health centres. 261

Appendix 11.2   Technical and scale efficiency scores for maternal,
child health, and family planning clinics 261

Appendix 11.3   Technical and scale efficiency score for community
health centres (CHCs) 262

Appendix 11.4   Technical and scale efficiency score for community
health posts (CHP) 263

Appendix 11.5   Output increases needed to make inefficient maternal
and child health posts efficient 263

Appendix 11.6   Output increases needed to make inefficient
community health centres efficient 264

Appendix 11.7   Output increases needed to make inefficient
community health posts efficient 265

Appendix 12.1   Health centre efficiency scores 283

Appendix 12.2   Summary of cost minimising input quantities 284

Appendix 12.3   Input reductions or increases needed to make
inefficient facilities efficient 285

Appendix 13.1   Descriptive statistics of inputs/outputs 309

Appendix 13.2   Frequency distribution of technical and scale efficiency
                 scores... 309

Appendix 13.3   Total output increases and/or input reductions
                 needed to make inefficient public hospitals efficient............. 310

Appendix 13.4   Malmquist index summary of annual means......................... 310

Appendix 13.5   Malmquist index of hospitals 311

Appendix 14.1   Socio-economic, national health accounts, and health
                 indicators for 2002... 331

Appendix 14.2   Frequency distribution of technical and scale efficiency
                 scores... 332

Appendix 14.3   Health centres' technical and scale efficiency scores
                 during 2001-2002 332

Appendix 14.4   Health centres' technical and scale efficiency scores
                 during 2003-2004 333

Appendix 14.5   Output (input) increases (reductions) needed to make
                 individual inefficient health centres efficient during
                 2001-2002 333

Appendix 14.6   Output (input) increases (reductions) needed to make
                 individual inefficient health centres efficient during
                 2003-2004 334

Appendix 14.7   Output (input) increases (reductions) needed to make
                 inefficient health centres efficient 335

Appendix 14.8   Malmquist index summary of annual means (output
                 oriented) 335

Appendix 14.9   Malmquist index summary of firm means 336

Appendix 15.1   Comparison of health indicators and health services
                 coverage of Benin with averages for the WHO African
                 Region 357

Appendix 15.2   Descriptive statistics of outputs and inputs of Benin
                 hospitals... 358

Appendix 15.3   Frequency distribution of technical and scale efficiency
                 scores... 359

Appendix 15.4   Hospitals' technical and scale efficiency during 2003-
                 2007 360

Appendix 15.5   Output (input) increases (reductions) needed to make
                 individual inefficient hospitals efficient................................... 363

Appendix 15.6   Output (input) increases (reductions) needed to make
                 inefficient hospitals efficient... 364

Appendix 15.7   Malmquist index summary of annual means......................... 364

Appendix 15.8   Malmquist index summary of firm geometric means............ 365

Appendix 16.1   Millennium Development Goals, health, and national
                 health accounts indicators.. 388

Appendix 16.2   Hospital technical and scale efficiency during 2006-
                 2008 390

Appendix 16.3   Output (input) increases (reductions) needed to make
                 individual inefficient hospitals efficient during 2006-
                 2008 391

Appendix 16.4   Total output (input) increases (reductions) needed to
                 make inefficient hospitals efficient 393

Appendix 16.5   Malmquist index summary of annual means (output-
                 oriented) 393

Appendix 16.6   Malmquist index summary of firm means 394

Appendix 17.1   Descriptive statistics of health outcome, per capita
                 health expenditure and adult literacy rate, by year 411

Appendix 17.2   Distribution of technical efficiency scores of national
                 health systems in Africa: 1999-2003 412

Appendix 17.3   Malmquist index summary of annual means (input
                 oriented) 413

Appendix 17.4   Malmquist index summary of annual means (input-
                 oriented) 414

Appendix 18.1   Health centres' inputs and outputs in a hypothetical
                 country called Muthuleni... 428

Appendix 18.2   Listing of the data file EG4.DTA 430

Appendix 18.3   Listing of the instruction file EG4.ins 430

Appendix 18.4   Listing of the output file EG4.OUT.. 431

Appendix 19.1   Health service outputs and inputs of private and
                 public hospitals in Njuri-Ncheke 461

Appendix 19.2   DEAP Data file called "eg4.dta" 469

Appendix 19.3   Listing of instruction file EG4.INS... 473

Appendix 19.4   Listing of output file EG4.OUT 473

Appendix 20.1   Male life expectancy, female life expectancy, per capita
                 total health expenditure, and adult literacy rates for
                 African countries during 1999 to 2003..................................... 485

Appendix 20.2   Listing of Malmquist Data File EG2.DTA 492

Appendix 20.3   Listing of Malmquist instruction file EG2.INS...................... 494

Appendix 20.4   Listing of Malmquist output file EG2.OUT 495

Preface

In May 2006, the African Union (AU) Ministers of Health adopted a decision calling upon all governments in the African continent to institutionalise national health systems (NHS) efficiency monitoring. In 2006, the fifty-sixth session of the World Health Organization (WHO) Regional Committee for Africa (RC56) adopted the health financing strategy for the African Region. The strategy urges Member States to institutionalise efficiency monitoring within their national health management information systems. The intention of both the African Union and the Regional Committee for Africa is to ensure that all current and future health systems resources are put to optimal use to enhance the achievement of national and international health development goals including the United Nations Millennium Development Goals (MDGs).

The aim of this book is to enable the reader acquire knowledge and skills for measuring the economic efficiency of health system decision-making units (DMUs) in the African context. The Data Envelopment Analysis (DEA) tool can assist in the process of identification of best practices relating to the use of health system resources among homogeneous groups of DMUs across the various levels of national health systems. DEA can also help to identify inefficiency in individual DMUs and the sources of such inefficiency. Acquiring this kind of information would be a prerequisite to the process of developing strategies for improving the efficiency of national health systems.

This book combines lecture notes, articles, and case studies to provide the reader with knowledge of the basic theory of health service production and efficiency analysis. The book will help the reader to develop the necessary skills for application of DEA in the measurement of relative economic efficiency of health system DMUs. The book contains fourteen of my previously published articles (with others) that have been reproduced with the permission of the original publishers. Except for alterations to suit the current publisher's presentation style and format and to enhance clarity, the articles appear as in the original publications. These articles are used to illustrate the application of DEA in measuring economic efficiency of actual health system DMUs in various countries in Africa. The book also contains case studies that I have developed and used in capacity strengthening workshops for health economists in various WHO country offices. Workshop participants who have absorbed the lectures and worked through the case studies diligently have been able to use DEA to successfully design and implement economic efficiency analyses of health system DMUs.

The book will be useful to health policy makers, planners, and managers (such as district, provincial, and tertiary hospital directors); university lecturers and students of economics, management science, operations research, medicine, and public health; and economics and public health consultants who require a versatile tool for measuring efficiency and productivity. There has been limited application of DEA in non-health sectors in Africa. However, experiences from Asia, Australia, Europe, and North America indicate that the technique has potential for application in all social and economic sectors in Africa. Indeed, researchers in agriculture, banking, commerce, education, environment, security, transport, and other sectors are encouraged to apply DEA in measurement of performance to guide the development of policies for obviating wastage of scarce resources.

Whereas DEA is a vital "first step" in the relative efficiency analysis of national health systems and their components, its weaknesses should not be overlooked. The limitations of DEA are highlighted in various chapters in the book. The theoretical predictions of DEA of potential efficiency gains may not, for instance, translate into actual gains when factors such as health service quality, fundamental differences between individual DMU's services, and the costs of implementing changes are fully accounted for. The implication is that governments will have to find ways of balancing efficiency benefits against non-efficiency social policy objectives such as equity. Nevertheless, I agree with Professor Anthony J. Culyer (my Ph.D. thesis supervisor at the University of York, UK) that efficiency is not necessarily an enemy of equity. Indeed, efficiency savings can always be used to advance the cause of equity, especially in resource-constrained settings.

STRUCTURE OF THE BOOK

The book consists of 21 chapters organised into four parts.

Part I: Health Systems and Economic Theory of Health Service Decision-Making Units (DMUs). Chapters 1 and 2 provide an introduction of the health development situation and challenges in Africa to enable the reader understand the context for the discussion on efficiency analysis of health system DMUs in subsequent chapters. Chapters 3 and 4 contain lecture notes on the goals and functions of health systems; definition of economic efficiency and the rationale for its measurement; the theory of health services production and cost; and how to measure technical, allocative, and cost efficiency of DMUs.

Part II: Application of DEA in Health Systems in Africa. The object of this part is to demystify measurement of technical efficiency, allocative efficiency, cost efficiency, and total factor productivity. Chapters 5-11 demonstrate the application of DEA in assessing technical efficiency of hospitals and health centres in Ghana, Kenya, Sierra Leone, and South Africa. Chapter 12 shows the application of DEA in analysing allocative and cost efficiency of a sample of private and public health centres in Zambia. In order to monitor the impact of health sector reform on efficiency of health system DMUs over time, it is often necessary to perform total factor productivity analysis. Chapters 13-16 show how Malmquist DEA has been used to decompose total factor productivity into technical efficiency, efficiency change, technical progress, and productivity growth among health facilities in Angola, Benin, Botswana, and Seychelles. Chapter 17 demonstrates the application of Malmquist DEA in estimating technical efficiency, efficiency change, technical progress, and productivity growth among national health systems in continental Africa.

Part III: Case Studies for Skills Development in Economic Efficiency Analysis. Chapters 18-20 contain case studies that are aimed at enabling the reader to develop skills for using DEA in the measurement of technical efficiency, allocative efficiency, cost efficiency, and Malmquist total factor productivity. The reader is encouraged to repeat the case studies as many times as necessary to polish the skills of estimating the efficiency of DMUs and interpreting the results.

Part IV: Continuing Education in Health Systems Efficiency Analysis. Chapter 21 explains how the reader can advance his or her knowledge and skills in efficiency measurement through a number of complementary approaches.

I am optimistic that this book will enable you to acquire the necessary skills for designing and conducting efficiency and productivity change analyses of health and non-health DMUs using Data envelopment analysis. I do hope that this book will encourage you to join the growing army of academics waging intellectual and advocacy "war" against wastage of scarce resources in Africa's social and economic sectors. I welcome your suggestions for improvement of the material presented here for future revisions.

Joses Muthuri Kirigia
Editor

Acknowledgements

I am grateful to my mentor Professor Germano Mwabu for introducing me to econometrics and the interesting sub-discipline of health economics and for continuing to inspire many with his economics articles and books on Africa.

I would like to express my thanks to Professor Gavin Mooney (Chief of Tromso Tribe) of the Aberdeen University (Scotland) and the Curtin University of Technology (Australia) for enrolling me for free in the distant postgraduate diploma course in health economics at the Tromso University (Norway); for introducing me to health economics; and for sharing with me his health economics lecture notes and textbooks. I am grateful to Professor Mooney for reviewing my initial economic evaluation papers that were subsequently published. His continuing academic and advocacy work against wastage of scarce health systems resources and health (and healthcare) inequities have inspired me greatly.

I am indebted to Professor Tony Culyer, my Ph.D. thesis supervisor at the University of York (UK), for the commendable guidance and encouragement throughout the very challenging process of thesis writing; for teaching me that efficiency and equity are not necessarily enemies; for continuing to inspire me through his numerous health economics and social policy articles and books; and for reminding me, when we met at the Inaugural Conference of International Health Economics Association at Vancouver in Canada in 1996, to publish in order to bequeath the knowledge and skills that God has blessed me with to current and future generations.

I would like to thank Dr. Luis Gomes Sambo (WHO/AFRO), Dr. Eyob Zere Asbu (WHO/AFRO), and Dr. Ali Emrouznejad (Aston University, UK) for labouring with me on various health systems DMUs efficiency analyses over the years. The collaboration has greatly enhanced my understanding of the versatility of DEA in cross-sectional and panel analysis of the efficiency of decision-making units.

I thank the publishers who gave me the permission to reproduce some of my previously published articles that constitute fourteen chapters of this book. The following articles are reproduced:

Chapter 2: "Health challenges in Africa and the way forward" from *International Archives of Medicine* 2008;1(27):1-4 by Kirigia JM, Barry SP. Reproduced with permission from BioMed Central.

Chapter 5: "Technical efficiency of public hospitals and health centres in Ghana: a pilot study" from *Cost Effectiveness and Resource Allocation*

2005;3(9):1-13 by Osei D, d'Almeida S, George MO, Kirigia JM, Mensah AO, Kainyu LH. Reproduced with permission from BioMed Central.

Chapter 6: "Measurement of technical efficiency of public hospitals in Kenya: using Data envelopment analysis" from *Journal of Medical Systems* 2002;26(1):39-45 by Kirigia JM, Emrouznejad A, Sambo LG. Reproduced with permission from Plenum Publishing.

Chapter 7: "Using Data envelopment analysis to measure the technical efficiency of public health centres in Kenya" from *Journal of Medical Systems* 2004;28(2):155-166 by Kirigia JM, Emrouznejad A, Sambo LG, Munguti N, Liambila W. Reproduced with permission from Plenum Publishing.

Chapter 8: "Technical efficiency of peripheral health units in Pujehun district of Sierra Leone: a DEA application" from *BMC Health Services Research* 2005;5(77):1-11 by Renner A, Kirigia JM, Zere EA, Barry SP, Kirigia DG, Kamara C, Muthuri LHK. Reproduced with permission from BioMed Central.

Chapter 9: "Are public hospitals in Kwazulu-Natal Province of South Africa technically efficient?" from *African Journal of Health Sciences* 2007;3-4: 25-32 by Kirigia JM, Lambo E, Sambo LG. Reproduced with permission from the Kenya Medical Research Institute (KEMRI).

Chapter 10: "Technical efficiency of public clinics in Kwazulu-Natal Province of South Africa" from *East African Medical Journal* 2001;78(3): S1-S13 by Kirigia JM, Sambo LG, Scheel H. Reproduced with permission from the East African Medical Journal (EAMJ).

Chapter 11: "Technical Efficiency of Primary Health Units in Kailahun and Kenema Districts of Sierra Leone" from *International Archives of Medicine 2011;4(15):1-14* by Kirigia JM, Sambo LG, Renner A, Alemu W, Seasa S, Bah Y. Reproduced with permission from BioMed Central.

Chapter 12: "Efficient management of health centres human resources in Zambia" from *Journal of Medical Systems* 2006;30:473-481 by Masiye F, Kirigia JM, Emrouznejad A, Sambo LG, Mounkaila A, Chimfwembe D, Okello D. Reproduced with permission from Plenum Publishing.

Chapter 13: "A performance assessment method for hospitals: the case of municipal hospitals in Angola" from *Journal of Medical Systems* 2008;32: 509-519 by Kirigia JM, Emrouznejad A, Cassoma B, Asbu EZ, Barry SP. Reproduced with permission from Plenum Publishing.

Chapter 14: "A comparative assessment of performance and productivity of health centres in Seychelles" from *International Journal of Productivity and Performance Management* 2008;57(1):72-92 by Kirigia JM, Emrouznejad A,

Vaz RG, Bastiene H, Padayachy J. Reproduced with permission from Emerald Group Publishing.

Chapter 15: "Productivity changes in Benin Zone hospitals: a nonparametric Malmquist approach" from *African Journal of Health Economics* 2011; 3: 1-13. Reproduced with permission from West African Health Economics Network.

Chapter 16: "Assessment of productivity of hospitals in Botswana: a DEA application" from *International Archives of Medicine* 2010;3(27):1-20 by Naomi Tlotlego, Justice Nonvignon, Luis G. Sambo, Eyob Z. Asbu, Joses M. Kirigia. Reproduced with permission from BioMed Central.

Chapter 17: "Technical efficiency, efficiency change, technical progress and productivity growth in the national health systems of continental African countries" from *Eastern Africa Social Science Research Review* 2007;23(2): 19-40 by Kirigia JM, Asbu EZ, Greene W, Emrouznejad A. Reproduced with permission from Organisation for Social Science Research in Eastern and Southern Africa (OSSREA).

Finally, I am grateful to my wife Lenity Honesty Kainyu Muthuri and daughter Rose-nabi Deborah Karimi Muthuri for their love, encouragement, unwavering support, and prayers during the entire process of putting this book together. I am indebted to my parents Josphat Kirigia M'Aburi and Rose Gakii Kirigia for making an indelible impression upon me that reverence of God and a good education are the keys to human prosperity. Lastly, I am immensely grateful to my heavenly father *Jehovah Jireh* for meeting all my household needs during the entire process of writing this book.

List of Contributors

Abdou Bilo Mounkaila	United States Agency for International Development, Maputo, Mozambique
Ade Renner	World Health Organization Country Office, Freetown, Sierra Leone
Ali Emrouznejad	Aston University, Aston, UK
Ayaye Omar Mensah	World Health Organization Regional Office for Africa, Brazzaville, Congo
Bassilio Cassoma	Formerly with the Ministry of Health, Luanda, Angola
Chris Ngenda Mwikisa	World Health Organization Regional Office for Africa, Brazzaville, Congo
Clifford Kamara	Formerly with the Ministry of Health, Freetown, Sierra Leone
Daniel Osei	Ministry of Health, Accra, Ghana
David Okello	World Health Organization Country Office, Nairobi, Kenya
Davis Chimfwembe	Ministry of Health, Lusaka, Zambia
Doris Gatwiri Kirigia	University of New South Wales, Sydney, Australia
Eitayo Lambo	Formerly Minister for Health with the Ministry of Health, Abuja, Nigeria
Eyob Zere Asbu	World Health Organization Regional Office for Africa, Harare, Zimbabwe
Felix Masiye	Department of Economics, University of Zambia, Lusaka, Zambia
Helger Scheel	University of Dortmund, Germany
Henry Bastiene	World Health Organization Country Office, Seychelles
Joses Muthuri Kirigia	World Health Organization Regional Office for Africa, Brazzaville, Congo
Jude Padayachy	Ministry of Health, Seychelles
Justice Nonvignon	School of Public Health, University of Ghana, Legon, Ghana
Lenity Honesty Kainyu	African Health Education and Economics Research Associates, Nairobi, Kenya
Luis Gomes Sambo	World Health Organization Regional Office for Africa, Brazzaville, Congo
Melvin George	Formerly with the World Health Organization Country Office, Accra, Ghana
Naomi Tlotlego	Department of Economics, University of Botswana, Gaborone, Botswana

Nzoya Munguti	Ministry of Health, Nairobi, Kenya
Patrick Makoudode	IRSP, Cotonou, Benin
Rui Gama Vaz	World Health Organization Regional Office for Africa, Brazzaville, Congo
Saidou Pathe Barry	World Health Organization Regional Office for Africa, Brazzaville, Congo
Sellassie D'Almeida	World Health Organization Country Office, Accra, Ghana
Santigie Seasay	Ministry of Health and Sanitation, Freetown, Sierra Leone
Yankuba Bah	Ministry of Health and Sanitation, Freetown, Sierra Leone
William Greene	New York University, New York, USA
Wilson Liambila	Ministry of Health, Nairobi, Kenya
Wondi Alemu	World Health Organization Country Office, Freetown, Sierra Leone
Abdou Bilo Mounkaila	United States Agency for International Development, Maputo, Mozambique
Ade Renner	World Health Organization Country Office, Freetown, Sierra Leone
Ali Emrouznejad	Aston University, Aston, UK
Ayaye Omar Mensah	World Health Organization Regional Office for Africa, Brazzaville, Congo
Bassilio Cassoma	Formerly with the Ministry of Health, Luanda, Angola
Chris Ngenda Mwikisa	World Health Organization Regional Office for Africa, Brazzaville, Congo
Clifford Kamara	Formerly with the Ministry of Health, Freetown, Sierra Leone
Daniel Osei	Ministry of Health, Accra, Ghana
David Okello	World Health Organization Country Office, Nairobi, Kenya
Davis Chimfwembe	Ministry of Health, Lusaka, Zambia
Doris Gatwiri Kirigia	University of New South Wales, Sydney, Australia
Eitayo Lambo	Formerly Minister for Health with the Ministry of Health, Abuja, Nigeria
Eyob Zere Asbu	World Health Organization Regional Office for Africa, Harare, Zimbabwe
Felix Masiye	Department of Economics, University of Zambia, Lusaka, Zambia
Helger Scheel	University of Dortmund, Germany
Henry Bastiene	World Health Organization Country Office, Seychelles

Joses Muthuri Kirigia	World Health Organization Regional Office for Africa, Brazzaville, Congo
Jude Padayachy	Ministry of Health, Seychelles
Justice Nonvignon	School of Public Health, University of Ghana, Legon, Ghana
Lenity Honesty Kainyu	African Health Education and Economics Research Associates, Nairobi, Kenya
Luis Gomes Sambo	World Health Organization Regional Office for Africa, Brazzaville, Congo
Melvin George	Formerly with the World Health Organization Country Office, Accra, Ghana
Naomi Tlotlego	Department of Economics, University of Botswana, Gaborone, Botswana
Nzoya Munguti	Ministry of Health, Nairobi, Kenya
Patrick Makoudode	IRSP, Cotonou, Benin
Rui Gama Vaz	World Health Organization Regional Office for Africa, Brazzaville, Congo
Saidou Pathe Barry	World Health Organization Regional Office for Africa, Brazzaville, Congo
Sellassie D'Almeida	World Health Organization Country Office, Accra, Ghana
Santigie Seasay	Ministry of Health and Sanitation, Freetown, Sierra Leone
Yankuba Bah	Ministry of Health and Sanitation, Freetown, Sierra Leone
William Greene	New York University, New York, USA
Wilson Liambila	Ministry of Health, Nairobi, Kenya
Wondi Alemu	World Health Organization Country Office, Freetown, Sierra Leone

Abbreviations and Acronyms

AE	allocative efficiency
AU	African Union
CAEHSP	Council for Assessment and Enhancement of Health Systems Performance
CAMHS	child and adolescent mental health service
CBoH	Central Board of Health
CE-	cost efficiency
CEPA	Centre for Efficiency and Productivity Analysis
CHC	community health centre
CHO	community health officer
CHP	community health post
CMTE	Centre for Management of Technology and Entrepreneurship
CRS	constant returns to scale
CRSTE	constant returns to scale technical efficiency
DALE	disability-adjusted life years
DEA	data envelopment analysis
DHBs	district health boards
DHMBs	district health management boards
DHMTs	district health management teams
DMUs	decision-making units
DOTS	directly observed treatment short course
DRC	Democratic Republic of Congo
DRS	decreasing returns to scale
ECA	Economic Commission for Africa
EFFCH	efficiency change
EMS	Efficiency Measurement Systems
ERS	efficiency reference set
FDH	Free Disposal Hall
FHGs	family health groups
FHN	family health networks
FHSA	family health service authorities
FLE	female life expectancy
FTE	full-time equivalent
GBP	Great Britain Pound

GDP	gross domestic product
GNHI	Ghana National Health Insurance
GNI	gross national income
HALE	health-adjusted life expectancy
HCs	health centres
HDI	human development index
HEWs	health extension workers
HHCs	hospital health centres
HIV/AIDS	Human Immuno-Deficiency Virus/ Acquired Immune Deficiency Syndrome
HMB	Hospital Management Board
HMIS	Health Management Information System
HSOs	health service organisations
IEC	Information, Education and Communication
IMCI	Integrated Management of Childhood Illness
IMF	International Monetary Fund
IRS	increasing returns to scale
LPM	linear probability model
MCH	maternal and child health
MCHP	maternal and child health post
MDGS	Millennium Development Goals
MLE	male life expectancy
MMR	maternal mortality ratio
MoH	Ministry of Health
MoHS	Ministry of Health and Sanitation
MPI	Malmquist productivity index
MPSS	most productive scale size
MTFP	Malmquist total factor productivity index
MTHS	medium-term health strategy
NEPAD	New Partnership for Africa's Development
NGO	Non-governmental Organisation
NHA	national health accounts
NHS	national health systems
NHSSP	National Health Sector Strategic Plan
NPHIS	non-profit health insurance schemes
ORT	oral rehydration therapy

OSSREA	Organisation for Social Science Research in Eastern and Southern Africa
PCTHE	per capita total health expenditure
PECH/PEFFCH	pure efficiency change
PF	production function
PHC	Primary Health Care
PHUs	public health units
PMTCT	prevention of mother-to-child transmission
PNC	postnatal care
QALY	quality-adjusted life years
QC	quality change
SD/STDEV	standard deviation
SE	scale efficiency
SECH/SCH	scale efficiency change
SECHNs	state enrolled community health nurses
SERC	Scientific and Ethical Review Committee
SSA	sub-Saharan Africa
TE	technical efficiency
TECHCH/TECH	technical change
TEE	total economic efficiency
TFP	total factor productivity
TQIP	Taiwan Quality Indicator Project
UNDP	United Nations Development Programme
UNICEF	United Nations Children's Fund
VRS	variable returns to scale
VRSTE	variable returns to scale technical efficiency
WHA	World Health Assembly
WHO AFR	WHO African Region
WHO AMR	WHO Region of the Americas
WHO EMR	WHO Eastern Mediterranean Region
WHO EUR	WHO European Region
WHO SEAR	WHO South-East Asia Region
WHO WPR	WHO Westerm Pacific Region
WHO	World Health Organization
WHO/AFRO	World Health Organization Regional Office for Africa
WHR	World Health Report

Part I

Health Systems and Economic Theory of
Health Service Decision-Making Units

Learning Objectives

By the end of Part 1 you should have a good understanding of the following issues:

1. Current health situation in Africa.

2. Health challenges in Africa.

3. Health system building blocks and goals.

4. Motivation for efficiency analysis of health facilities.

5. Concepts of production and cost functions for single and multiple product health system DMUs.

6. Differences between technical efficiency, allocative efficiency, cost efficiency, and Malmquist total factor productivity.

7. How to measure technical efficiency, allocative efficiency, cost efficiency, and Malmquist total factor productivity of health system DMUs.

-1-

Overview of Health Situation in Africa

Joses Muthuri Kirigia

INTRODUCTION

This chapter gives an overview of Africa's performance in health-related indicators of the Millennium Development Goals (MDGs) and other indicators of global health including mortality and morbidity, health service coverage, risk factors, health workforce and infrastructure, and health expenditure. The chapter compares the performance of the African Region (AFR) with that of the other five regions of the World Health Organization (WHO) namely Region of the Americas (AMR), Western Pacific Region (WPR), European Region (EUR), South-East Asia Region (SEAR) and Eastern Mediterranean Region (EMR). This comparison will enable the reader to appreciate the enormity of the African region's disease burden and unmet health needs vis a vis the scarcity of health systems resources.

HEALTH-RELATED MILLENNIUM DEVELOPMENT GOALS

Health is at the heart of the MDGs [1]. Three of the eight MDGs specifically focus on health: Goal 4, reduce child mortality; Goal 5, reduce maternal mortality; and Goal 6, combat HIV/AIDS, malaria, and other diseases (Appendix 1.1). However, it will be impossible to achieve the health goals in the African Region (AFR) without making progress in such critical areas as food security, gender equality, empowerment of women, wider access to education, better housing, adequate water and sanitation, and better environmental stewardship thereby underlining the importance of addressing hunger and extreme poverty as well as the promotion of environmental sustainability as articulated in goals 1 and 7 respectively. According to the sixty-second World Health Assembly - Looking to 2015 and Beyond - the challenges presented by weak health systems, epidemiological transition from communicable to non-communicable diseases, demographic transition to relatively lower fertility and mortality rates, and emerging health threats such as pandemic Influenza H1N1 and Ebola will become more prominent in the AFR [2,3].

Reducing Child Mortality

The indicators for MDG 4 on reducing child mortality are under-five mortality rate, infant mortality rate, the proportion of one-year-old children immunised against measles, and percentage of under-five children receiving treatment for acute respiratory infections and diarrhoea.

Under-five mortality rate

In 2007, the under -five mortality rate per 1,000 live births was less than 51 in 5 countries of AFR; 51-100 in 10 countries; 101-150 in 17 countries; and over 150 in the remaining 14 countries of the region [4]. Thus, 67 per cent of the countries in AFR had an under-five mortality rate exceeding 100 per 1,000 live births. The under-five mortality rate for AFR exceeded that of AMR by 7.6 times, that of EUR by 9.7 times, that of EMR by 1.8 times, that of SEAR by 2.2 times, and that of WPR by 6.6 times. Seychelles experienced the lowest under-five mortality rate (16 per 1,000 live births) in AFR while Sierra Leone had the highest (262 per 1,000 live births). The range of the under-five mortality rate values was 246 in AFR, 70 in AMR, 65 in EUR, 249 in EMR, 106 in SEAR, and 88 in WPR. The average under-five mortality rate of 145 per 1,000 live births in AFR was the highest among the WHO regions (Appendix 1.2). In 2007, the AFR average measles immunisation coverage among one-year-olds was comparable to that of SEAR but lower than those recorded in AMR, EUR, EMR, and WPR. The difference between the maximum and minimum immunisation coverage (i.e., the range) was also higher in AFR than the other five regions. The low immunisation coverage might partially account for the relatively high under-five mortality rate.

In 2004, the average neonatal mortality ratio varied from a maximum of 40 to a minimum of 20 per 1,000 live births in AFR and EUR respectively (Appendix 1.3). The average neonatal mortality ratio for AFR was higher than that of AMR by 29; EUR by 30; EMR by 2; SEAR by 5; and WPR by 23 [4]. In 2004, neonatal conditions were responsible for 21% of the total number of deaths among children under five years of age in AFR; HIV/AIDS accounted for 5% of the deaths in this category; diarrhoea, 16.3%; measles, 3.9%; malaria, 15.6%; pneumonia, 20.4%; injuries, 2.4%; and other causes, 15.4% [5]. During the same year, neonatal conditions were the leading cause of death among children below five years of age in all the WHO regions of the world (Appendix 1.4).

A negative correlation exists between neonatal mortality rates and coverage of neonatal tetanus immunisation. In 2007, the percentage of neonates protected, through vaccination at birth, against neonatal tetanus varied from a maximum of 59% in SEAR to a minimum of 10% in EUR. Only one-third of neonates in AFR are protected against neonatal tetanus at birth. In 2008, an estimated 309,649 children in AFR died of childhood vaccine-preventable diseases such as pertussis (28.5%), poliomyelitis (0.1%), diphtheria (0.6%), measles (51.3%), and tetanus (19.5%) [5].

Infant mortality rate

The average infant mortality rate (i.e., probability of dying between birth and age 1 per 1,000 live births) varied from 88 to 13 deaths per 1,000 live births in AFR and EUR respectively. The average infant mortality rate for AFR, which was the highest globally, was higher than for AMR by 72 deaths; EUR by 75 deaths; EMR by 28 deaths; SEAR by 39 deaths; and WPR by 69 deaths [4].

Immunisation

Many children in the AFR are not fully immunised against vaccine-preventable diseases such as measles, hepatitis B, pertussis, tetanus, polio, diphtheria, yellow fever, rotavirus, meningococcus, and pneumococcus among others. For example, in 2007 nine countries of the AFR had measles immunisation coverage of 91-99% among one-year-olds; eleven countries had coverage of 81-90%; eight countries had coverage of 71-80%; thirteen countries had coverage of 61-70%; and four countries had coverage of 61% and below. Rwanda, Seychelles, Mauritius, Eritrea, Ghana, and Liberia had measles immunisation coverage of 95% and above [4]. The measles immunisation coverage was 71% and above in 62% of the countries in the AFR.

In 2007, immunisation coverage among one-year-olds was 74% for measles and DPT3; 69% for HepB3; and 34% for Hib3 in AFR. Globally, measles immunisation coverage ranged from a maximum of 93 in AMR to a minimum of 73% in SEAR; DPT3 coverage varied from a maximum of 96% in EUR to a minimum of 69% in SEAR; HepB3 coverage ranged from 88% in AMR to 30% in SEAR; and Hib3 coverage ranged from 91% in AMR to 3% in WPR. The proportion of children aged 6-59 months who received vitamin A supplementation was 47.9% in AFR; 38.9% in SEAR; and 34.7% in WPR [4]. Comparing measles vaccine coverage across the WHO regions, SEAR had the lowest coverage followed by AFR, EMR, WPR, AMR, and EUR. The AFR had the greatest variation in measles immunisation coverage among infants (Appendix 1.5).

Prevention and treatment of acute respiratory infections and diarrhoea

While only 36.9% of under-five children with symptoms of acute respiratory infections (ARI) were taken to a health facility in AFR; 63.2% and 62.3% of children manifesting ARI symptoms in EMR and SEAR respectively were taken to a health facility (Appendix 1.5). Generally, the proportion of under-five children who received oral rehydration therapy (ORT) for diarrhoea was low in various WHO regions (e.g., 35.7% in AFR, 47.3% in EMR, and 34.7% in SEAR) [4].

The Integrated Management of Childhood Illness (IMCI), the major strategy for reducing child morbidity and mortality in the African region, is being implemented in 44 of the 46 Member States of AFR. The Regional Child Survival Strategy developed by WHO, UNICEF, and the World Bank builds upon and broadens the IMCI approach [6]. It advocates for the scaled-up implementation of cost-effective interventions including newborn care; infant and young child feeding including micronutrient supplementation; prevention of malaria using insecticide-treated nets; immunisation; management of common childhood illnesses; prevention of mother-to-child transmission of HIV, and care and treatment of HIV-exposed or infected children.

Improving Maternal Health

The MDG 5 aims to improve maternal health. One of the two targets of this goal is to reduce by three quarters, between 1990 and 2015, the maternal mortality ratio. The two indicators of this target are maternal mortality ratio (MMR) and the proportion of births attended by skilled health personnel. The second target of MDG 5 is to have achieved universal access to reproductive health by 2015. The indicators for this target are contraceptive prevalence rate; adolescent birth rate; antenatal care coverage (at least one visit and at least four visits); and unmet need for family planning.

In 2005, eight countries of the AFR had an MMR of less than 401 per 100,000 live births; thirteen countries had 401-800; twelve countries had 800-1,000; and eleven countries had an MMR of over 1,000 per 100,000 live births [4]. Thus, 25% of the countries of the AFR had a very high average MMR of over 1,000 although this index varied from a minimum of 15 in Mauritius to a maximum of 2,100 in Sierra Leone. The MMR of AFR was 33 times higher than that of EUR, 11 times that of WPR, 9 times that of AMR, and 2 times that of EMR and SEAR (see Appendix 1.2).

In 2008, a number of health conditions resulted in 229,238 maternal deaths in AFR as follows: maternal haemorrhage (23.8%), maternal sepsis (11.7%), hypertensive disorders (8.6%), obstructed labour (5.2%), abortion (13.8%), and other maternal conditions (36.9%). In AFR, perinatal conditions caused 988,943 deaths including prematurity and low birth weight (31.6%), birth asphyxia and birth trauma (29.2%), and neonatal infections and other conditions (39.2%) [5].

In 2005, skilled personnel attended to less than 46% of births in eight countries in AFR (see Appendix 1.2). Skilled personnel attended 41-50% of births in ten countries; 51-60% of births in nine countries; 61 -70% of births in six countries; and more than 70% of births in twelve countries [4]. The proportion of births attended by skilled personnel varied from 6% in Ethiopia to 99% in Mauritius. Worldwide, the AFR had the lowest percentage of births attended by skilled personnel compared to the other WHO regions. The highest coverage of births attended by skilled health personnel occurred in EUR at about 96% while AFR had the lowest coverage at about 46%. There is a high correlation between maternal mortality ratio and attendance of skilled health personnel during birth [7, 8]. Thus, the African region, which has the lowest attendance of skilled personnel during birth in the world also has the highest maternal mortality ratio.

Contraceptive prevalence rate

In 2006, the contraceptive prevalence rate in AFR was less than 10% in 9 countries, 10-20% in 9 countries, 21-30% in 9 countries, 31-40% in 5 countries, 41-50% in 5 countries, and over 50% in 5 countries [4]. On average contraceptive prevalence rate is very low in the AFR varying from about 76% in Mauritius to 3% in Chad. In terms of regional comparisons, the average contraceptive prevalence is lowest in AFR with 24.4% followed by EMR with 43%, SEAR with 57.2%, AMR with 70%, and WPR with 85.5% (see Appendix 1.5).

Adolescent fertility rate

The adolescent fertility rate per 1000 girls aged 15-19 years was less than 50 in four countries; 50-100 in thirteen countries; 101-150 in seventeen countries; and over 150 in ten countries [4]. The African region's average adolescent fertility rate of 117 was 11 times that of WPR; 5 times that of EUR; 3 times that of EMR; and 2 times that of AMR and SEAR.

Antenatal care coverage

In 2007, the antenatal care coverage of at least one visit was less than 50% in three countries; 50-70% in four countries; 70-90% in twenty-three countries; and over 90% in fourteen countries of the AFR. The average antenatal care coverage in AFR was 73% [4]. However, this index varied from a maximum of 98% in Cape Verde to a minimum of 28% in Ethiopia. The average antenatal care coverage in the other WHO regions was 51% in EMR, 74% in SEAR, 89% in WPR, and 94% in AMR. All the WHO regions have antenatal care coverage of over 60% for the first visit [4,5]. However, antenatal care coverage declines dramatically by the fourth visit. For example, in AFR and EMR only 45% of pregnant mothers made four visits to an antenatal care clinic but SEAR recorded even lower coverage of only 42%. The AMR had the highest coverage of both first and fourth antenatal clinic visits (Appendix 1.5).

Unmet need for family planning

In 2007, AFR's unmet need for family planning was less than 20% in six countries; 20-30% in sixteen countries; and 31-41% in seven countries [4]. The average unmet need for family planning was 24.4% in AFR and varied widely from a maximum of 40.6% in Uganda to a minimum of 3.3% in Mauritius. Similarly, contraceptive use prevalence ranged from a maximum of 85.5% in WPR to a minimum of 24.4% in AFR. The prevalence of contraceptive use in AFR was 46 percentage points lower than in AMR; 19 percentage points lower than in EMR; 33 percentage points lower than in SEAR; and 61 percentage points lower than in WPR (see Appendix 1.5).

In 2005, the World Health Assembly adopted a resolution entitled "Working towards universal coverage of maternal, newborn and child health interventions" [9]. Additionally, the WHO Regional Committee for Africa's "Roadmap for accelerating the attainment of the millennium development goals (MDGs) related to maternal and newborn health in Africa" [10] outlines the interventions that Member States should implement to curb maternal, newborn, and child mortality.

Combating HIV/AIDS, Malaria and Other Diseases

The three indicators related to HIV/AIDS under MDG 6 on combating HIV/AIDS, malaria, and other diseases include HIV prevalence among pregnant women aged 15-24 years; condom use rate of the contraceptive prevalence rate; and ratio of school attendance of orphans to school attendance of non-orphans aged 10-14 years [1]. In 2005, the estimated number of adults and children living with HIV/AIDS in Africa was 29,973,851. In the same year, about 2,732,397 people lost their lives to AIDS-related illness on the continent [5].

Prevalence of HIV

In 2007 the prevalence of HIV among adults aged ≥15 years per 100,000 of the population was less than 1,000 in seven countries in AFR; 1,001-2,000 in thirteen countries; 2001-4,000 in seven countries; 4,001-6,000 in five countries; and 11,367-24,301 in nine countries [4,5]. The average prevalence of HIV in AFR was 4,735 but varied widely from less than 40 in Comoros to 24,301 in Swaziland (see Appendix 1.2). Comparatively, the average HIV prevalence was highest in AFR compared to the other regions.

The high prevalence of HIV in AFR is partly attributed to dearth of comprehensive correct knowledge of HIV/AIDS. For example, in 2007 the proportion of males aged 15-24 years with comprehensive correct knowledge of HIV/AIDS was greater than 40% in five countries; 31-40% in eleven countries; 20-30% in eight countries; and less than 20% in four countries [4].

The average proportion of males aged 15-24 years with comprehensive correct knowledge of HIV prevalence in AFR was 30% with a maximum of 62% in Namibia and a minimum of 16% in Niger. Similarly, the proportion of females aged 15-24 years with comprehensive correct knowledge of HIV/AIDS in the AFR was greater than 40% in six countries; 31-40% in six countries; 20-30% in ten countries; and less than 20% in sixteen countries.

In 2007, the average proportion of females with comprehensive correct knowledge of HIV prevalence in AFR was 23% varying from a maximum of 65% in Namibia to a minimum of 4% in Equatorial Guinea. The average proportion of females with comprehensive correct knowledge of HIV was only 21% in SEAR. Information regarding this indicator was unavailable for other WHO regions. The high HIV prevalence in AFR could also be attributed to low percentage (19%) of young women and men (24%) aged 15-49 years who had more than one sexual partner in the past 12 months and who reported the use of a condom during their last sexual intercourse.

Antiretroviral therapy coverage among people with advanced HIV infection in AFR was greater than 50% in four countries; 41-50% in five countries; 31-40% six countries; 20-30% in seventeen countries; and less than 20% in ten countries [4]. In AFR the average coverage of antiretroviral therapy was 30% with a maximum of 88% in Namibia and a minimum of 4% in Madagascar. The average coverage of antiretroviral therapy in other regions was as follows: 5% in EMR, 17% in EUR, 25% in SEAR, 28% in WPR, and 62% in AMR (Appendix 1.5).

In 2007, the coverage of 34% of prevention of mother-to-child transmission (PMTCT) antiretroviral therapy among pregnant women in AFR was higher than in EMR (1%), SEAR (24%), and WPR (13%). However, PMTCT coverage of the AFR was lower than that of AMR (36%) and EUR (71%) [4]. During the same year, the coverage of antiretroviral therapy among people with advanced HIV infection was 30% in AFR; which was higher than that of all other WHO regions except AMR. The World Health Assembly resolutions [11,12] and the WHO African Region resolutions [13] outline strategies for accelerating, scaling-up, and sustaining adequate response to the HIV/AIDS epidemic.

Contraceptive prevalence rate

On average, contraceptive prevalence rate is very low in the AFR and varies from about 76% in Mauritius to 3% in Chad. In 2007, the contraceptive prevalence rate in AFR was less than 10%, 10-20%, and 21-30% in nine countries each while it was 31-40%, 41-50%, and over 50% in five countries each [4]. In terms of regional comparisons, the average contraceptive prevalence during the 2002-2006 period was lowest in AFR with 24.4%

followed by EMR with 43%, SEAR with 57.2%, AMR with 70%, and WPR with 85.5% (see Appendix 1.5).

Malaria mortality rate and treatment

In 2008, malaria resulted in a total of 724,900 deaths in the AFR. The malaria mortality rate per 100,000 of the population in AFR was less than 50 and 50-100 in eleven countries each; 101-150 in ten countries; and 151-229 in eleven countries [5]. During the same year, the average malaria mortality rate in AFR was 104 per 100,000 of the population. It ranged from 0 in Algeria to 229 per 100,000 of the population in Niger. The average malaria mortality rates were less than 1 per 100,000 of the population in AMR and WPR; 1 per 100,000 of the population in EMR; and 2 per 100,000 in SEAR. Thus, the average malaria mortality rate for AFR exceeded that of the other WHO regions by more than 100 times.

The most cost-effective preventive intervention against malaria infection in endemic areas is the use of insecticide-treated bed nets [6]. In AFR, the proportion of children under the age of five years sleeping under insecticide-treated bed nets was less than 10% in fifteen countries; 10-20% in nine countries; 21-30% in four countries; and over 30% in six countries [4]. The average proportion of children under five years sleeping under insecticide-treated bed nets was 14% in AFR; which varied from 0% in Swaziland to 56% in Niger.

In AFR, the proportion of children aged less than five years who received antimalarial treatment for fever was greater than 60% in four countries; 51-60% in seven countries; 41-50% in six countries; 31-40% and 20-30% in seven countries each; and less than 20% in six countries [4]. In AFR, the average proportion of under-fives who received any antimalarial treatment for fever was 36% from a maximum of 63% in Comoros and Gambia to a minimum of 4% in Eritrea. Comparatively, the average proportion of the under-five children who received any antimalarial treatment for fever in SEAR was 10%. The proportion varied from a maximum of 47% in Timor-Leste to a minimum of 1% in Indonesia.

The 2005 United Nations General Assembly resolution entitled "2001-2010: decade to roll back malaria in developing countries, particularly Africa", calls upon the international community to meet the financial needs of the Global Fund to Fight AIDS, Tuberculosis and Malaria (GFATM) through country-led initiatives to create conditions for insecticide-treated mosquito nets, insecticides for indoor residual spraying for malaria control, and effective antimalarial combination treatments to be fully accessible, including free distribution of such nets where appropriate. The resolution appeals to the international community to assist states, in particular malaria-endemic countries, to implement sound national plans to control malaria in a sustained and equitable way that contributes to health system development [14]. The Roll Back Malaria Partnership global strategic plan for roll-back malaria: 2005-2015 [15] details the actions that malaria-endemic countries ought to implement to prevent and control the disease.

Tuberculosis-related mortality and treatment under DOTS

In 2007, the WHO recorded a total of 1,251,737 new and relapse cases of tuberculosis from AFR countries. During the same year a total of 734,890 tuberculosis-related deaths were reported from the region [5]. In 2007, the prevalence of TB was highest in AFR at 475 per 100,000 of the population and lowest in AMR at 38 per 100,000 of the population [4]. The prevalence of TB in AFR was 437 higher than in AMR; 424 higher than in EUR; 336 higher than in EMR; 195 higher than in SEAR; and 278 higher than in WPR. In the same year, the AFR had the highest incidence of tuberculosis estimated at 363 per 100,000 of the population, which is 331 higher than AMR; 314 higher than EUR; 258 higher than EMR; 182 higher than SEAR; and 255 higher than WPR.

The tuberculosis detection rate under DOTS ranged from a maximum of 77% in WPR to a minimum of 47% in AFR in 2007 [4]. The AFR detection rate was 26% lower than that of AMR; 4% lower than EUR; 13% lower than EMR; 22% lower than SEAR; and 30% lower than WPR. In AFR, tuberculosis treatment success under DOTS was over 90% in two countries; 71-90% in twenty-five countries; 51-70% in seven countries; and less than 51% in four countries. The average tuberculosis treatment success under DOTS was 75% in AFR ranging from a maximum of 92% in Mauritius to 18% in Angola. Comparatively, the average tuberculosis treatment success rate under DOTS was 75% in AMR; 70% in EUR; 86% in EMR; 87% in SEAR; and 92% in WPR. The African Region's tuberculosis treatment success rate under DOTS was equal to that of AMR but lower than that of EMR, SEAR, and WPR. The WHO tuberculosis programme framework for effective tuberculosis control [16] and the expanded DOTS framework for effective tuberculosis control [17] contain the interventions that endemic countries need to implement to curb tuberculosis (see Appendix 1.5).

Non-communicable diseases and injuries

In AFR in 2004, 80% of years of life lost resulted from communicable diseases; 13% from non-communicable diseases (NCD); and 7% from injuries. However, in AMR, EMR, and WPR over 54% of years of life lost are caused by non-communicable diseases. In 2008, about 3,039,220 deaths resulted from non-communicable diseases in the AFR and were attributed to various causes as follows: cardiovascular diseases (41.58%), malignant neoplasms or cancers (18.04%) respiratory diseases (11.24%), digestive diseases (7.37%), diabetes mellitus (6.43%), neuropsychiatric conditions (4.39%), genitourinary diseases

(3.54%), congenital anomalies (3.16%), endocrine disorders (2.33%), and other NCDs (1.92%) [5]. In the same year, a total of 852,072 deaths resulted from injuries; 65.4% from unintentional injuries, and 34.6% from intentional injuries [5].

Compared to the other WHO regions, AFR had the highest age-standardised mortality rate due to non-communicable diseases of 841 per 100,000 of the population and AMR the least with 499 deaths per 100,000 of the population. The mortality rate of AFR from non-communicable diseases was 342 higher than that of AMR; 251 higher than EUR; 51 higher than EMR; 140 higher than SEAR; and 284 higher than WPR. The highest cardiovascular-related mortality of 458 per 100,000 of the population occurred in EMRO while the least, at 202 deaths per 100,000 of the population occurred in AMR. The cardiovascular-related mortality of the EMR was higher than that of AFR by 68 deaths; AMR by 256 deaths; EUR by 126 deaths; SEAR by 93 deaths; and WPR by 215 deaths. The AFR had the highest age-standardised cancer mortality rate of 147 per 100,000 of the population while EMR had the lowest estimated at 101 per 100,000 of the population. Intentional and unintentional injuries were another major cause of premature mortality. For example, SEAR had the highest injury-related mortality of 131 per 100,000 of the population while AMR had the lowest at 66 per 100,000 of the population. The injury-related mortality reported in AFR of 126 per 100,000 of the population was the second highest globally.

Some of the non-communicable disease burden could be attributed to excessive consumption of alcohol and the use of tobacco. For instance, alcohol consumption among adults aged ≥ 15 years varied from a minimum of 0.19 litres per person per year in EMR to a maximum of 8.84 litres per person per year in EUR. The prevalence of current tobacco use ranged from a minimum of 10.6% in AFR to a maximum of 35.3% in EUR. Also, the prevalence of current tobacco use among adolescents (13-15 years) varied from a minimum of 7.3% in WPR to 22.3% in AMR (Appendix 1.6).

At the global level, the WHO World Health Assembly resolution WHA32.40 on development of the WHO programme on alcohol-related problems [18]; WHA36.12 on alcohol consumption and alcohol-related problems: development of national policies and programmes [19]; WHA42.20 on prevention and control of drug and alcohol abuse [20]; WHA55.10 on mental health: responding to the call for action [21]; WHA57.10 on road safety and health [22]; WHA57.16 on health promotion and healthy lifestyles [23]; WHA57.17 on the Global Strategy on Diet, Physical Activity and Health [24]; and WHA58.26 on public-health problems caused by harmful use of alcohol [25] detail actions that countries need to implement in order to combat the growing trend of NCDs. In addition, the WHO Regional Committee for Africa has provided strategic orientations on how countries should combat non-communicable diseases [26], cardiovascular diseases [27], diabetes [28], cancer [29], and mental health problems [30]. Furthermore, the WHO Regional Committee for Africa adopted a regional strategy on health promotion [31] and discussed implementation of the WHO Framework Convention on Tobacco Control [32].

All the above-mentioned resolutions and strategies of the WHO governing bodies contain public health interventions that would, if made universally accessible to populations that can benefit from them, enable countries to successfully prevent and control the exponential growth of the incidence and prevalence of NCDs and dramatically reduce the quantity and quality of life lost. Inefficient use of the available scarce health system resources, however, partly explains why countries have not been able to scale up the coverage of the proven public health interventions contained in those resolutions and regional strategies.

Eradicating Extreme Poverty and Hunger

One of the indicators for eradicating extreme poverty and hunger under MDG 2 is the prevalence of underweight children under five years of age. In 2007, out of 42 countries in the African region for which data were available, the proportion of under-fives who were underweight for age was <11% in 6 countries; 11-20% in 22 countries; 21-30% in 12 countries; and over 31% in 7 countries [4, 5]. The WHO region with the highest percentage of under-fives who were underweight was SEAR with a minimum of 7% in Thailand and a maximum of 43.5% in India. The AFR was next with the percentage of underweight children below five years ranging from a minimum of 6.1% in Swaziland to a maximum of 39.9% in Niger. Clearly, a wide variation exists across countries in all regions but the difference is especially marked in AFR, SEAR, and WPR. The public health challenge of low birth weight could be ameliorated through breastfeeding. Unfortunately, the proportion of infants who are exclusively breastfed for the first six months is low in all regions. For example, the proportion of infants who were exclusively breastfed for the first six months of life varied from a maximum of 43.2% in SEAR to a minimum of 17.7% in EUR (Appendix 1.6). In AFR, only 29.5% of infants were exclusively breastfed for the first six months of life [4,5].

Ensuring Environmental Sustainability

There are two indicators for MDG 7 on ensuring environmental sustainability: proportion of the population with sustainable access to improved water sources (both urban and rural) and proportion of the population with access to improved sanitation. Appendix 1.6 contains the region-by-region access to improved drinking water and access to improved sanitation. Limited access to potable water and hygienic human waste disposal systems is responsible for the heavy burden of diarrhoeal diseases.

In 2008, diarrhoeal diseases resulted in a total of 872,145 deaths in the African region [5] and enormous economic loss. For example, it was estimated that the 110,837 cases of cholera reported to WHO by countries of the African Region in 2007 resulted in economic loss of US$43.3 million, US$60 million, and US$72.7 million assuming life expectancies of 40, 53, and 73 years respectively [33]. Most of the disease burden due to diarrhoea and related economic losses could have been prevented through provision of clean drinking water and hygienic sanitation facilities for populations living in both rural and urban areas.

Access to improved drinking water sources

In 2006, the proportion of people with access to improved drinking water sources in AFR was greater than 80% in eleven countries; 71-80% and 61-70% in seven countries each; 50-60% in eleven countries; and under 50% in eight countries [4]. The average proportion of people with access to improved drinking water sources in AFR was 59%, which means that the remaining 41% had no access. It is important to note that access to improved drinking water sources varies widely in the AFR from 100% in Mauritius to 42% in Niger. Compared to AFR, the average proportion of the population with access to improved drinking water sources was 94% in AMR; 97 in EUR; 82% in EMR; 87% in SEAR; and 89% in WPR. Thus, access to improved drinking water sources was much lower in the African region compared to the other WHO regions.

The proportion of urban population with access to improved drinking water sources varied from a maximum of 100% in EUR to a minimum of 82% in AFR [4]. Compared to AFR, access to improved drinking water sources by the urban population was 16% higher in AMR, 18% higher in EUR, 11% higher in EMR, 12% higher in SEAR, and 16% higher in WPR. In contrast, the proportion of the rural population with access to improved water sources ranged from a maximum of 92% in EUR to a minimum of 46% in AFR. Once again, compared to AFR, rural population access to improved drinking water sources was 35% higher in AMR, 46% higher in EUR, 29% higher in EMR, 38% higher in SEAR, and 36% higher in WPR. Generally, there are more people without access to improved drinking water sources in rural areas than in urban areas. The variance between rural and urban population access to improved water supply is significantly higher in the African region.

Access to improved sanitation

In AFR in 2006, the proportion of people with access to improved sanitation was greater than 60% in two countries; 51-60% in six countries; 41-50% in seven countries; 31-40% in eleven countries; 20-30% in eight countries; and less than 20% in ten countries [4]. The average proportion of the population in AFR with access to improved sanitation was 33%, but this varied widely from a maximum of 94% in Mauritius to a minimum of 5% in Eritrea. Compared to AFR, the average access to improved sanitation was 87% in AMR; 93% in EUR; 60% in EMR; 37% in SEAR; and 69% in WPR. Thus, improved sanitation coverage in AFR was lower than that of the other WHO regions.

The proportion of urban population with access to improved sanitation ranged from a maximum of 97% in EUR to a minimum of 46% in AFR. Compared to AFR, urban population access to improved sanitation was 46% higher in AMR, 51% higher in EUR, 39% higher in EMR, 12% higher in SEAR, and 33% higher in WPR. On the other hand, the proportion of the rural population with access to improved sanitation varied from a maximum of 85% in EUR to a minimum of 26% in AFR. Compared to AFR, rural population access to improved sanitation was 42% higher in AMR, 59% higher in EUR, 17% higher in EMR, 1% higher in SEAR, and 35% higher in WPR.

In 1998, the fifty-first World Health Assembly discussed an agenda item entitled "Environmental matters: strategy on sanitation for high-risk communities" [34]. The Assembly argued that a new approach to sanitation was the best solution for the persistently low sanitation coverage, the high prevalence of diseases caused by poor environmental conditions, low investment in sanitation, and rapid population growth and urbanisation. The strategy on sanitation, among other actions, urged Member States, international development organisations, and non-governmental organisations to accord higher priority to sanitation in national planning for health and to invest in infrastructure by asking them to:

> ...begin a sanitation promotion programme to increase political will at every level; establish priorities in the preparation of national action plans for health and environment, and integrate them firmly into programmes for implementation; integrate sanitation with as many other aspects of development as possible, e.g. child survival, maternal and child health, communicable disease control, essential drugs and agricultural development [34, p. 5].

HEALTH WORKFORCE AND INFRASTRUCTURE

A country's chances of achieving the MDGs and national health development objectives largely hinge on the strength of its national health system. According to WHO [35], a health system consists of organisations, people, and actions whose primary intent is to promote, restore, or maintain health. For a health system to improve health and health equity in a responsive, financially fair, and efficient manner, its building blocks of leadership/governance, service delivery, health workforce, information, health technologies (medical products, vaccines, equipment, physical infrastructure), and financing ought to be strong.

Ideally, a country ought to have sufficient numbers and a mix of fairly distributed competent, responsive, and productive staff. Appendix 1.7 provides the distribution of physicians, nurses and midwives, dentistry personnel, other health service providers, and hospital beds across the six WHO regions. Firstly, out of the 8,404,351 physicians available globally, 1.79% of them are in AFR, 19.28% in AMR, 33.51% in EUR, 6.34% in EMR, 10.11% in SEAR, and 28.97% in WPR. The physician density varies from a minimum of 2% in AFR to 32% in EUR. Secondly, out of the 17,651,585 nursing and midwifery staff available globally, 4.49% of them are in AFR, 23.20% in AMR, 37.73% in EUR, 4.16% in EMR, 11.08 in SEAR, and 19.34% in WPR. The AFR has the lowest nursing and midwifery density of 11 per 10,000 while EUR has the highest density of 79 per 10,000 of the population.

Thirdly, of the 1,854,512 dentistry personnel available globally, 1.29% practice in AFR, 48.57% in AMR, 23.45% in EUR, 4.53% in EMR, 5% in SEAR, and 17.15% in WPR. The AFR and SEAR have the lowest density of dentistry personnel of 1 per 10,000 of the population while the AMR has the highest dentistry personnel density of 11 per 10,000 of the population. Fourthly, out of the 14,631,863 other health personnel available globally, 1.76% are in AFR, 40.35% in AMR, 22.81% in EUR, 3.42% in EMR, 13.69% in SEAR, and 17.97% in WPR. The AMR has the highest density of other health service providers estimated at 94 per 10,000 of the population and AFR has the lowest density of 4 health personnel per 10,000 of the population.

Lastly, the distribution of hospital beds (a proxy for infrastructure) varies from a maximum of 63 beds per 10,000 of the population in EUR to a minimum of 9 beds per 10,000 of the population in SEAR. The AFR, with 10 beds per 10,000 of the population, has the second lowest hospital bed density compared to the other WHO regions. The hospital bed density for AFR is 2.4 times lower than that of AMR, 6.3 times lower than that of EUR, 1.4 times lower than that of EMR, and 3.3 times lower than that of WPR. Thus, AFR is grossly under-resourced in terms of health workforce and infrastructure compared to most of the other WHO regions. The health workforce situation in the AFR has been exacerbated by the growing cost of emigration to developed countries [36,37].

HEALTH EXPENDITURE

A well-performing health financing system raises adequate funds for health development in ways that ensure people can access and use needed services and are also protected from financial catastrophes or the impoverishment associated with having to pay for these services [38]. Tracking of health expenditure sheds light on the performance of a national health financing system.

Appendix 1.8 compares various parameters of health expenditure over time across the six WHO regions [39]. In 2006, 21 out of 46 countries in the AFR, spent less than 5% of their GDP on health; 10 countries spent 5.0-6.0%; 9 countries spent 6.1-7.0%; and 6 countries spent over 7% [39]. The percentage of GDP spent on health ranged from a maximum of 12.8% in AMR to a minimum of 3.6% in SEAR. In 2006, the AFR spent a higher percentage of GDP on health than EMR and SEAR. However, AMR, EUR, and WPR spent a higher percentage of their GDP on health than AFR. Between years 2000 and 2006 the percentage of GDP spent on health remained constant in AFR; decreased in SEAR; and increased slightly in AMR, EUR, EMR, and WPR.

The general government expenditure on health as a percentage of total expenditure on health for AFR was less than 31% and 31-50% in 10 countries each; 51-70% in 17 countries; and over 70% in 9 countries. Thus, general government expenditure on health as a percentage of total expenditure on health was less than 51% in 20 countries in the AFR. In 2006, the general government expenditure on health as a percentage of total expenditure on health varied from a maximum of 75.6% in EUR to a minimum of 33.6% in SEAR [39]. Compared to EUR's general government expenditure on health as a percentage of total expenditure on health; the other regions had lower expenditure as follows: AFR, 28.5%; AMR, 27.9%; EMR, 24.7%; SEAR 42%; and WPR, 14.6%. Between 2000 and 2006, the percentage of total health expenditure from government sources increased by 2.3% in AFR, 2% in AMR and EUR, 3.8% in EMR, and 5.6% in SEAR, whilst the percentage of total health expenditure from government sources decreased by 2.9% in WPR. In EUR and WPR the government contribution to the total expenditure on health is significantly higher than the private expenditure on health whereas in AFR, AMR, and SEAR the percentage of total health expenditure from private sources is higher than the contribution from the general government expenditure.

In 2006, the private expenditure on health as a percentage of total expenditure on health was less than 31% in 11 countries; 31-40% in 6 countries; 41-50% in 10 countries; 51-60% in 5 countries; 61-70% in 4 countries; 71-80% in 7 countries; and over 80% in 3 countries of the AFR [39]. Thus, private spending accounted for less than 50% of total expenditure on health in 27 (59%) countries. In 2006, private expenditure on health as a percentage of total expenditure on health ranged from a maximum of 66.4% in SEAR to 24.4% in EUR. Compared to SEAR, the other regions realised lower private expenditure on health as a percentage of total expenditure on health by the following margins: AFR, 13.5%; AMR, 14.1%; EUR, 42%; EMR, 17.3%; and WPR, 27.4%. Between years 2000 and 2006 the percentage of total health expenditure from private sources decreased by 2.3% in AFR, 2% in AMR, 1.4% in EUR, 3.8% in EMR, and 5.6% in SEAR. However, the private contribution to total health expenditure increased by 2.9% in WPR.

The general government expenditure on health as a percentage of total government expenditure varied from a maximum of 16.8% in EUR to a minimum of 4.7% in SEAR. The average for this index for AFR was 8.7%; which was much lower than the 15% pledged by African Heads of State in 2001. Between years 2000 and 2006 the general government expenditure on health as a percentage of total government expenditure increased by 0.5% in AFR, AMR, and SEAR; by 1.1% in EUR; by 0.3% in EMR; and by 0.1% in WPR. In 2006, external resources for health as a percentage of total expenditure on health varied from a maximum 10.7% in AFR to 0.1% in AMR and EUR [39]. Between years 2000 and 2006, the contribution of donor funding to total expenditure on health increased by 3.9% in AFR and 0.8% in EMR; decreased by 0.1% in EUR and 0.5% in SEAR; and remained constant in AMR and WPR.

Social security expenditure on health as a percentage of general government expenditure on health ranged from a maximum of 63.1% in WPR to a minimum of 7.6% in AFR [39]. Compared to AFR, the other regions incurred higher social security expenditure on health as a percentage of general government expenditure on health by the following margins: AMR, 20.1%; EUR, 41.6%; EMR, 12.1%; SEAR, 0.9%; and WPR, 55.5%. Between years 2000 and 2006 the social security expenditure on health as a percentage of general government expenditure on health decreased by 0.6% in AFR, 4.5% in AMR, 0.8% in EUR, and 2.5% in WPR but increased by 4.7% in EMR and 2.2% in SEAR.

Out-of-pocket expenditure as a percentage of private expenditure on health varied from a maximum of 88.3% in SEAR to a minimum of 30.6% in AMR [39]. Compared to AFR's out-of-pocket expenditure as a percentage of private expenditure on health of 49.8%, the AMR recorded a lower proportion by 19.2%. The other regions' out-of-pocket expenditure as a percentage of private expenditure on health exceeded that of AFR by the following margins: EUR, 21%; EMR, 37.2%; SEAR, 38.5%; and WPR, 30.9%. Between years 2000 and 2006 the out-of-pocket expenditure as a percentage of private expenditure on health decreased by 6.1% in AFR, 3.1% in AMR, 0.4% in EMR, 0.4% in SEAR, and 8.2% in WPR but increased by 2.2% in EUR.

The private prepaid plans as a percentage of private expenditure on health varied from a maximum of 60.4% in AMR to a minimum of 2.8% in SEAR [39]. The AFR's private prepaid plans as a percentage of private expenditure on health of 39% were lower than those of AMR of 21.4% but higher than those of EUR, EMR, SEAR, and WPR of 16.9%, 30.9%, 36.2%, and 29.7% respectively. Between years 2000 and 2006 the private prepaid plans as a percentage of private expenditure on health increased by 2.8% in AFR, 3.7% in AMR, 0.7% in EMR, 0.3% in SEAR, and 5.1% in WPR; whilst that of EUR decreased by 0.3%.

In 2006, six out of 46 countries in the AFR had a per capita total expenditure on health of less than US$11 at average exchange rate. The per capita total expenditure on health has US$11-20 for 9 countries; US$21-30 for 8 countries; US$31-40 for 6 countries; US$41-50 for 5 countries; and over US$50 for 12 countries [39]. It is clear that per capita total expenditure on health was less than US$34 in 27 (59%) countries. In the same year, the per capita total expenditure on health at average exchange rate ranged from a maximum of US$2,636 in AMR to US$31 in SEAR. The per capita total expenditure on health at average exchange rate for the other regions exceeded that of AFR as follows: AMR 45 times, EUR 30 times, EMR 2 times, and WPR 6 times. The per capita total expenditure on health of SEAR, however, was less than that of AFR. Between 2000 and 2006 the per capita total expenditure on health at average exchange rate increased by US$25 in AFR; US$837 in AMR; US$820 in EUR; US$47 in EMR; US$12 in SEAR; and US$71 in WPR. Thus, the nominal per capita total expenditure on health increased in all the regions by varying magnitudes.

In 2006, the per capita government expenditure on health at average exchange rate was less than US$10 in 16 countries; US$10-20 in 14 countries; US$21-30 in 2 countries; US$31-40 in 2 countries; and over US$40 in 12 countries [39]. Similarly, the per capita government expenditure on health at average exchange rate varied from a maximum of US$815 in AMR to a minimum of US$6 in SEAR. The per capita government expenditure on health at average exchange rate for the other WHO regions exceeded that of AFR as follows: AMR 46 times, EUR 50 times, EMR 2 times, and WPR 9 times. The per capita government expenditure on health of SEAR was less than that of AFR. Between years 2000 and 2006 the per capita government expenditure on health at average exchange rate was US$12 in AFR; US$437 in AMR; US$648 in EUR; US$29 in EMR; US$5 in SEAR; and US$34 in WPR.

The fifty-sixth WHO Regional Committee for Africa, in its health financing strategy [40], has recommended interventions that countries ought to implement in order to strengthen the health financing functions of revenue collection, revenue pooling and resource allocation, and purchasing. The fifty-ninth WHO Regional Committee for Africa implementation framework of the Ouagadougou Declaration [41] details how countries can translate the strategic interventions recommended in the health financing strategy into action at the country level.

CONCLUSION

Several conclusions emanate from the analysis contained in this chapter as follows:

1. In 2008, an estimated 11.14 million deaths occurred in the AFR. About 65.1% of those deaths resulted from communicable, maternal, perinatal, and nutritional conditions; 27.3% were due to non-communicable diseases; and 7.6% resulted from intentional and unintentional injuries.

2. The prevalence of underweight children below five years is higher in the AFR than in AMR, EUR, EMR, and WPR. Thus, many African countries are far from achieving MDG 1 on eradicating poverty and hunger.

3. The under-five mortality rate is still very high in many African countries. Africa's average under-five mortality rate of 145 per 1,000 live births is much higher than that of all the other WHO regions.

4. Africa's average maternal mortality ratio of 900 per 100,000 live births is the highest among the six WHO regions. The high number of maternal deaths could be attributed to the fact that on average, 54% of births are not attended by skilled health personnel. The other related factors are low contraceptive prevalence, low antenatal care coverage, and a high fertility rate among adolescents.

5. The prevalence of HIV among adults (aged 15 years and above) was much higher in Africa than in all other WHO regions. This could be attributed to such factors as lack of comprehensive correct knowledge of HIV/AIDS among an average of 70% of males and 77% of females and to lack access to antiretroviral therapy by 70% of the people with advanced HIV infection.

6. In 2007, Africa's tuberculosis prevalence of 475 per 100,000 of the population and disease incidence of 363 per 100,000 people was the highest among the WHO regions. This could be attributed to the fact that tuberculosis detection rate under DOTS was only 47% with the tuberculosis treatment success rate under DOTS being 75%.

7. Africa's malaria mortality rate of 104 per 100,000 of the population is more than 100 times above that of any other WHO region. The region's high mortality due to malaria could be explained by the low percentage of people sleeping under insecticide-treated nets in endemic areas. For example, in 2007 the proportion of children under five years who did not sleep under insecticide-treated nets was 86% while 64% of those with fever did not receive treatment with any antimalarials; 63.1% of those with acute respiratory infection symptoms were not taken to a health facility;

and 64.3% of those with diarrhoea did not receive oral rehydration therapy.

8. The AFR has the highest burden of non-communicable diseases compared to the other five regions of the WHO. The heavy burden of non-communicable diseases, which includes cardiovascular disease, diabetes, mental illnesses, and cancer, can be effectively addressed using relatively low-cost interventions, especially preventative actions relating to diet, smoking, alcohol, and lifestyle.

Currently, cost-effective interventions are available for tackling the above-mentioned contributors to disease burden, but these interventions are not reaching the poor and hence the need for substantial scaling up. Regrettably, available health systems resources are not adequate to assure universal coverage of essential health services. For instance, even though African Heads of State agreed on the target of allocating at least 15% of their annual budget towards improving the health sector in 2001, forty-four countries were far from reaching this target by end of 2006. In 2001, the WHO Commission for Macroeconomics and Health (CMH) [42] called for minimum health expenditure of US$34 to US$40 per person per year with the caveat that much of that sum ought to be covered using government budgetary allocation rather than private-sector financing. Sadly, by the end of 2006 the per capita total expenditure on health was less than US$34 in 27 (59%) countries of AFR.

As countries strive to expand the effective coverage of strategies and interventions geared towards reducing child mortality; improving maternal health; combating HIV/AIDS, malaria and TB; and ensuring environmental sustainability through reduction in the use of solid fuels and expansion of sustainable access to both improved water sources and sanitation, such improvement should be done in a manner that redresses the inequalities in various MDG indicators [43].

In order to achieve the health-related MDGs, national health development objectives, and expanded coverage of health services especially targeting the poor, countries in the AFR urgently need increased funding, greater equity in financing and access to health services, and improved efficiency in the use of health resources [40]. In addition, there is need for intersectoral action to improve daily living conditions (where people are born, grow, live, work, and age); tackle the inequitable distribution of power, money, and resources; and develop the requisite human and institutional capacities for measuring health inequity and assessing the impact of action [44].

REFERENCES

1. United Nations. *Millennium development declaration, Resolution A/55/L.2.* New York: United Nations; 2000.

2. World Health Organization. *Monitoring of the achievement of the health-related Millennium Development Goals, Document A62/10.* Geneva: World Health Organization; 2009.

3. Organization of African Unity. *Abuja declaration on HIV/AIDS, tuberculosis and other related infectious diseases.* Addis Ababa: Organization of African Unity; 2001.

4. World Health Organization. *World health statistics 2009.* Geneva: World Health Organization; 2009.

5. World Health Organization. *Health statistics and health information systems: global burden of disease.* Available at http://www.who.int/healthinfo/global_burden_disease/en/

6. World Health Organization Regional Office for Africa. *Child survival: a strategy for the African Region, Document AFR/RC56/13.* Brazzaville: World Health Organization; 2006.

7. United Nations. *The Millennium Development Goals report 2009.* New York: United Nations; 2009.

8. Bryce J. Countdown to 2015 for maternal, newborn, and child survival: the 2008 report on tracking coverage of interventions. *Lancet* 2008;371:1247-1258.

9. World Health Organization. *Working towards universal coverage of maternal, newborn and child health interventions, World Health Assembly Resolution WHA58.31.* Geneva: World Health Organization; 2005.

10. World Health Organization Regional Office for Africa. *Roadmap for accelerating the attainment of the Millennium Development Goals (MDGs) related to maternal and newborn health in Africa.* Brazzaville: World Health Organization; 2004.

11. World Health Organization. *HIV/AIDS: strategies for sustaining an adequate response to the epidemic, World Health Assembly Resolution A52/DIV/7.* Geneva: World Health Organization; 1999.

12. World Health Organization. *Scaling up the response to HIV/AIDS, Fifty-fourth World Health Assembly Resolution WHA54.10.* Geneva: World Health Organization; 2001.

13. World Health Organization Regional Office for Africa. *Tuberculosis and HIV/AIDS: a strategy for the control of a dual epidemic in the WHO African region, Document AFR/RC57/10.* Brazzaville: World Health Organization; 2007.

14. United Nations. 2001-2010: *Decade to roll back malaria in developing countries, particularly Africa, General Assembly Resolution A/60/L.44.* New York: United Nations; 2005.

15. World Health Organization. *Roll back malaria partnership: global strategic plan for roll back malaria: 2005-2015.* Geneva: World Health Organization; 2005.

16. World Health Organization. *WHO tuberculosis programme: framework for effective tuberculosis control.* Geneva: World Health Organization; 1994.

17. World Health Organization. *An expanded DOTS framework for effective tuberculosis control.* Geneva: World Health Organization; 2002.

18. World Health Organization. *Development of the WHO programme on alcohol-related problems, World Health Assembly Resolution WHA32.40.* Geneva: World Health Organization; 1979.

19. World Health Organization. *Alcohol consumption and alcohol-related problems: development of national policies and programmes, World Health Assembly Resolution WHA36.12.* Geneva: World Health Organization; 1983.

20. World Health Organization. *Prevention and control of drug and alcohol abuse, World Health Assembly Resolution WHA42.20.* Geneva: World Health Organization; 1989.

21. World Health Organization. *Mental health: responding to the call for action. World Health Assembly Resolution WHA55.10.* Geneva: World Health Organization; 2002.

22. World Health Organization. *Road safety and health, World Health Assembly Resolution WHA57.10.* Geneva: World Health Organization; 2004.

23. World Health Organization. *Health promotion and healthy lifestyles, World Health Assembly Resolution WHA57.16.* Geneva: World Health Organization; 2004.

24. World Health Organization. *The global strategy on diet, physical activity and health, World Health Assembly Resolution WHA57.17.* Geneva: World Health Organization; 2004.

25. World Health Organization. *Public-health problems caused by harmful use of alcohol, World Health Assembly Resolution WHA58.26.* Geneva: World Health Organization; 2005.

26. World Health Organization Regional Office for Africa. *Non-communicable diseases: a strategy for the African Region, Document AFR/RC50/10.* Brazzaville: World Health Organization; 1990.

27. World Health Organization Regional Office for Africa. *Cardiovascular diseases in the African Region: current situation and perspectives, Document AFR/RC55/12.* Brazzaville: World Health Organization; 2005.

28. World Health Organization Regional Office for Africa. *Diabetes prevention and control: a strategy for the WHO African Region, Document AFR/RC57/7.* Brazzaville: World Health Organization; 2007.

29. World Health Organization Regional Office for Africa. *Cancer prevention and control in the WHO African Region, Document AFR/RC57/RT/1.* Brazzaville World Health Organization; 2007.

30. World Health Organization Regional Office for Africa. *Regional strategy for mental health 2000-2010, Document AFR/RC49/9.* Harare: World Health Organization; 2000.

31. World Health Organization Regional Office for Africa. *Health promotion: a strategy for the African Region, Document AFR/RC51/12 Rev.1.* Brazzaville: World Health Organization; 2003.

32. World Health Organization Regional Office for Africa. *Implementation of the framework convention on tobacco control, Document AFR/RC55/13.* Brazzaville: World Health Organization; 2005.

33. Kirigia JM, Sambo LG, Yokouide A, Soumbey E, Muthuri LK, Kirigia DG. Economic burden of cholera in the WHO African Region. *BMC International Health and Human Rights* 2009; 9:8. Available at: http://www.biomedcentral.com/1472-698X/9/8.

34. World Health Organization. *Environmental matters: strategy on sanitation for high-risk communities, World Health Assembly Document A51/20.* Geneva: World Health Organization; 2001.

35. World Health Organization. *World health report 2000 – Health systems: improving performance.* Geneva: World Health Organization; 2000.

36. Kirigia JM, Gbary AR, Muthuri LK, Nyoni J, Seddoh A. The cost of health professionals' brain drain in Kenya. *BMC Health Services Research* 2006;6:89. Available at: http://www.biomedcentral.com/1472-6963/6/89

37. Kirigia JM, Gbary AR, Kainyu LM, Nyoni J, Seddoh A. The cost of health-related brain drain to the WHO African Region. *African Journal of Health Sciences* 2006;13(3-4):1-12.

38. World Health Organization. *Everybody's business. Strengthening health systems to improve health outcomes: WHO's framework for action.* Geneva: World Health Organization; 2007.

39. World Health Organization. *National health accounts database.* Geneva: World Health Organization; 2009. Available at: http://www.who.int/nha/country/en/index.html

40. World Health Organization Regional Office for Africa. *Health financing: a strategy of the African Region, Document AFR/RC56/10.* Brazzaville: World Health Organization; 2007.

41. World Health Organization Regional Office for Africa. *Framework for the implementation of the Ouagadougou declaration on primary health care and*

health systems in Africa: achieving better health for Africa in the new millennium, Document AFR/RC59/4. Brazzaville: World Health Organization; 2009.

42. World Health Organization. *Macroeconomics and health: investing in health for economic development.* Geneva: World Health Organization; 2001.

43. Kirigia DG, Kirigia JM. Inequalities in selected health-related Millennium Development Goal indicators in all WHO Member States. *African Journal of Health Sciences* 2007;14(3-4):171-186.

44. World Health Organization. *Closing the gap in a generation: health equity through action on the social determinants of health.* Geneva: World Health Organization; 2008.

Appendix 1.1   Health in the Millennium Development Goals

Goal	Health targets	Health indicators
1. Eradicate extreme poverty and hunger	Halve, between 1990 and 2015, the proportion of people who suffer from hunger	- Prevalence of underweight children under five years of age - Proportion of population below level of dietary energy consumption
4. Reduce child mortality	Reduce by two-thirds, between 1990 and 2015, the under-five mortality rate	- Under-five mortality rate - Infant mortality rate - Proportion of one-year-old children immunised against measles
5. Improve maternal health	Reduce by two-thirds, between 1990 and 2015, the maternal mortality ratio	- Maternal mortality ratio - Proportion of births attended by skilled health personnel
6. Combat HIV/AIDS, malaria and other diseases	Have halted by 2015 and begun to reverse the spread of HIV/AIDS	- HIV prevalence among pregnant women aged 15-24 years - Condom use rate of the contraceptive prevalence rate - Ratio of school attendance of orphans to school attendance of non-orphans aged 10-14 years
	Have halted by 2015 and begun to reverse the incidence of malaria and other major diseases	- Prevalence and death rates associated with malaria - Proportion of population in malaria-risk areas using effective malaria prevention and treatment measures - Prevalence and death rates associated with tuberculosis - Proportion of tuberculosis cases detected and cured under DOTS (directly observed treatment short-course)
7. Ensure environmental sustainability	Halve by 2015 the proportion of people without sustainable access to safe drinking water and sanitation	- Proportion of population with sustainable access to an improved water source, urban and rural - Proportion of population with access to improved sanitation, urban and rural

Source: United Nations [1]

Appendix 1.2. Health-related Millennium Development Goals indicators

Indicator		World Health Organization Regions					
		AFR	AMR	EUR	EMR	SEAR	WPR
1. Children aged <5 years underweight for age (%)	Mean						
	Range	6.1 (Swaziland) to 39.9 (Niger)	0.6 (Chile) to 18.9 (Haiti)	1.3 (Belarus) to 14.9 (Tajikistan)	3.6 (Jordan) to 38.4 (Sudan)	7.0 (Thailand) to 43.5 (India)	3.3 (Singapore) to 36.4 (Leo People's Democratic Republic)
2. Under-5 mortality rate (Probability of dying by age 5 per 1000 live births)	Mean	145	19	15	82	65	22
	Range	16 (Seychelles) to 262 (Sierra Leone)	6 (Canada) to 76 (Haiti)	2 (San Marino) to 67 (Tajikistan)	8 (United Arab Emirates) to 257 (Afghanistan)	7 (Thailand) to 113 (Myanmar)	3 (Singapore) to 91 (Cambodia)
3. Measles immunisation coverage among 1-year-olds (%)	Mean	74	93	94	84	73	92
	Range	99 (Rwanda) to 23 (Chad)	99 (Antigua & Barbuda) to 55 (Venezuela)	99 (Belarus) to 79 (Malta)	99 (Bahrain) to 34 (Somalia)	99 (Democratic People's Republic of Korea) to 63 (Timor-Leste)	99 (Nauru) to 40 (Leo People's Democratic Republic)
4. Maternal mortality ratio (per 100,000 live births)	Mean	900	99	27	420	450	82
	Range	15 (Mauritius) to 2100 (Sierra Leone)	7 (Canada) to 670 (Haiti)	1 (Ireland) to 170 (Tajikistan)	4 (Kuwait) to 1800 (Afghanistan)	58 (Sri Lanka) to 830 (Nepal)	4 (Australia) to 660 (Leo People's Democratic Republic)
5. Births attended by skilled health personnel (%)	Mean	46	92	96	59	48	92
	Range	99 (Mauritius) to 6 (Ethiopia)	100 (Antigua & Barbuda) to 26 (Haiti)	100 (Albania & 25 other countries) to 83 (Turkey)	100 (Kuwait, Libya, Qatar, UAE) to 14 (Afghanistan)	99 (Sri Lanka) to 18 (Bangladesh)	100 (Cook Islands, Malaysia, Niue, Palau, Republic of Korea, Samoa, Tuvalu, Japan, Brunei Darussalam, Singapore) to 20 (Leo People's Democratic Republic)
6. Contraceptive prevalence (%)	Mean	24.4	70.0		43.0	57.2	85.5
	Range	75.9 (Mauritius) to 2.8 (Chad)	78.2 (Colombia) to 32.0 (Haiti)	82 (UK) to 32 (The former Yugoslav Republic of Macedonia)	73.8 (Iran) to 7.6 (Sudan)	71.5 (Thailand) to 10 (Timor-Leste)	90.2 (China) to 32.2 (Leo People's Democratic Republic)

.../cont.

Efficiency Analysis of Health Systems in Africa

Appendix 1.2 (cont.)

7. Adolescent fertility rate (per 1,000 girls aged 15-19 years)	Mean	117	61	24	35	56	11
	Range	4 (Algeria) to 199 (Niger)	14 (Canada) to 109 (Nicaragua)	1 (San Marino) to 51 (Turkey)	4 (Libya) to 151 (Afghanistan)	8 (Maldives) to 127 (Bangladesh)	2 (Republic of Korea) to 110 (Leo People's Democratic Republic)
8. Antenatal care coverage (%): at least 1 visit	Mean	73	94	100	51	74	89
	Range	98 (Cape Verde) to 28 (Ethiopia)	100 (Antigua & Barbuda, Barbados, Dominica, Saint Kitts and Nevis) to 77 (Bolivia)	100 (Kazakhstan) to 77 (Tajikistan)	100 (Oman) to 16 (Afghanistan)	100 (Maldives) to 44 (Nepal)	99 (Mongolia) to 35 (Leo People's Democratic Republic)
9. Unmet need for family planning (%)	Mean	24.4				12.4	
	Range	40.6 (Uganda) to 3.3 (Mauritius)	37.5 (Haiti) to 5.0 (Ecuador)	16.4 (Georgia) to 1.2 (Albania)	50.9 (Yemen) to 10.0 (Morocco)	37.0 (Maldives) to 3.8 (Timor-Leste)	39.5 (Leo People's Democratic Republic) to 4.6 (Mongolia)
10. Prevalence of HIV among adults aged $\geq$ 15 years per 100,000 population	Mean	4735	448	336	202	295	89
	Range	<40 (Comoros) to 24301 (Swaziland)	67 (Cuba) to 2508 (Bahamas)	<11 (Slovakia) to 1082 (Ukraine)	18 (Egypt) to 2870 (Djibouti)	11 (Bangladesh) to 1191 (Thailand)	9 (Japan) to 1395 (Papua New Guinea)
11. Proportion of males aged 15-24 years with comprehensive correct knowledge of HIV/AIDS (%)	Mean	30					
	Range	62 (Namibia) to 16 (Niger) N=28	47 (Guyana) to 18 (Bolivia) N=4	43 (Ukraine) to 5 (Azerbaijan) N=3	N=0	44 (Nepal) to 36 (India) N=2	50 (Vietnam) to 18 (Philippines) N=4
12. Proportion of females aged 15-24 years with comprehensive correct knowledge of HIV/AIDS (%)	Mean	23			21		
	Range	65 (Namibia) to 4 (Equatorial Guinea) N=38	60 (Jamaica) to 15 (Bolivia) N=11	48 (Bosnia and Herzegovina) to 3 (Tajikistan) N=13	18 (Djibouti) to 3 (Iraq) N=5	46 (Thailand) to 16 Bangladesh N=4	50 (Cambodia) to 12 (Philippines) N=5

.../cont.

Appendix 1.2 (cont.)

13. Antiretroviral therapy coverage among people with advanced HIV infection (%)	Mean	30	62	17	5	25	28
	Range	88 (Namibia) to 4 (Madagascar) N=42	>95 (Costa Rica) to 22 (Paraguay) N=23	73 (Romania) to 6 (Tajikistan) N=16	31 (Morocco) to 1 (Sudan) N=8	61 (Thailand) to 0 (Democratic People's Republic of Korea) N=7	>95 (Leo People's Democratic Republic) to 19 (China) N=7
14. Malaria mortality rate per 100,000 population	Mean	104	<1		1	2	<1
	Range	0 (Algeria) to 229 (Niger) N=43	0 (Argentina to 10 (Guyana) N=20	0 (Armenia, Azerbaijan, Turkmenistan) to <1 (Tajikistan) N=8	0 (Egypt, Iraq, Morocco, Oman, Saudi Arabia, Syria) to 85 (Sudan) N=13	0 (Democratic People's Republic of Korea) to 93 (Timor-Leste) N=10	0 (Republic of Korea) to 45 (Papua New Guinea) N=10
15. Children aged <5 years sleeping under insecticide treated bed-nets (%)	Mean	14	3	1	28	8	18
	Range	56 (Niger) to 0 (Swaziland) N=34	3 Suriname N=1	1 (Azerbaijan, Tajikistan) N=2	28 (Sudan) to 0 (Iraq) N=4	8 (Timor-Leste) to 0 (Indonesia) N=2	18 (Leo People's Democratic Republic) to 4 (Cambodia) N=3
16. Children aged <5 years who received any antimalarial treatment for fever (%)	Mean	36	5	2	50	10	9
	Range	63 (Comoros, Gambia) to 4 (Eritrea) N=37	5 (Haiti) to 1 (Honduras) N=3	2 (Tajikistan) to 1 (Azerbaijan) N=2	50 (Sudan) to 1 (Iraq) N=4	47 (Timor-Leste) to 1 (Indonesia) N=3	9 (Leo People's Democratic Republic) to 0 (Cambodia) N=3
17. Tuberculosis treatment success under DOTS (%)	Mean	75	75	70	86	87	92
	Range	92 (Mauritius) to 18 (Angola) N=38	100 (Barbados, Saint Kitts and Nevis) to 41 (Jamaica) N=29	100 (Malta) to 30 (Croatia) N=38	91 (Tunisia) to 69 (Qatar) N=21	92 (Bangladesh) to 77 (Thailand) N=11	100 (Nauru, Tonga) to 48 (Malaysia) N=24

.../cont.

Efficiency Analysis of Health Systems in Africa

Appendix 1.2 (cont.)

18. Access to improved drinking water sources (%)	Mean	59	94	97	82	87	89
	Range	100 (Mauritius) to 42 (Niger) N=44	100 (Barbados, Canada, Uruguay) to 58 (Haiti) N=28	100 (Andorra & 23 other countries) to 67 (Tajikistan) N=44	100 (Lebanon, Qatar, UAE) to 22 (Afghanistan) N=15	100 (Democratic People's Republic of Korea) to 62 (Timor-Leste)	100 (Australia, Japan, Niue, Tonga) to 40 (Papua New Guinea) N=20
19. Access to improved sanitation (%)	Mean	33	87	93	60	37	69
	Range	94 (Mauritius) to 5 (Eritrea) N=44	100 (Uruguay, Canada, USA, Bahamas) to 19 (Haiti) N=29	100 (Andorra & 13 other countries) to 72 (Romania) N=39	100 (Qatar) to 23 (Somalia) N=15	96 (Thailand) to 27 (Nepal) N=10	100 (Niue, Japan, Australia, Cook Islands, Samoa) to 25 (Micronesia) N=20

Source: WHO [4]

Appendix 1.3   *Global mortality and burden of disease*

Indicators	AFR	AMR	EUR	EMR	SEAR	WPR
Life expectancy at birth (years)2007	52	76	74	64	65	74
Healthy life expectancy (HALE) at birth (years) 2007	45	67	67	56	57	67
Neonatal mortality ratio (per 1,000 life births) 2004	40	11	10	38	35	17
Infant mortality rate (probability of dying between birth and age 1 per 1,000 live births) MDG4	88	16	13	60	49	19
Under-5 mortality rate (probability of dying between birth and age 5 per 1,000 live births) MDG4	145	19	15	82	65	22
Adult mortality rate (probability of dying between 15 and 60 years per 1,000 population)	401	127	159	203	220	115

Source: WHO [4]

Appendix 1.4   Cause-specific mortality and morbidity

Indicators		AFR	AMR	EUR	EMR	SEAR	WPR
Mortality rate per 100,000 population -2007	HIV/AIDS	198	11	10	10		4
	Malaria	104	<1		7	2	<1
	TB among HIV-negative people	45	4	6	17	28	16
	TB among HIV-positive people	47.6	0.9	0.9	1.4	2.3	0.8
Age-standardised mortality rate (per 100,000 population)	Non-communicable	841	499	590	790	701	557
	Cardiovascular	390	202	332	458	365	243
	Cancer	147	130	142	101	130	135
	Injuries	126	66	79	109	131	68
Distribution of years of life lost by broader causes (%)	Communicable	80	25	56	12	52	24
	Non-communicable	13	55	30	70	31	57
	Injuries	7	20	15	18	17	19
Distribution of causes of death among children aged <5 years (%) – 2004	Neonatal	21.0	37.7	37.8	32.6	39.0	46.2
	HIV/AIDS	5.0	0.7	0.7	0.3	0.4	0.3
	Diarrhoea	16.3	12.7	14.0	16.7	19.5	12.0
	Measles	3.9	0.0	0.1	3.0	5.5	0.8
	Malaria	15.6	0.2	0.0	2.3	0.4	0.3
	Pneumonia	20.4	12.7	14.9	19.6	13.7	9.8
	Injuries	2.4	5.9	5.7	3.5	5.3	7.5
	Other	15.4	30.0	26.7	21.9	16.2	23.1
Morbidity-2007	Prevalence of tuberculosis (per 100,000 population)	475	38	51	139	280	197
	Incidence of tuberculosis (per 100,000 population)	363	32	49	105	181	108
	Prevalence of HIV among adults aged >=15 years (per 100,000 population)	4735	448	336	202	295	89

Source: WHO [4]

Appendix 1.5   *Health service coverage*

Indicators		AFR	AMR	EUR	EMR	SEAR	WPR
Antenatal care coverage (%) (MDG5)	At least 1 visit	73	94		61	74	89
	At least 4 visits	45	83		45	42	
Births attended by skilled health personnel (%)		46	92	96	59	48	92
Births by caesarean section (%)-2000-2008		3.3	31.3	19	11.9	7.5	34.1
Neonates protected at birth against neonatal tetanus (%)		31	42	10	39	59	28
Immunisation coverage among 1-year olds (%) – 2007	Measles	74	93	94	84	73	92
	DPT3	74	93	96	87	69	92
	HepB3	69	88	78	85	30	85
	Hib3	34	91	57	20		3
Children aged 6-59 months who received vitamin A supplementation (%)-2000-2007		47.9			38.9	34.7	
Children aged <5 years (%)	Sleeping under insecticide treated nets	14					
	With fever who received treatment with any antimalarials	36				10	
	With ARI symptoms taken to facility	36.9			63.2	62.3	
	With diarrhoea receiving ORT	35.7			47.3	34.7	
Unmet need for family planning (%) – 2000-2006		24.4				12.4	
Contraceptive prevalence (%) – 2000-2006		24.4	70		43.0	57.2	85.5
Antiretroviral therapy coverage (%) 2007	Pregnant women (PMTCT)	34	36	71	1	24	13
	People with advanced HIV infection	30	62	17	5	25	28
Tuberculosis detection rate under DOTS (%) -2007		47	73	51	60	69	77
Tuberculosis treatment success under DOTS (%) - 2006		75	75	70	86	87	92

Source: WHO [4]

Appendix 1.6   Risk factors

Indicators		AFR	AMR	EUR	EMR	SEAR	WPR
MDG 7: Access to improved drinking water sources (%) -2006	Urban	82	98	100	93	94	98
	Rural	46	81	92	75	84	82
	Total	59	94	97	82	87	89
MDG 5: Access to improved sanitation (%)-2006	Urban	46	92	97	85	58	79
	Rural	26	68	85	43	27	61
	Total	33	87	93	60	37	69
Low birth-weight newborns (%)		14	9	6			5
Infants exclusively breastfed for the first 6 months of life (%)		29.5	30.9	17.7	34.2	43.2	
Alcohol consumption among adults aged $\geq$ 15 years (litres per person per year)		4.09	6.66	8.84	0.19	0.51	5.18
Prevalence of current tobacco use (%)	Adults ($\geq$ 15 years)	10.6	24.8	35.3	18.3	22.2	30.8
	Adolescents (13-15 years)	16.4	22.3	18.4	15.2	13.0	7.3

Source: WHO [4]

Appendix 1.7   Health workforce and infrastructure

Indicators		AFR	AMR	EUR	EMR	SEAR	WPR
Physicians	Number	150,708	1,620,329	2,816,481	532,486	849,324	2,435,023
	Density (per 10,000 population)	2	19	32	10	5	14
Nursing and midwifery	Number	792,361	4,095,757	6,659,394	734,949	1,955,203	3,413,921
	Density (per 10,000 population)	11	49	79	15	12	20
Dentistry personnel	Number	23,964	900,702	434,972	84,033	92,759	318,082
	Density (per 10,000 population)	1	11	5	2	1	2
Other health service providers	Number	257,520	5,904,376	3,338,011	499,977	2,002,575	2,629,404
	Density (per 10,000 population)	4	94	38	9	12	15
Hospital beds (per 10,000 population)		10	24	63	14	9	33

Source: WHO [4]

Appendix 1.8   Health expenditure

Indicators		AFR	AMR	EUR	EMR	SEAR	WPR
Total expenditure on health as % of gross domestic product	Year 2000	5.5	11.3	8.0	4.3	3.6	6.0
	Year 2006	5.5	12.8	8.4	4.5	3.4	6.1
General government expenditure on health as % of total expenditure on health	Year 2000	44.8	45.7	73.6	47.1	28.0	63.9
	Year 2006	47.1	47.7	75.6	50.9	33.6	61.0
Private expenditure on health as % of total expenditure on health	Year 2000	55.2	54.3	25.8	52.9	72.0	36.1
	Year 2006	52.9	52.3	24.4	49.1	66.4	39.0
General government expenditure on health as % of total government expenditure	Year 2000	8.2	16.3	13.7	7.0	4.2	13.7
	Year 2006	8.7	16.8	14.8	7.3	4.7	13.8
External resources for health as % of total expenditure on health	Year 2000	6.8	0.1	0.2	1.2	2.4	0.2
	Year 2006	10.7	0.1	0.1	2.0	1.9	0.2
Social security expenditure on health as % of general government expenditure on health	Year 2000	8.2	32.2	50.0	15.0	6.3	65.6
	Year 2006	7.6	27.7	49.2	19.7	8.5	63.1
Out-of-pocket expenditure as % of private expenditure on health	Year 2000	55.9	33.7	68.6	88.0	88.7	88.9
	Year 2006	49.8	30.6	70.8	87.0	88.3	80.7
Private prepaid plans as % of private expenditure on health	Year 2000	36.2	56.7	22.4	7.4	2.5	4.2
	Year 2006	39.0	60.4	22.1	8.1	2.8	9.3
Per capita total expenditure on health at average exchange rate (US$)	Year 2000	33	1,799	936	69	19	290
	Year 2006	58	2,636	1,756	116	31	361
Per capita total expenditure on health (PPP Int.$)	Year 2000	83	1,935	1,197	184	58	297
	Year 2006	111	2,788	1,719	259	85	461
Per capita government expenditure on health at average exchange rate (US$)	Year 2000	15	815	704	36	6	212
	Year 2006	27	1,252	1,350	65	11	246
Per capita government expenditure on health (PPP Int.$)	Year 2000	37	855	881	87	16	190
	Year 2006	52	1,329	1,299	132	29	282

Source: WHO [39]

-2-

Health Challenges in Africa and the Way Forward*

Joses M. Kirigia and Saidou P. Barry

ABSTRACT

Africa is confronted by a heavy double burden of communicable and non-communicable diseases. Cost-effective interventions that can prevent the disease burden exist but coverage is too low due to health systems weaknesses. This editorial reviews the challenges related to leadership and governance; health workforce; medical products, vaccines and technologies; information; financing; and services delivery. It also provides an overview of the orientations provided by the WHO Regional Committee for Africa for overcoming those challenges. It cautions that it might not be possible to adequately implement those orientations without a concerted fight against corruption, sustained domestic and external investment in social sectors, and an enabling macroeconomic and political (i.e., internally secure) environment.

OVERVIEW OF DISEASE BURDEN

Out of 58.03 million people who died globally in 2005, 10.9 million (18.8%) were from the WHO African Region [1]. Majority of deaths (64%) that occurred in the region resulted from HIV/AIDS (19%), lower respiratory infections (10%), malaria (8%), diarrhoeal diseases (7%), cerebrovascular disease (4%), ischaemic heart disease (3%), tuberculosis (3%), measles (3%), low birth weight (2%), birth asphyxia and birth trauma (2%), and maternal conditions (2%). Even though cost-effective interventions that could have prevented most of the deaths exist, coverage is low due to weak and under-resourced health systems. Some of the weaknesses can be attributed to challenges related to leadership and governance; health workforce; medical

---

* The original artile appeared in *International Archives of Medicine* 2008; 1(27): 1-4. Reproduced with permission of BioMed Central Ltd.

products, vaccines and technologies; information; financing; and services delivery [2].

CHALLENGES

Firstly, there are serious leadership and governance challenges that include weak public health leadership and management [3]; inadequate health-related legislations and their enforcement; limited community participation in planning, management and monitoring of health services; weak inter-sectoral action; horizontal and vertical inequities in health systems [4]; inefficiency in resource allocation and use [5]; and weak national health research systems [6]. Secondly, extreme shortages of health workers exist in 57 countries of which 36 are in Africa [7]. The crisis has been exacerbated by inequities in workforce distribution and brain drain. Thus, the delivery of effective public health interventions to people in need is compromised particularly in remote rural areas.

Thirdly, there is rampant corruption in medical products and technologies procurement systems, unreliable supply systems, unaffordable prices, irrational use, and wide variance in quality and safety [2]. This has contributed to the current situation where 50% of the population in the Region lacks access to essential medicines [6]. Fourthly, there is a dearth of information and communications technology (ICT) and mass Internet connectivity compounded by a paucity of ICT-related knowledge and skills limiting capacities of national health management information systems (HMIS) to generate, analyse, and disseminate information for use in decision-making [8].

Fifthly, health financing systems in the region are characterised by low investment in health, lack of comprehensive health financing policies and strategic plans, extensive out-of-pocket payments, lack of social safety nets to protect the poor, weak financial management, inefficient resource use, and weak mechanisms for coordinating partner support [9]. Finally, in terms of service delivery, the lack of effective organisation and management of health services combined with the abovementiond challenges have in tandem led to the current situation where 47% of the population have no access to quality health services and 59% of pregnant women deliver babies without the assistance of skilled health personnel. In relation to water and sanitation, which contribute to reducing the burden of communicable diseases, 64% of the population lack sustainable access to improved sanitation facilities and 42% lack sustainable access to an improved water source [6].

THE WAY FORWARD

Orientations for Strengthening National Health Systems

Cognisant of the above-mentioned challenges, the 46 Ministers of Health from the African Region adopted and signed the Ouagadougou Declaration [10] that proposes ways of addressing health system challenges. The Ouagadougou Declaration urges Member States to update their national health policies and plans according to the primary health care (PHC) approach; promote inter-sectoral collaboration and public-private partnership to address broad determinants of health; improve health workforce production and retention; set up mechanisms for increasing availability and accessibility of essential medicines, health technologies and infrastructure; strengthen health information systems; develop and implement strategic health financing policies and plans; promote health awareness; and build behavioural change capacities among communities.

Subsequently, the fifty-eighth WHO Regional Committee for Africa endorsed a framework for implementing the Ouagadougou Declaration [11]. The framework proposes to countries generic interventions for addressing the health systems challenges. Firstly, regarding leadership and governance, it proposes updating national health policy and strategic plan; updating and enforcing public health laws; and strengthening mechanisms for transparency and accountability and intersectoral collaboration [10]. Secondly, concerning human resources for health (HRH), it recommends generation and use of evidence in HRH policy development, planning and management; reinforcing health training institutions' capacity; strengthening HRH leadership and management capacities; implementing HRH retention strategies; and increasing fiscal space for HRH development [10].

Thirdly, with regard to medical products and technologies, it proposes development of formulae for determining the requirements and forecasting for medicines, commodities, essential technologies and infrastructure; and creation of a transparent and accountable procurement system [10]. Fourthly, relating to health information and research, the Declaration on Primary Health Care and Health Systems suggests development and implementation of a comprehensive HMIS policy and strategic plan; and establishment of a functional national HMIS by leveraging ICT [10]. In addition, the Algiers Declaration [12] recommends development and retention of a critical mass of human resources for health research; updating of national health research policies and strategic frameworks; strengthening of South-South and North-South research cooperation; establishment of mechanisms for scientific and ethical oversight of research; acquisition of ICT for research and information; and allocation of at least 2% of national health expenditure and at least 5% of external aid for health to research.

Fifthly, pertaining to health financing, it recommends development of a comprehensive health financing policy and a strategic plan; institutionalisation of national health accounts and efficiency monitoring; strengthening of financial management skills at all levels; allocation of at least 15% of the national budget to health development; implementation of the Paris Declaration on aid effectiveness; and development of social protection mechanisms [10].

Finally, as regards service delivery, the Ouagadougou Declaration proposes building on the elements of essential health services, mode of delivery and costs; development of norms, standards and procedures for service provision and health infrastructure construction and maintenance; formulation of integrated service delivery model at all levels of the referral system; development of mechanisms to involve all private health providers in provision of essential health services; and development and implementation of multi-sectoral health promotion policies and strategies to optimise community involvement in health development [10].

CONCLUSIONS

Effective public health interventions are available to curb the heavy disease burden in Africa. Unfortunately, health systems are too weak to efficiently and equitably deliver those interventions to people who need them, when, and where they are needed. Fortunately, health policy makers know what actions ought to be implemented to strengthen health systems. However, it might not be possible to adequately implement those actions without a concerted and coordinated fight against corruption, sustained domestic and external investment in social sectors (e.g., health, education, water, sanitation), and enabling macroeconomic and political (i.e., internally secure) environment.

ACKNOWLEDGEMENTS

We are grateful to our colleagues at the DSD/AFRO for their suggestions. We are grateful to Professor Manuel Menendez Gonzalez and the anonymous peer reviewers for their suggestions that helped to improve the Editorial. We are immensely grateful to Jehovah for multifaceted support. This article contains the views of the authors only and does not represent the decisions or the stated policies of the World Health Organization.

REFERENCES

1. http://www.who.int/healthinfo/bod/en/index.html

2. World Health Organization. *Strengthening health systems to improve health outcomes: WHO's framework for action.* Geneva: World Health Organization; 2007.

3. Brinkerhoff DW, Bossert TJ. *Health governance: concepts, experience, and programming options.* Bethesda: Abt Associates; 2008.

4. McIntyre D, Mooney G. *The economics of health equity.* Cambridge: Cambridge University Press; 2007.

5. Kirigia JM, Asbu Z, Greene W, Emrouznejad A. Technical efficiency, efficiency change, technical progress and productivity growth in the national health systems of continental African countries. *Eastern Africa Social Science Research Review* 2007;23(2):19-40.

6. Kirigia JM, Wambebe C.Status of resources for health research in ten African countries. *BMC Health Services Research* 2006;6:135.

7. World Health Organization. *The world health report 2006 - working together for health.* Geneva: World Health Organization; 2006.

8. Gething PW, Noor AM, Gikandi PW, Ogara E, Hay SI, Nixon MS, Snow RW, Atkinson, PM. Improving imperfect data from health management information systems in Africa using space-time geostatistics. *PLoS Medicine* 2006;3(6):e271.

9. Preker A, Langenbrunner JC. *Spending wisely: buying health services for the poor.* Washington, D.C.: The World Bank; 2005.

10. World Health Organization Regional Office for Africa. Ouagadougou declaration on primary health care and health systems in Africa: achieving better health for Africa in the new millennium. Brazzaville: World Health Organization; 2008.

11. World Health Organization Regional Office for Africa. *Framework for implementation of the Ouagadougou declaration on primary health care and health systems in Africa: achieving better health for Africa in the new millennium.* Brazzaville: World Health Organization; 2008.

12. World Health Organization Regional Office for Africa. *The Algiers Declaration.* Brazzaville: World Health Organization; 2008c.

-3-

Lecture Notes on Efficiency Analysis of Health Systems

Joses M. Kirigia

HEALTH SYSTEM CONCEPTUAL FRAMEWORK

A health system includes all activities whose primary purpose is to promote, restore, or maintain an individual's physical, mental, and social well-being [1]. Thus, the activities of a health system include health promotion, disease prevention, treatment, rehabilitation, and nursing that includes both community and home-based care. The *World Health Report 2000* [2] defines overall health system goals as follows:

> improving health and health equity, in ways that are responsive, financially fair, and make the best, or most efficient, use of available resources. There are also important intermediate goals: the rout from inputs to health outcomes is through greater access to and coverage for effective health interventions, without compromising efforts to ensure provider quality and safety. [p.2]

Health System Goals

The WHO [2] health system framework consists of four overall goals or outcomes (Fig.3.1). Firstly, a health system aims at improving the health of the population; where health refers to both length of life and health-related quality of life. Secondly, a health system must enhance its responsiveness to the legitimate expectations of the population it serves. The two dimensions of responsiveness are respect for persons and client orientation. Respect for persons has three aspects: dignity (courtesy and sensitivity to patients during diagnosis and treatment); individual autonomy (whereby competent individuals or their agents have the right to choose interventions); and confidentiality (privacy and non-disclosure of personal health information). Client orientation covers four aspects: prompt attention to health needs (through physical, social, and financial access); clean and adequate basic amenities (such as waiting rooms, beds, and food); access to social support networks (including family and community) for individuals receiving care; and choice of the institution and individual providing care [1].

Thirdly, a health system must work towards ensuring fairness in financial contribution. Fairness implies that households should not become impoverished nor should they pay an excessive share of their income towards obtaining needed health care and poor households should pay less towards the health system than rich households [1]. Lastly, a health system must aim at improved efficiency in all its processes through the use of health system inputs and production of health services without waste.

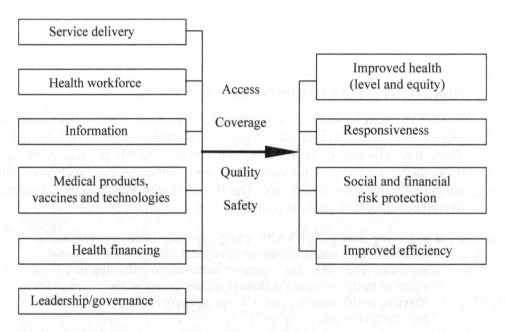

Figure 3.1   The WHO health system framework

HEALTH SYSTEM BUILDING BLOCKS

The six building blocks of a health system include service delivery; health workforce; information; medical products, vaccines and technologies; financing; and leadership and governance.

Service Delivery

This refers to the process through which a decision-making unit combines human resources, physical capital, and consumable inputs at its disposal to deliver effective, safe, and quality personal health services (e.g., therapeutic, rehabilitative, or preventive services) and non-personal health services (e.g., mass health education and sanitation) to those in need. The provision of health services encompasses delivery of integrated health service packages (prevention, promotion, and treatment); service delivery models that leverage all networks of public, private-not-for-profit, and private-for-profit providers; and improved management of health system inputs (human resources, finances, logistics, physical infrastructure, medicines, time, and information). Service provision by health systems also includes health services and partners; infrastructure and logistics; patient safety (systems and procedures that improve safety) and quality of care (treatment protocols, clinical management schedules, supervision and assessment, continuing education, registration or licensing, and inspection); and activities to influence demand for care through use of media to promote health and engage civil society in service delivery planning and oversight [2, 3]. Faced with acute resource constraints, African countries must deploy and use health system inputs optimally and also build appropriate incentives within organisational structures so as to maximise the quantity and quality of health service outputs.

Health Workforce

The *World Health Report 2006* [4, p.1] defines health workers as all people engaged in actions whose primary intent is to enhance health. A country's health workforce consists of health service providers (e.g., physicians, dentists, pharmacists, clinical officers, nurses, diagnosticians, community health workers, and environmental health workers) and health management and support workers (e.g., accountants, planners, carpenters, and storekeepers). Africa has only 17% of the global workforce and the lowest health workforce density per 1,000 of the population compared to other WHO regions (Table 3.1). In addition, 83% and 17% of the total health workforce in Africa consists of personnel directly involved in provision of health services (i.e., health service providers) and health management and support workers respectively.

Thirty-six of the 57 countries experiencing critical shortages of doctors, nurses, and midwives globally are in Africa (Table 3.2). It is estimated that Africa has a shortage of 817,992 health workers (i.e., doctors, nurses, and midwives). The scarcity of health personnel in the African region underscores the importance of more efficient utilisation of the available human resources for health.

The object of this building block is to ensure that the health workforce is available, competent, responsive, and productive. The *World Health Report 2006* lays out a "working lifespan" approach to the dynamics of the health workforce through modulation of the roles of both labour markets and state action in preparing the workforce through strategic investment in education and effective and ethical recruitment practices (entry); enhancing worker performance through better management in both the public and private sectors (workforce); and managing migration and attrition to reduce wasteful loss (exit) of human resources.

Table 3.1   Distribution of global health workforce across the six WHO regions (2006)

WHO Region	Total health workforce		Health service providers		Health management and support workers	
	No.	Density (per 1,000 population)	No.	% of total health workforce	No.	% of total health workforce
Africa	1,640,000	2.3	1,360,000	83	280,000	17
Eastern Mediterranean	2,100,000	4.0	1,580,000	75	520,000	25
South-East Asia	7,040,000	4.3	4,730,000	67	2,300,000	33
Western Pacific	10,070,000	5.8	7,810,000	78	2,260,000	23
Europe	16,630,000	18.9	11,540,000	69	5,090,000	31
Americas	21,740,000	24.8	12,460,000	57	9,280,000	43
World	59,220,000	9.3	39,480,000	67	19,730,000	33

Source: WHO [4]

Table 3.2   Estimated critical shortages of doctors, nurses, and midwives by WHO region (2006)

WHO Region	Number of countries		In countries with shortages		
	Total	With shortages	Total stock	Estimated shortage	% increase required
Africa	46	36	590,198	817,992	139
Eastern Mediterranean	21	7	312,613	306,031	98
South-East Asia	11	6	2,332,054	1,164,001	50
Western Pacific	27	3	27,260	32,560	119
Europe	52	0	NA	NA	NA
Americas	35	5	93,603	37,886	40
World	192	57	3,355,728	2,358,470	70

Source: WHO [4]

The entry aspect, which aims at provision of sufficient numbers of skilled workers with appropriate technical competencies, requires active planning and management of the production of health workforce. The focus here should be on building strong training institutions; strengthening of health sciences education institutions, and accreditation and professional regulation (licensing, certification, or registration) to assure quality, responsiveness, and ethical practice; and revitalising recruitment and placement capabilities. The workforce dimension is geared towards maximising the availability, competence, responsiveness, and productivity of available human resources for health. This goal can be achieved through firm and fair supervision (including on-the-job training); fair and reliable financial and non-financial compensation; enabling work environments (e.g., clean water, adequate lighting, heating, vehicles, drugs, working equipment, and other supplies); and lifelong learning in the workplace (e.g., through short-term training, innovation, sharing of ideas, and teamwork).

In Africa, exit of health workers occurs through worker illness, deaths, migration (internal and external), and retirement. Attrition could be attenuated through managing migration (as is the case in the Eastern Mediterranean region), making health a career of choice, establishing programmes for promoting the health and safety of workers, and retirement. Unplanned migration can be reduced through tailoring education and recruitment to rural realities, improving working and living conditions, entering into bilateral agreements with recipient countries, and advocating for compensation of the opportunity cost by recipient countries. Appropriate human resource policies in countries can elicit succession planning, reduce incentives for early retirement, decrease the cost of employing older people, recruit retirees back to work, and improve conditions for older workers.

Information

The information building block of a health system involves development of health information and surveillance systems, development of standardised tools and instruments, and collation and publication of health statistics on health determinants, health systems performance, and health status. According to WHO [5, p.18], "a well-functioning health information system is one that ensures the production, analysis, dissemination and use of reliable and timely health information by decision-makers at different levels of the health system, both on regular basis and in emergencies". Such a system should generate population and facility-based data; detect, investigate, and communicate events that threaten public health security; and have the capacity to synthesise information and promote the availability and application of that knowledge. Many countries in Africa need to strengthen their national surveillance and response capacity with up-to-date technologies and dedicated competent staff; establish a set of core and additional health systems indicators to track health system performance; adapt global standards, methods, and tools (e.g., the International Classification of Diseases and MDG monitoring tools); and promote a single reporting system instead of inefficient parallel reporting by development partners.

Medical Products, Vaccines and Technologies

Health technologies are the drugs, devices, procedures, and organisational support systems for delivering health care [6]. The scope of this building block includes development, implementation, and monitoring of national policies, strategies, and programmes for improving use of health technologies; establishment or strengthening of a national health technologies regulatory authority to assure quality, effectiveness, and safety; and ensuring evidence-based selection of essential technologies for inclusion in the essential technologies lists. This component of a health system also includes development or strengthening of existing training programmes on rational use of technologies in the curricula of all health professionals; enactment of new laws or enforcement of existing legislation to ban inaccurate, misleading, or unethical promotion of health technologies; development or strengthening of the capacity of hospital health technologies committees to promote the rational use of health technologies; and strengthening of health technologies procurement, supply, and distribution systems to avoid wastage of resources. The health technologies component of a health system also covers the establishment or strengthening of post-marketing surveillance, pharmaco-vigilance, ensuring blood safety, monitoring prescription, and communicating the outcomes to all stakeholders in order to promote patient safety and ensure adequate supply of health technologies of assured quality [7].

Health Financing

Health financing has been defined as raising or collection of revenue to pay for the operation of the health system [8]. Health financing has the three functions of revenue collection from various sources, pooling of funds and spreading of risks across larger population groups, and allocation or use of funds to purchase services from public and private providers of health care [2]. The revenue base of a health system depends on the gross national product, efficiency of the tax system, the labour market, natural resources, and external aid. Some forms of revenue collection include out-of-pocket payments, co-payments, voluntary prepayment, mandatory prepayment, indirect taxes, and direct taxes.

With the exception of out-of-pocket payment, the revenue from the other forms of collection are pooled through various institutions such as central government, local government, quasi-public agencies, public insurance agencies, private insurance companies, and non-governmental organisations. Households leverage their resources to purchase services from providers directly; otherwise, the pooled resources are allocated by inputs (e.g., salaries and traditional budgets), by outputs (e.g., fee for service) or by covered individuals (e.g., capitation) [9]. Health financing systems ought to be designed such that they contribute to optimising or maximising the achievement of health system goals.

Leadership and Governance

Leadership and governance involves overseeing and guiding the whole health system (public plus private) and health development partners (including donors, civil society organisations, and non-governmental organisations among others) in order to protect the public interest. Leadership and governance are primarily the prerogative of the government. However, the government can delegate (but not abrogate the responsibility) some of the tasks to other institutions. Some functions of this building block include policy guidance (development of policies, strategies, priority setting, and definition of roles and responsibilities of various partners in health development); intelligence and oversight (generation, analysis and use of intelligence on trends and differentials in health system inputs, processes, outputs, and outcomes); and collaboration and coalition building with pertinent stakeholders including promotion of policies in other social and productive sectors to advance health goals.

Leadership and governance as a key component of a health system also involves designing, implementing (enforcing), and monitoring health-related laws, regulations, and standards; system design (ensuring a fit between strategy and structure and reducing duplication and fragmentation of a health system); transparency and accountability among all stakeholders; and consumer protection all of which promote and safeguard the life, health, privacy, and dignity of patients [10].

HEALTH SERVICE PRODUCTION PROCESS

A health system consists of institutions (e.g., tertiary hospitals, regional/provincial hospitals, district hospitals, health centres, dispensaries, health posts, programmes, community-based health activities, and households) that leverage their entrepreneurial acumen to transform inputs (e.g., buildings, medical equipment, beds, vehicles, medicines, non-pharmaceutical supplies, human resources for health, food, and health education) into health service outputs (e.g., outpatient visits and inpatient discharges) and ultimately into health outcomes (e.g., improved life expectancy and health-related quality of life). The extent to which the above-mentioned health institutions utilise their inputs without waste (i.e., efficiency) determines the quantity and quality of health services produced and eventually the degree to which a health system achieves its goals.

Every institution combines health system inputs within its process to produce health services that ultimately sustain or improve health outcomes (health-related quality of life and life expectancy). An example of the input-process-output production function is a health promoting schools programme (Figure 3.2). Figure 3.3 illustrates an input-process-output production process of a health institution. The main economic problem facing health decision-makers is how to use scarce health system inputs (resources used in production) to satisfy unlimited population health needs for promotive, preventive, curative, rehabilitative, and cosmetic surgery services. The scarcity of health system inputs calls for their efficient use economically where efficiency means obtaining the maximum health benefits for a given cost or minimising the cost of a given health benefit. In other words, economic efficiency is getting the most health output from available resources.

Efficiency Analysis of Health Systems in Africa

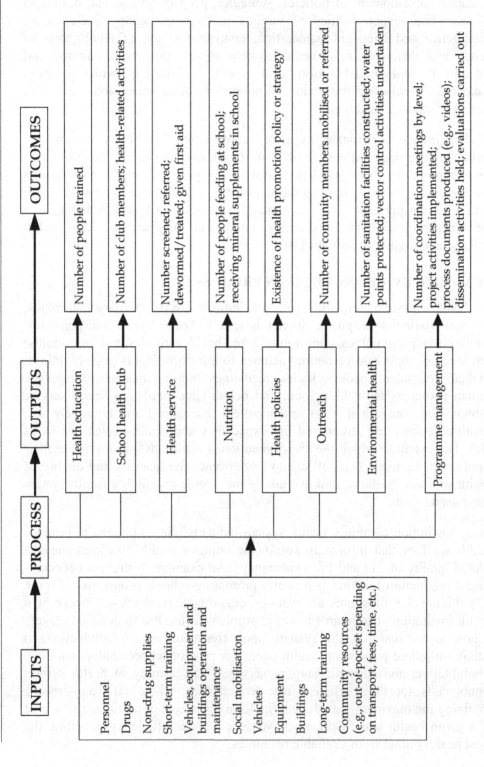

Figure 3.2   Health promoting schools programme

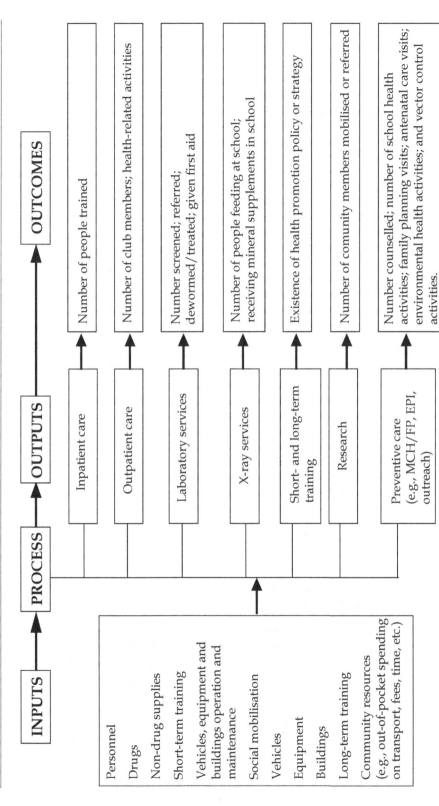

Figure 3.3 Production process for a health institution

Why Should Health Policy Makers Emphasise Efficiency and Efficiency Analysis?

There are several reasons why policy makers in sub-Saharan Africa should be concerned with health systems efficiency monitoring:

(a) Health systems of countries in the region are facing severe resource constraints [11].

(b) Health institutions and programmes are large consumers of scarce health sector resources. For instance, hospitals in developing countries consume an average of 50-80 per cent of the public health sector resources [12].

(c) Inefficiencies lead to inflated costs of service delivery and in the process undermine cost recovery ratios and any other stated benefits of cost-sharing schemes [13]. Indeed, inefficiencies in service provision leads to inflation of unit costs thus undermining the sustainability of health financing schemes and systems.

(d) Inefficiency is unethical and immoral because it denies people an opportunity to improve their health status at no extra cost to providers [14]. Inefficiencies undermine the extent to which countries are able to achieve both national and internationally agreed health development goals.

(e) Efficiency analysis enables the policy makers and healthcare managers to identify the magnitudes by which some inputs could be reduced without lowering output or the extent to which health service outputs could be increased without altering the current input/resource endowments.

(f) Much of the attention of policy makers, healthcare managers, health systems researchers, and donors is focussed on mobilising additional resources and not on efficiency of application of these resources.

(g) There is growing evidence that health institutions and programmes in SSA are inefficient [13, 15-23].

(h) There is need for identification of "best practice" that should be emulated by inefficient health decision-making units (DMU) and identification of "poor practice" that should be avoided by all DMUs.

(i) Efficiency analysis will guide the reallocation of resources from the inefficient to the efficient DMUs.

(j) Efficiency analysis will help to set performance targets and monitor efficiency changes over time with a view to implementing interventions for curbing or curtailing wasteful allocation and use of resources.

In August 2005, the fifty-fifth session of the WHO Regional Committee for Africa (consisting of Ministers of Health of 46 Member States) recommended that the WHO and the World Bank should support countries to institutionalise mechanisms for monitoring efficiency in the use of health sector resources [24]. Subsequently, at a special session of the African Union in May 2006 the Ministers of Health of countries in the African continent agreed to undertake measures to strengthen the health financing function of their health systems [25] with a view to mobilising more domestic resources for massive expansion of the coverage of health interventions envisaged in the United Nation's MDGs [26].

The Health Ministers undertook to institutionalise efficiency monitoring within the national health information management systems. In August 2006, the fifty-sixth session of the WHO Regional Committee for Africa adopted a strategy for health financing with the specific objective of ensuring efficiency in the allocation and use of health sector resources [27]. Thus, there is a growing awareness among the African Ministers of Health that as they attempt to mobilise more domestic and external resources, it is also important to ensure that available and future health-related sector resources are optimally used to produce health outcomes.

What is Efficiency?

Efficiency refers to the extent to which a health decision-making unit (DMU) uses the available health resources (inputs) to produce the maximum possible health-related outputs of a given quality [28]. According to Farrell [28], the efficiency of a firm consists of three components, namely, technical, allocative, and total economic or cost efficiency. Technical efficiency reflects the capability of a health-related DMU to produce optimal or maximum outputs from the available health system inputs. Alternatively, technical efficiency can be viewed as a situation in which a DMU produces a given level of outputs with the least quantities of inputs. Skaggs and Carlson [29] define technical efficiency as operating on the production possibilities frontier (PPF); that is, producing without waste. Estimation of technical efficiency requires information on quantities of both outputs and inputs.

Allocative efficiency refers to a situation where for any level of production of a DMU inputs are used in the proportions that minimise the cost of production given input prices. Skaggs and Carlson [29] define allocative efficiency as using resources to produce goods and services with the highest possible value. Estimation of allocative efficiency requires data on quantities of outputs and inputs and input prices. Total economic or cost efficiency is a product of technical efficiency and allocative efficiency. In other words, economic efficiency combines productive efficiency (producing without waste on the PPF) with allocative efficiency (allocating resources to their most highly valued uses) [29].

A DMU, for example a health unit, is regarded as technically efficient if it is operating on the best-practice production frontier in the industry. Conversely, a DMU is relatively inefficient under the following two conditions: (*a*) it is posssible to increase one output without either increasing any input or decreasing another output or (*b*) it is possible to decrease one input without either increasing another input or decreasing any output [30]. The basic ideas underlying Farrell's [28] concepts of technical and allocative efficiency (under the assumption of constant returns to scale) are illustrated in Figure 3.4. A household health education visits (HHEV) programme produces its output (one health education visit) from a combination of two inputs (community health nurse time and household time).

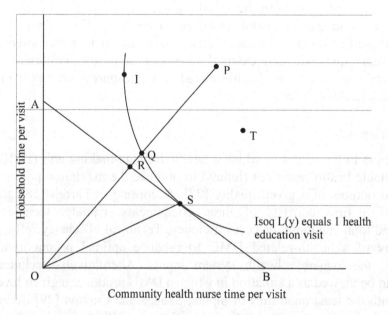

Figure 3.4   Technical, allocative, and cost efficiencies of a household health education visits programme

A technically efficient HHEV programme is one that is "located on an isoquant" (IS), that is, on the frontier. Thus, HHEV programmes operating at points *I*, *Q*, and *S* are technically efficient while those operating at points *P* and *T* are technically inefficient. The measure of technical efficiency (*TE*) of the HHEV programme *P* can be depicted as follows:

$$TE_P = OQ/\ OP \tag{1}$$

The equation denotes the ratio of the minimum input required to the actual input used given the input mix used by programme *P*. The ratio QP/OP represents the magnitude by which all inputs could be reduced without a corresponding reduction in output. For the HHEV programme P to be efficient, it has to relocate to point Q. Technical efficiency takes values between zero and one $(0 \leq TE_i \leq 1)$. Technically inefficient production HHEV programmes have a TE_i value less than one while the efficient ones have a TE_i value of 1.

Considering input prices, the isocost line AB represents the minimum cost of producing one unit of output (i.e., one household health education visit in our hypothetical example above). Allocative efficiency demands that production takes place at the point where the isoquant is tangential to the isocost line. Given this definition, the HHEV programmes I and Q are technically efficient but allocatively inefficient. However, the HHEV programme S is both technically and allocatively efficient [30]. The allocative efficiency for the HHEV programme P is given as $AE_P = OR/OQ$. The ratio RQ/OQ represents the magnitude of the reduction in production cost required if HHEV programme P were to operate at an allocatively efficient point like programme S. In his seminal paper, Farrel proposes that overall economic or cost efficiency *(EE)* be measured as $EE_P = OR/OP$. The advantage of overall economic efficiency is that it readily decomposes into technical (TE) and allocative (AE) efficiencies such that $EE = TE \times AE$.

How Do We Measure Efficiency?

The two methods found in the literature for measuring efficiency are parametric approaches that employ econometric (statistical) modelling [31] and non-parametric approaches that use mathematical linear programming techniques such as Data envelopment analysis *(DEA)* [32]. Measurement of the concept of efficiency is best illustrated using an example. If health service-producing units, for instance, had a single input and a single output the efficiency of transforming inputs into outputs for each health unit would be defined simply as:

Efficiency = output/input

Let us assume that a hypothetical country called Kibari has ten health districts. Each district has an innovative house-to-house health education programme for teaching citizens the causes of diabetes mellitus and cardiovascular disease, symptoms, and how to prevent these diseases through lifestyle behavioural change. The programme is operated by community health nurses with training in health promotion strategies for lifestyle behavioural change. During a household visit, a nurse will do a quick blood sugar test and a massive blood pressure test for all individuals in a household; analyse and advise on healthy diet; and maintain accurate records. For monitoring purposes, the Kibari Ministry of Health (MoH) has decided that the performance indicators for each health district will be the number of household health education visits. The data for the number of community health nurses, number of household education visits, and the ratio of household visits to nurses are contained in Table 3.3.

Nyanche health district has the highest number of household visits per nurse of 218 and is, therefore, the most efficient facility among the ten health districts. Isinya, by contrast, is the least efficient health district with only 32 visits per nurse per month. The efficiency of the health districts relative to Nyanche can be determined by dividing the ratio of "visits/nurse" (in column C) for each district by a similar ratio for Nyanche (i.e., 218). The outcome of those calculations is presented in column D of Table 3.3.

Table 3.3   Relative efficiency of health districts in Kibari State with one input and one output

Health district	Input=Nurses (A)	Output=Visits per month (B)	Output/Input= Visits/Nurse C=(B/A)	Relative efficiency (D)=(C/218)	Efficiency scores (E)= (D)x100
Kanyakine	4	858	215	0.99	99
Bissel	3	171	57	0.26	26
Enkorika	1	165	165	0.76	76
Kathera	11	374	34	0.16	16
Isinya	9	289	32	0.15	15
Mbale	3	394	131	0.60	60
Ndeiya	7	940	134	0.62	62
Kiambere	12	586	49	0.22	22
Nyanche	2	435	218	1.00	100
Simba	4	819	205	0.94	94

Note: Values in column D are obtained by dividing the values in column C by the value for the health district with the highest number of visits per nurse, that is, Nyanche.

The values in column *E* were obtained by multiplying each health district's relative efficiency value by 100. Since Nyanche has a value of 100%, it is said to be efficient. All the other health districts are inefficient. On the basis of the relative efficiency scores in column *E*, the health districts can be ranked as follows: 1=Nyanche, 2=Kanyakine, 3=Simba, 4=Enkorika, 5=Ndeiya, 6=Mbale, 7=Bissel, 8=Kiambere, 9=Kathera, and 10=Isinya. Isinya is, therefore, the least efficient health district with an efficiency score of 15%.

In terms of "visits/nurse" Nyanche is an example of "best-achieved performance" and is the health district whose practice all the other districts should strive to emulate. Nyanche can be used as a reference health district to set targets for improving the performance of the other health districts. In order to become efficient like Nyanche, for example, Isinya has two options. One alternative for Isinya would be to reduce the number of nurses by 85% (i.e.,

100% minus its score of 15%). That means [9 nurses minus (9 nurses times 0.15)] = 1.328 nurses. This would yield a performance ratio of 218, which is 289 visits divided by 1.328 nurses. Isinya also has the option of working to increase the number of household education visits from 289 to 1962, which would yield a visits/nurse ratio of 218 that is equivalent to that of Nyanche's.

The Director of Medical Services (DMS) for Kibari presented these results to District HHEV programme managers who appreciated the scoring and the policy implication. However, they brought to the attention of the DMS that the community health nurses not only provide health education but also immunise children during their visits. Thus, they agreed that the HHEV had two outputs: number of health education visits and number of children immunised. Therefore, the Kibari MoH economist was instructed by the DMS to re-evaluate the performance of the ten health districts based on how efficiently they used their single input of community health nurses to produce the two categories of health outputs. Table 3.4 shows the number of nurses, health education visits, and number of children immunised per health district.

The Kibari MoH economist obtained the efficiency of each health district in producing the two outputs by dividing each output by the corresponding input and determining the district with the highest ratios (presented in columns (D) and (E) of Table 3.4). Nyanche health district had the highest number of health education visits per nurse and was, therefore, the most efficient in producing health education visits. Similarly, Kanyakine had the highest number of children immunised per nurse and was, therefore, more efficient than other districts in immunising children. Thus, from Table 3.4 the picture of efficiency is not clear if we consider two outputs. However, an efficiency frontier graph can get us out of this predicament if we plot health education visits per nurse against number of children immunised per nurse (Figure 3.5).

Table 3.4   Relative efficiency of health districts in Kibari State with one input and two outputs

Health district	Input= nurses (A)	Output1= visits (B)	Output2= No. immunised (C)	Visits/ Nurse D=(B)/(A)	No. immunised/ Nurse E=(C)/(A)
Kanyakine	4	858	1,333	215	**333**
Bissel	3	171	427	57	142
Enkorika	1	165	36	165	36
Kathera	11	374	2,050	34	186
Isinya	9	289	260	32	29
Mbale	3	394	441	131	147
Ndeiya	7	940	1,287	134	184
Kiambere	12	586	698	49	58
Nyanche	2	435	257	**218**	129
Simba	4	819	428	205	107

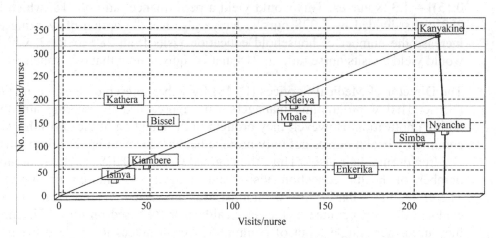

Figure 3.5 *Relative efficiency of health districts in Kibari State with one input and two outputs*

The efficiency frontier is the cornerstone of data envelopment analysis (DEA). The efficiency frontier has been derived using the performance ratios (in columns (D) and (E) of Table 3.4) for Kainyakine and Nyanche, the most efficient health districts in our data set. The two districts represent the standard of best performance. The efficiency frontier "envelops" the inefficient units within it and clearly shows the relative efficiency of each health district. Any health district on the frontier is considered 100% efficient and any district below it is inefficient and has an efficiency score of less than 100%. In our hypothetical example, except for Kanyakine and Nyanche, the other eight health districts are inefficient since they are not on the efficiency frontier.

Data envelopment analysis

This book focuses on the use of DEA in the measurement of efficiency of health systems DMUs. Therefore, in this subsection an overview of the DEA framework, its estimation, interpretation of results, and strengths and weaknesses will be given.

What is DEA?

Data envelopment analysis is a linear programming method for measuring the relative efficiencies of a set of DMUs. As demonstrated in the Kibari example, DEA measures the efficiency of a DMU relative to the efficiency of similar DMUs in the group subject to the restriction that all DMUs are situated on or below the production frontier [33-35]. Data envelopment analysis performs this feat by solving as many linear programming problems as the number of DMUs in the study sample. As mentioned earlier, the efficiency of a DMU that uses one input to produce one output would be obtained as follows [36]:

Efficiency = output/input (1)

Usually, health systems DMUs (hospitals and health centres) wil employ multiple inputs (e.g., different cadres of human resources for health, medicines, non-medical supplies, and capital inputs) to produce multiple outputs (e.g., curative, preventive, and rehabilitative services). In such a scenario, the efficiency of a DMU could be expressed as follows [36]:

Efficiency = weighted sum of outputs/weighted sum of inputs (2)

According to Charness *et al.* [36], the efficiency of a target DMU from the set "*j*" can then be obtained by solving the following model:

$$Max \quad h_0 = \sum_{R=1}^{s} U_r Y_{r0} \bigg/ \sum_{I=1}^{m} V_i X_{i0}$$

(3)

$$Subject \quad to: h_j \leq 1, \quad j = 1,...,n$$

$$u_r, v_r \geq 0$$

where Y_{rj} is the amount of output r from DMU j; X_{ij} is the amount of input i in j^{th} DMU; u_r is the coefficient of output r to be generated; v_i is the coefficient of input i to be generated; and n is the number of DMUs.

Charness et al [34] convert the fractional programming model (3) into the following constant returns to scale (CRS) linear programming model:

$$Max \quad h_0 = \sum u_r y_{rj0} = 1$$

(4)

$$s.t.: \sum_{r=1}^{s} v_i x_{ij0} = 1$$

$$\sum_{i=1}^{m} u_r y_{rj} - \sum v_i x_{ij} \leq 0, \quad j = 1,...,N.$$

where Y_r is the amount of output r ($r = 1,..., s$); X_i is the amount of input i ($i = 1,..., m$); u_r is the weight given to output r; and v_i is a weight given to input i. The latter constraint means that all DMUs are either on or below the frontier. When variable returns to scale are assumed, the linear programming problem to be estimated is:

$$Max\, h_o = \sum u_r y_{rj0} = 1 \qquad (5)$$

$$s.t.: \sum_{r=1}^{s} v_i x_{ij0} = 1$$

$$\sum_{i=1}^{m} u_r y_{rj} - \sum v_i x_{ij} + U_0 \le 0,\, j = 1,...,N$$

$$U_r, V_i \ge 0.$$

From equation (5) it is possible to derive scale efficiency; that is, whether or not the DMUs are operating on an optimal scale of production.

When is it appropriate to conduct a DEA?

Data envelopment analysis is the preferred method of efficiency analysis in the non-profit sector where [35]:

(a)   random noise is less of a problem;

(b)   multiple-output production is relevant;

(c)   price data is difficult to find;

(d)   setting behavioural assumptions such as profit (cost) maximisation (minimisation) is difficult.

There is a very strong case for application of DEA in the efficiency analysis of health systems and their components in Africa. Firstly, in most African countries different levels of health systems (e.g., teaching hospitals, provincial hospitals, district hospitals, health centres, dispensaries, or health posts) are fairly homogeneous in design and staffing. Secondly, health systems employ multiple inputs to produce multiple outputs. Thirdly, price data are either difficult to find or when available they do not reflect the true opportunity cost of the inputs concerned. Fourthly, majority of health services are provided by not-for-profit government or non-government owned hospitals and health centres.

What are the requirements and sources of data for estimating DEA models?

1. Health service inputs

The factors of production that health systems entrepreneurs use to produce health services fall under the following broad categories:

(a)   Labour, which may be measured in terms of, for example, number of full-time equivalent physicians, clinical officers, nurses, diagnostic staff, administrative/management staff, and support staff. This information can be obtained from the health facility level, the health management information systems (HMIS) office at the Ministry of Health headquarters, or the human resource department of the Ministry of Health.

(b) Supplies, transport, and maintenance, which may be measured in terms of, for example, monetary values of pharmaceuticals and non-pharmaceutical supplies. Here, one could use the total amount of money spent by a DMU to purchase medicines or the total monetary value of medicines supplied to a DMU from the central medical stores. One could also have another input variable consisting of expenditure on all other items such as non-pharmaceutical supplies; utilities (e.g., water, postage, telephone, and electricity); fuel and maintenance of buildings, equipment, and vehicles. These kinds of data might be obtained from the printed government annual expenditure and health facility expenditure records.

(c) Capital, which may be proxied by, for example, number of beds or volume of facility space expressed in square metres for buildings, number of functional equipment, and number of vehicles. This kind of information might be available from the HMIS or departments of the Ministry of Health dealing with health facilities infrastructure and transport.

2. Health service outputs

A health facility may produce two or more of the following outputs depending on its level:

(a) Inpatient treatment, which may be measured in terms of number of admissions or number of discharges.

(b) Outpatient treatment, which may be measured in terms of number of curative visits.

(c) Preventive services provided, which may be measured in terms of number of infant and child growth monitoring visits, number of fully immunised children, number of people undergoing voluntary counselling and testing (VCT) for HIV, number of contraceptive products distributed, number of health education sessions, number of water sources protected, number of households with clean water, number of households with hygienic human excreta disposal facilities, and number of public facilities inspected among others.

(d) Teaching, which may be measured in terms of number of different cadres of health workers graduating.

(e) Research, which may be measured in terms of number of health-related research outputs (books, monographs, articles, and policy briefs) published.

(f)   Supervision, which may be measured in terms of number of supervisory visits to health centres and health posts.

The choice of inputs and outputs will depend on preferences of the client who has commissioned the study, purpose of the study, and availability of data. Thus, it is worthwhile to have discussions with the client, those in charge of national health services (e.g., DMS) and health management information systems (HMIS) managers before settling on a set of variables. It is also advisable to review the relevant national, regional, and global literature to determine the types of conceptual frameworks, variables, and data sources that have been employed by other researchers. The possible sources of output data are the Ministry of Health HMIS office, medical records of health facilities (hospitals and health centres), and programme offices. The latter is relevant if the aim of the study is to measure performance of a specific programme; for example, HIV/AIDS, malaria, maternal and child health, and family planning among others.

3. Health outcomes

The two main health outcomes are changes in life expectancy and changes in health-related quality of life. Various indices have been used to measure health outcomes in a combined manner including quality-adjusted life years (QALY) [37]; health-adjusted life years (HALE) [38]; disability-adjusted life years (DALY) [36]; and disability-adjusted life expectancy (DALE) [38]. It is beyond the scope of this book to go into the details of how these indices are calculated, but the reader is encouraged to look at the references provided in Kirigia [37] in order to acquire an understanding of these indices, how they are quantified, and data sources. Very few studies have estimated the efficiency of producing health outcomes [31]. There are several explanations for this:

(a)   it takes a while for health impact to be noticed for many health interventions;

(b)   health outcomes are influenced by many factors not related to health systems [39];

(c)   calculation of health indices is data-intensive and costly;

(d)   health interventions are often implemented in combinations and permutations making it difficult to isolate the effects of individual interventions. Thus, efficiency studies usually employ health service indicators as measures of outputs.

How do we interpret results of DEA?

You will gain a deeper understanding of how to interpret DEA results as you read the contents of various chapters in this book. Nevertheless, the efficiency scores range from 1 (100%) to 0 (0%). A score of 1 indicates that a health service DMU is relatively efficient compared to its peers, but this does not mean that such a DMU cannot increase its efficiency further. On the other extreme, a zero value implies that the DMU in question is totally inefficient compared to its peers.

The Frontier Analyst software was used to estimate the efficiency of the ten health districts mentioned earlier (see Table 3.4) in our hypothetical example and the output is contained in Table 3.5. Nyanche and Kanyakine health districts have technical efficiency scores of 100% suggesting that they are efficient compared to their peers. Since there is no evidence that the two health facilities have an allocative efficiency of 100%, it is impossible to tell from the available information whether or not they are economically efficient. The other eight health districts are technically inefficient since their scores are less than 100%. However, the degree of inefficiency varies widely from 94.14% in Simba to 14.83% in Isinya. Thus, in order to become efficient Isinya would need to reduce its inputs by about 85%.

Table 3.5   Technical efficiency of Kibari health districts

Health District (DMU)	Technical efficiency score
Nyanche	100.00
Kanyakine	100.00
Simba	94.14
Enkorika	75.86
Ndeiya	62.44
Mbale	60.85
Kathera	55.92
Bissel	42.71
Kiambere	22.65
Isinya	14.83

What are the strengths of DEA?

Data envelopment analysis has the following attributes that make it appealing [35, 40]:

(a)   focuses on each decision-making unit (DMU) in contrast to population averages;

(b)   produces a single efficiency measure for each DMU in terms of input-output relationships;

(c)   can simultaneously handle multiple inputs and multiple outputs without the requirement for homogeneous measurement units;

(d)   can adjust for exogenous variables that are beyond the control of the decision-making unit;

(e)   does not require assigning a priori knowledge of prices for the inputs and outputs;

(f)   does not require the assumption of a functional form relating inputs to outputs;

(g)   produces estimates for the desired changes in inputs and outputs for moving the inefficient DMUs to the efficient frontier;

(h)   inputs and outputs can have very different units (e.g., X_1 could be in disability-adjusted life years and X_2 in shillings or another currency) without the need for an a priori trade-off between the two;

(i)   it is pareto-optimal;

(j)   focuses on observed best-practice frontiers rather than on central tendency properties of frontiers.

What are the weaknesses of DEA?

(a)   It is *non*-stochastic. It does not capture random noise (e.g., epidemics, weather, strikes, or civil strife). Any deviation from the estimated efficiency frontier is interpreted as being due to inefficiency.

(b)   It is non-statistical in the sense that it is not possible to conduct statistical tests of hypotheses regarding the inefficiency and structure of the production technology [35].

(c)   It is good at estimating "relative" efficiency of a DMU but it converges very slowly to "absolute" efficiency. In other words, it can tell you how well you are doing compared to your peers but not compared to a "theoretical maximum" [40].

(d)   Since a standard formulation of DEA creates a separate linear programme for each DMU, large problems can be computationally intensive [40].

REFERENCES

1. Murray CJL, Frenk J. A framework for assessing the performance of health systems. *Bulletin of the World Health Organization 2000*;78(6):717-731.

2. World Health Organization. *The world health report 2000 – improving performance of health systems*. Geneva: World Health Organization; 2000.

3. Adams OB, Shengella B, Stilwell B, Larizgoitia I, Issakov A, Kwankam SY, Tjam FS. Provision of personal and non-personal health services: proposal for monitoring. In: In: Murray CJL, Evans DB, editors. *Health systems performance assessment: debates, methods and empiricism*. Geneva: World Health Organization; 2003.p 235-249.

4. World Health Organization. *The world health report 2006 – working for health*. Geneva: World Health Organization;; 2006.

5. World Health Organization. *Strengthening health systems to improve health outcomes: WHO's framework for action*. Geneva: World Health Organization; 2007.

6. World Health Organization Regional Office for Europe. *European Observatory on health systems and policies.* Copenhagen:World Health Organization; 2010. Available at: http://www.euro.who.int/observatory/Glossary/

7. World Health Organization. *Progress in the rational use of medicines, World Health Assembly Resolution WHA60.16.* Geneva: World Health Organization; 2007.

8. Mills AJ, Ranson MK. The design of health systems. In: Merson MH, Black RE, Mills AJ, editors. *International public health - diseases, programmes, systems, and policies.* Gaithersburg: Aspen; 2001. p 515-557.

9. Savedoff WD, Carrin G, Kawabata K, Mechbal A. Monitoring the health financing function. In: Murray CJL, Evans DB, editors. *Health systems performance assessment: debates, methods and empiricism.* Geneva: World Health Organization; 2003.p 205-210.

10. Kirigia JM, Wambebe C, Baba-Moussa A. Status of national research bioethics committees in the WHO African Region. *BMC Medical Ethics* 2005;6:10. Available at: http://www.biomedcentral.com/content/6/1/10.

11. Kirigia JM, Preker A, Carrin G, Mwikisa CN, Diarra-Nama AJ. An overview of health financing patterns and the way forward in the WHO African Region. *East African Medical Journal* 2006;83(9 Suppl):S1-S28.

12. Barnum H, Kutzin J. *Public hospitals in developing countries: resource use, cost, financing.* Baltimore: Johns Hopkins University Press for the World Bank; 1993.

13. Zere EA, Addison T, McIntyre D. Hospital efficiency in sub-Saharan Africa: evidence from South Africa. *South African Journal of Economics* 2000;69(2):336-358.

14. Culyer AJ. The morality of efficiency in health care: some uncomfortable implications. *Health Economics* 1992;1(1):7-18.

15. Kirigia JM, Emrouznejad A, Cassoma B, Asbu EZ, Barry SP. A performance assessment method for hospitals: the case of municipal hospitals in Angola. *Journal of Medical Systems* 2008;32(6):509-519.

16. Osei D, D'Almeida S, George MO, Kirigia JM, Mensah AO, Kainyu LH. Technical efficiency of public district hospitals and health centres in Ghana: a pilot study. *Cost Effectiveness and Resource Allocation* 2005;3:9. Available at: *http://www.resource-allocation.com/ content/3/1/9.*

17. Kirigia JM, Emrouznejad A, Sambo LG, Munguti N, Liambila W. Using Data envelopment analysis to measure the technical efficiency of public health centers in Kenya. *Journal of Medical Systems* 2004;28(2):155-166.

18. Kirigia JM, Emrouznejad A, Sambo LG. Measurement of technical efficiency of public hospitals in Kenya: using Data envelopment analysis. *Journal of Medical Systems* 2002; 26(1):39-45.

19. Zere E, Mbeeli T, Shangula K, Mandlhate C, Mutirua K, Tjivambi B, Kapenambili W. Technical efficiency of district hospitals: evidence from Namibia using Data envelopment analysis. *Cost Effectiveness and Resource Allocation* 2006;4:5. Available at: *http://www.resource-allocation.com/content/4/1/95*.

20. Renner A, Kirigia JM, Zere AE, Barry SP, Kirigia DG, Kamara C,Muthuri HK. Technical efficiency of peripheral health units in Pujehun district of Sierra Leone: a DEA application. *BMC Health Services Research* 2005;5:**77**. Available at: *www.biomedcentral.com/1472-6963/5/77*.

21. Kirigia JM, Sambo LG, Scheel H.Technical efficiency of public clinics in Kwazulu-Natal Province of South Africa. *East African Medical Journal* 2001;78(3 Suppl):S1-S13.

22. Kirigia JM, Sambo LG, Lambo E. Are public hospitals in Kwazulu/Natal province of South Africa technically efficient? *African Journal of Health Sciences* 2000;7(3/4):24-31.

23. Masiye F, Kirigia JM, Emrouznejad A, Sambo LG, Mounkaila AB, Chimfwembe D, Okello D. Efficient management of health centres human resources in Zambia. *Journal of Medical Systems* 2006;30:473–481.

24. World Health Organization Regional Office for Africa. *Fifty-fifth WHO Regional Committee for Africa final report.* Brazzaville: World Health Organization; 2005.

25. African Union. *Universal access to HIV/AIDS, tuberculosis and malaria services by a united Africa by 2010, Resolution Sp/Assembly/ATM/5(I) Rev. 3 of the Ministers of Health on health financing in Africa.* Addis Ababa: African Union; 2006.

26. United Nations. *Millennium Development Declaration, Resolution A/55/L.2.* New York: United Nations; 2000.

27. World Health Organization Regional Office for Africa. *Health financing: a strategy for the African Region, Document AFR/RC56/10.* Brazzaville: World Health Organization; 2006.

28. Farrel MJ. The measurement of productive efficiency. *Journal of Royal Statistical Society* 1957;120(3):283-281.

29. Skaggs NT, Carlson JL. *Microeconomics: individual choices and its consequences.* Oxford: Blackwell; 1996.

30. Coelli TJ. *A Guide to DEAP Version 2.1: a Data envelopment analysis (computer) program,* Centre of Efficiency and Productivity Analysis (CEPA) Working Paper 96/08. Department of Econometrics, University of New England, Armidale, NSW Australia; 1996.

31. Evans DB, Lauer JA, Tandon A, Murray CJL. Determinants of health systems performance: second stage efficiency analysis. In: Murray CJL, Evans EB, editors. *Health systems performance assessment: debates, methods and empiricism.* Geneva: World Health Organization; 2003.p 692-698.

32. Tandon A, Lauer JA, Evans DB, Murray CJL. Health system efficiency: concepts.In: Murray CJL, Evans EB, editors. *Health systems performance assessment: debates, methods and empiricism.* Geneva: World Health Organization; 2003.p 683-691.

33. Fare R, Grosskopf S, Lovell CAK. *Production frontiers.* Cambridge: Cambridge University Press; 1994.

34. Thanassoulis E. *Introduction to the theory and application of Data envelopment analysis: a foundation text with integrated software.* Boston: Kluwer Academic Publishers; 2001.

35. Coelli T, Rao DSP, Battese G. *An introduction to efficiency and productivity analysis.* Boston: Kluwer Academic Publishers; 1998.

36. Charness A, Cooper WW, Rhodes E. Measuring the efficiency of decision making units.*European Journal of Operational Research* 1978;2(6):429-444.

37. Kirigia JM, editor. *Economic evaluation of public health problems in sub-Saharan Africa.* Nairobi: University of Nairobi Press; 2009.

38. Mathers CD, Salomon JA, Murray CJL, Lopez AD. Alternative summary measures of average population health. In: Murray CJL, Evans EB, editors. *Health systems performance assessment: debates, methods and empiricism.* Geneva: World Health Organization; 2003.p 319-334.

39. Anand S, Ammar W, Evans T, Hasegawa T, Kissimova-Skarbek K, Langer A, Lucas AO, Makubalo L, Marandi A, Meyer G, Podger A, Smith P, Wibulpolprasert S. Report of the scientific peer review group on health systems performance assessment. In:Murray CJL, Evans EB, editors. *Health systems performance assessment: debates, methods and empiricism.* Geneva: World Health Organization; 2003.p 839-913.

40. http://www.emp.pdx.edu/dea/homedea.html.

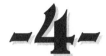

Introduction to Health Services Production and Cost Theory

Joses M. Kirigia

INTRODUCTION

The ultimate objective of health decision-making units (DMUs) is to equitably promote, restore, and maintain the individual's physical, mental, and social well-being [1]. This objective must be pursued in a responsive and financially fair manner that maximises the impact of the health systems resources of a country on its population [2]. Consequently, each DMU must strive to maximise the production and provision of quality (intensity) health services subject to allocated and available health system resources; that is, DMUs must produce health services efficiently and at minimal cost. This chapter presents the essential aspects of health services production theory.

HEALTH SYSTEMS INPUTS

Our health needs are satisfied by promotive, preventive, curative, and rehabilitative health services. The quantity of health services provided depends largely on the amount of productive resources at our disposal. In the context of health systems, a productive resource is a natural substance or manufactured good used in the production of health services. Such resources are also called factors of production since they are used as inputs in the process of producing health services. The factors of production for health systems include the following:

(a) **Labour:** This refers to the productive persons and their skills and knowledge (human capital). In health systems, labour includes both technical and support human resources. Technical human resources in health systems include physicians, dentists, pharmacists, nurses, midwives, community health workers, field health educators, laboratory technologists and technicians, and radiologists. Support human resources in health systems include administrators, personnel managers, clerks, accountants, secretaries, cleaners, storekeepers, and security guards.

(b) **Medicines**: These refer to the pharmaceutical products used in prevention of illnesses (e.g., vaccines) or the treatment of diseases (e.g., antiretrovirals and antimalarials). They include both conventional and traditional medicines, which are proven to be effective in curing or ameliorating illnesses.

(c) **Non-pharmaceutical materials and supplies:** These refer to non-medical materials used in health facilities or programmes such as bedding, cleaning materials, and stationery.

(d) **Utilities:** These refer to water, electricity, and information and communications technology.

(e) **Capital goods:** These consist of manufactured tools of production and the technology embodied in them, for example, land, buildings, furniture, medical equipment used in diagnosis and treatment, computers, computer software, insecticide-treated bed nets, and beds. Capital inputs have a useful life of more than one year.

(f) **Entrepreneurial ability:** This refers to the ability to envision, organise, and plan the production of health services.

Inputs are usually expressed or measured in flow units such as amount of physician or nursing time, number of magnetic resonance imaging hours per week, quantity of medicine used per week, and litres of water per hour or week among others. Health systems' inputs are in very limited supply especially in Africa [3]. Given the heavy burden of both communicable and non-communicable diseases [4] and the poor health conditions, such as maternal mortality in Africa, it is not possible to meet all of the health needs of the region's popuation. Therefore, society (or policy makers) must determine those health needs that must be addressed with the available health systems' inputs.

Each decision entails an opportunity cost; that is, the value of the next best opportunity forgone because a decision has been made to allocate the resources to a particular need. For example, if a poor country decides to acquire an organ transplant unit costing USD1 million, the opportunity cost would be the number of children who would have been immunised instead using that money. If the cost of immunising one child is USD1.50, for instance, then it means that the USD1 million used to buy the organ transplant unit could have been used to immunise 666,667 children (1,000,000/1.5). If health policy makers are rational decision-makers, they would be expected to have the capacity of setting health development goals and acting purposefully towards achieving these goals. Since health systems resources are scarce, health decision-makers ought to choose health policies, programmes, interventions, or services for which there is evidence that the net health gains are greatest.

HEALTH SYSTEM OUTPUTS

The ultimate object of health systems DMUs is to improve health. Health is a "state of complete physical, mental, and social well-being and not merely the absence of disease or infirmity" [1]. Social scientists define individual health as the ability to perform one's expected societal roles or functions such as moving around unaided; participating in social activities including cultural, religious, and leisure functions; performing usual activities like work or schooling; and caring for oneself, for example, by bathing, cleaning one's house and clothes, and feeding and toileting oneself.

Health is a product of longevity and health-related quality of life [3,4,5,6]. Health is a function of multiple non-health systems' factors such as information and technology, communication, cultural practices, education, employment, personal hygiene, environment, food, security, shelter, water, and sanitation. Health is also the result of health systems' factors such as goods and services [5,7]. It is important to note that health systems DMUs do not produce health but health services. This chapter delves mainly into the economic theory that underpins the behaviour of such DMUs as they endeavour to produce and provide effective health services. Like inputs, the outputs of health services are measured in flow units such as the number of children immunised per year against measles, tuberculosis, diphtheria, or hepatitis; the number of family planning visits per year; and the number of maternal and child health visits per year among others.

PRODUCTION FUNCTION FOR A SINGLE HEALTH SERVICE

Production Function with One Variable Input

Production technology refers to the process through which health systems' inputs are turned into health services (or outputs) so as to maintain or enhance health-related quality of life and longevity. The production theory of a health DMU such as a hospital, health centre, or programme examines the physical process of production of health services. The technical relationship between the quantity of health systems' inputs required to produce a health service and the quantity of health services produced is called a production function. The production function determines the maximum health services output that can be produced from a given quantity of inputs (and a given level of technology). Therefore, the production function embodies productive efficiency, which is the process of getting the maximum health services outputs from a given quantity of health systems' inputs [8].

For any type of health service, the production function is expressed in the form of a table, a graph, or an equation showing the maximum output rate of the health service that can be attained from any specified set of usage rates of health system inputs. The production function summarises the characteristics of existing health technology at a given time and shows the technological constraints that a DMU must reckon with [9]. Consider, for example, the short-run production function for child immunisation at Kathera Health Centre with one input of fixed quantity and another input whose quantity is variable. Suppose that the fixed input ($\overline{K}$) is the health centre's building space (300 sq. ft.), the variable input is the number of community health nurses (N), and the output is the number of children immunised (Q_{IC}). The short-run production function for Kathera Health Centre would be expressed as $Q_{IC} = f(\overline{K}, N)$. In the short run, the number of children immunised at Kathera Health Centre is determined by the number of nurses employed within a fixed stock of building space.

Suppose that the nurse in charge of Kathera Health Centre, Mrs Lenity Muthuri, decides to determine the effect on annual output of varying the number of nurses during the year for the same building space (and if she maximises output). The results in Table 4.1 represent the short-run production function in this situation if Kathera Health Centre is maximising the health service output of the nurses and the health centre space it uses.

Table 4.1   Output of children immunised when various
            numbers of nurses are applied to a fixed health
            centre space of 300 sq. ft.

Number of nurses used per year	Total number of children immunised
0	–
1	270
2	600
3	1,300
4	2,800
5	3,500
6	4,000
7	4,000
8	3,400

Mrs Muthuri discovers that as more nurses are added to the production process, the number of children immunised (output) increases but eventually the magnitude of the increase declines. Alternatively, a line graph depicting the relationship between output (total number of children immunised) and input (nurses) can be regarded as the production function for the health centre (Figure 4.1).

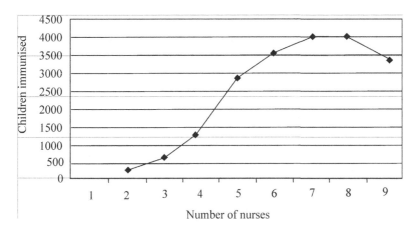

Figure 4.1   *Relationship between number of children immunised and*
number of nurses at Kathera Health Centre

Table 4.2 shows the average product and the marginal physical product of a variable input (in this case nurse labour). Average product is defined as the level of health service output per unit of the variable health system input employed. In this case, the average product of nurses (input) equals the total number of children immunised (Q_{CI}) divided by the number of full-time nurses (N) used to immunise them; that is, $AP_N = Q_{CI} \div N$. In our example, the average product of two nurses equals 300 fully immunised children per nurse per year (i.e., $600 \div 2$). Note that the average number of children immunised per nurse increases to a maximum of 700 and decreases thereafter.

The marginal physical product (MP) of an input is the change in total health service output (∂Q) resulting from the addition of the last unit of the health system input (∂N) when the levels of other health system inputs are held constant; that is, $MP = \partial Q \div \partial N$. For Kathera Health Centre, the marginal physical product of nurses (MP_N), as shown in the fourth column (Table 4.2) was obtained using the formula $MP_N = \partial Q_{CI} \div \partial N$. For example, the marginal physical product of the fifth nurse is $MP_{N=5} = (3{,}500 - 2{,}800) \div (5\text{-}4) = 700 \div 1 = 700$. Figure 4.2 shows the average and marginal product curves for labour for the Kathera Health Centre.

Table 4.2   Average and marginal product of labour (nurses) at Kathera Health Centre

Number of nurses (N)	Total output (Q_{CI})	Average product of labour (AP_N)	Marginal product of labour (MP_N)
0	0	-	-
1	270	270	270
2	600	300	330
3	1,300	433	700
4	2,800	700	1,500
5	3,500	700	700
6	4,000	667	500
7	4,000	571	0
8	3,400	425	-600

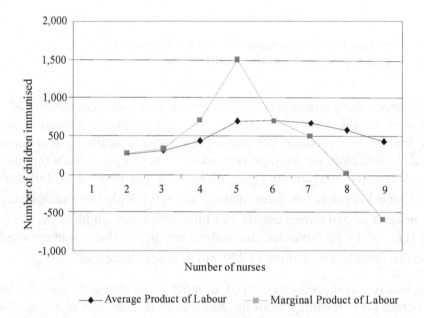

Figure 4.2   Average and marginal product curves for labour

Marginal product exceeds average product when the latter is increasing and vice versa. At its maximum (in this case at 700 children immunised per nurse), average product equals marginal product and this is the point at which the MP and the AP curves cross. When average product is at its maximum, marginal product, $\partial(Q_{IC}/N)/\partial N$, equals zero. This means that marginal product $\partial Q_{IC}/\partial N$ must be equal to average product Q_{IC}/N when average product is at its maximum [9]. Thus,

$$\frac{\partial(Q_{ic}/N)}{\partial N} = \frac{1}{N}\left(\frac{\partial Q_{ic}}{\partial N} - \frac{Q_{ic}}{N}\right) = \left(\frac{1}{5}\right) \times \left(700 - \frac{3500}{5}\right) = 0.$$

Table 4.2 also illustrates the law of diminishing marginal returns, which states that "if equal increments of an input are added, and the quantities of other inputs are held constant, the resulting increments of the product will decrease beyond some point; that is, the marginal product of the input will diminish" [10]. In the examples given, the marginal product of labour decreases beyond four units of nurses; this is because the health centre space would become overcrowded when more than this number of nurses is applied.

Note that the law of diminishing returns is an empirical generalisation and not a deduction from physical or biological laws. It assumes that health technology remains fixed, and also that the quantity of at least one health system input is being held constant [8]. Thus the law of diminishing returns does not apply to cases where there are increases in all health systems inputs or when health technology is allowed to change.

Production Function with Two Variable Inputs

All the inputs can be varied in the long term, for example, by expanding the building space, training more specialised human resources for health, and purchasing more organ transplant units. In a two-input situation, an isoquant curve is used to show the set of all technically efficient combinations of inputs which are just sufficient to produce a specific quantity of health services outputs [8]. Isoquants are labelled with the level of output they can produce and this is fixed by the technology employed. Table 4.3 depicts ten ways or production techniques of producing an output of 2,000 fully immunised children. This information was then used to generate an isoquant or equal output curve (Figure 4.3). The isoquant locates all the combinations of building space and number of nurses that yield the same level of total outputs. Note that the isoquant is convex to the origin (it is bowed toward the origin) indicating the diminishing of marginal productivity of nurses and health centre space.

Table 4.3 *Alternative combinations of two inputs that yield the same level of total output for a representative health centre*

Output: number of fully immunised children	Capital (S): health centre space (sq. ft)	Labour (N): number of nurses
2,000	100	1
2,000	90	2
2,000	80	4
2,000	70	7
2,000	60	11
2,000	50	16
2,000	40	22
2,000	30	29
2,000	20	39
2,000	10	50

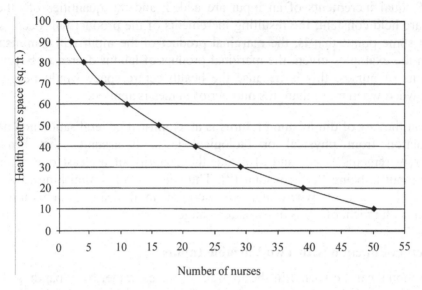

Figure 4.3   Alternative combinations of two inputs needed to immunise 2,000 children

There are two main properties of production functions (technology). First, they are monotonic suggesting that if a health DMU increases the level of at least one of its inputs, it should be possible to produce as much of the health service outputs as it was producing originally. This is sometimes referred to as the property of free disposal, which indicates that if a DMU can dispose of any input at no cost, then having extra inputs around cannot hurt [8]. Second, production functions are convex, which means that if a health DMU has two ways of producing y units of health services outputs, (x_1, x_2) and (k_1, k_2), then the weighted average of the two approaches will produce at least y units of outputs. If a DMU can conduct the production activities independently, then the weighted averages of the production plans will also be feasible and thus the isoquants will have a convex shape [8]. Health systems' production isoquants may assume various shapes depending on the degree to which health systems' inputs can be substituted [8,10].

Fixed proportions input–output or Leontief isoquant

Figure 4.4 shows a right-angled isoquant depicting zero substitutability (strict complementarity) of two factors of production of a health system. This is an extreme situation where it is impossible to make any substitution between the health system's inputs because each level of health services output requires a specific combination of the two inputs. Let us take an example of the Magnetic Resonance Imaging (MRI) Department at the Nairobi Private Hospital that specialises in producing films of the human body. The only way of getting a film is to use one radiologist (x_1) and one MRI unit hour (x_2). Therefore, the total number of human anatomy films that the MRI unit can produce depends on the minimum number of radiologists and the number of MRI hours that the unit has. The production function can be written as $f(x_1, x_2) = \min\{x_1, x_2\}$. Only one combination of MRI unit hours and radiologists can be used to efficiently produce a given number of films (e.g., point X on isoquant $q1$, point Y on isoquant $q2$, and point Z on isoquant $q3$). Adding more MRI units alone will not increase the number of films and neither will the addition of more radiologists alone. To produce a unit of output (e.g., MRI film), a fixed amount of each input is required. In this case, there is only one method of producing the films.

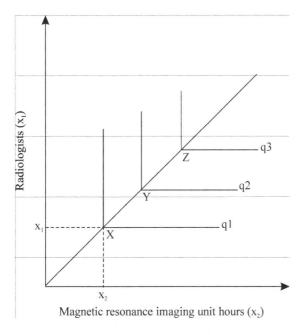

Magnetic resonance imaging unit hours (x₂)

Figure 4.4 *Fixed proportions input-output isoquants when inputs are used in fixed proportions*

Linear isoquant

Figure 4.5 shows a different kind of extreme situation where a health system's inputs are perfect substitutes of each other. Suppose, for example, that a community health programme in rural Africa is conducting health education activities for prevention of communicable and non-communicable diseases and two of its inputs, such as community health workers (x_1) and field health educators (x_2), are perfectly substitutable. Perfect substitutability means that a given level of output, say $q1$ may be produced using only x_1 or x_2 or an infinite combination of x_1 an x_2. Since the marginal rate of technical substitution

(MRTS) is constant at all points on the linear isoquant, the same health services output (e.g., $q3$) can be produced with mostly field health educators (at Z), mostly community health workers (at X), or an infinite combination of both (at Y). Thus, points X, Y, and Z represent three different combinations of community health workers and field health educators that produce the same level of health services outputs (in this case the number of persons reached with health education).

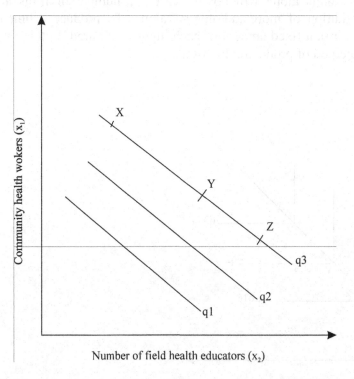

Figure 4.5   Linear isoquants when inputs are perfect substitutes of each other

This hypothetical example of perfect substitution is of particular interest to developing countries experiencing a crisis in human resources for health. For example, if clinical officers can perform all the functions of physicians, then it might be more cost-effective to train more clinical officers than physicians. Clinical officers take a shorter time to train, are less costly to produce, and are less prone to the problem of emigration since they are not in demand internationally. Likewise, if community health nurses can perform the same duties as registered nurses, the available scarce resources for producing nurses could instead be spent on producing this category of health workers.

Linear programming isoquant

It is also referred to as activity analysis or kinked isoquant. Figure 4.6 depicts a production function characterised by just a few processes of producing any one health service output. It applies in situations where substitutability of two health systems' inputs is only limited to the kinks [10]. An example of a kinked isoquant might be combinations of general physicians and surgeons where general physicians might substitute for surgeons especially for minor surgical operations. Another example is substitution of midwives for gynaecologists particularly in delivering babies of mothers without complications.

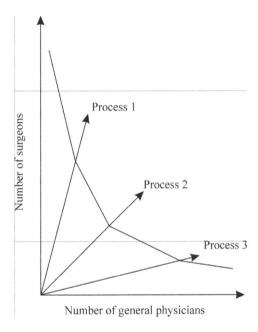

Figure 4.6   Linear programming isoquant

Smooth, convex isoquant

Figure 4.7 shows an isoquant that appears as a smooth curve convex to the origin. This isoquant assumes continuous substitutability of the two health systems' inputs over a certain range beyond which the inputs cannot be substituted for each other [10]. For example, suppose that a malaria prevention programme has the objective of distributing as many insecticide-treated bed nets (ITNs) as possible to the population living in a malaria-endemic catchment area. The ITNs can be distributed by either community health workers (x_1) or dedicated community-based ITN distributors (x_2).

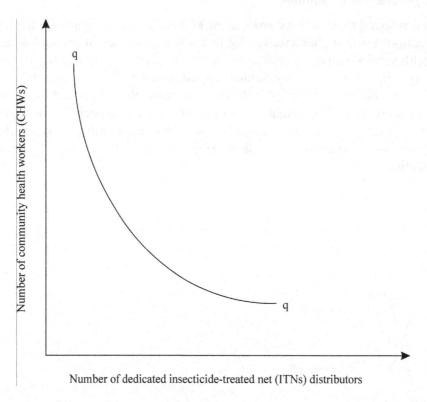

Figure 4.7   Smooth convex isoquant

Generally, a DMU production function describes not just a single isoquant but a set of isoquants (or an isoquant map) showing different levels of a health service output. As illustrated in Figure 4.8, individual isoquants correspond to different levels of health services output (in this case the number of children immunised) that increase as one moves outwards to the right. The output of number of children immunised increases from isoquant $q1$ with 500 to isoquant $q3$ with 1,500.

Marginal Productivity of the Health Systems' Factors of Production

In a two-input situation, in traditional economic theory, the production function of a health system's DMU in a two-input situation would assume the form:

$$Q = f(L, K, v, \gamma)$$

where Q is the quantity of a DMU's health services outputs per unit of time, L is the human resources for health hours per year, K is the physical capital (building space, health technologies, and vehicles), v is the returns to scale, and γ is entrepreneurial and organisational efficiency. Two health systems' DMUs with identical inputs and the same returns to scale may have different levels of health services output owing to differences in their entrepreneurial and organisational efficiency [10].

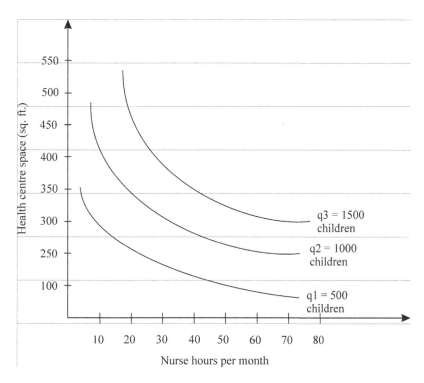

Figure 4.8   Isoquant map of a health centre immunisation of children

The marginal product (MP) of a health system's input or factor of production is the change in output of health services resulting from a very small change in this input or factor while keeping all other inputs or factors constant [10]. Even though the marginal product can take a positive, zero, or negative value, production theory focuses only on the range of health services output for which the marginal product of health systems' inputs is positive (i.e., the efficient part of the health system's production function). The marginal product of each health system's input is the partial derivative of the production function with respect to that factor and can be expressed as follows:

$$MP_L = \frac{\partial Q}{\partial L} \text{ and } MP_K = \frac{\partial Q}{\partial K}$$

where ∂ stands for change in variables as defined above. The marginal product of a health system's input or factor can be obtained by estimating a

Cobb-Douglas production function using the regression analysis $Q = b_0 L^{b_1} K^{b_2} \varepsilon$ where b_0, b_1, and b_2 are intercept, coefficient for labour, and coefficient for capital input respectively. The marginal product of human resources for health (MP_L) is

$$MP_L = b_1 \left(\frac{Q}{L_i} \right) = b_1 (AP_L)$$

where Q is the total health services output of a given DMU, L_i is the quantity of the ith category of human resources for health used within a given period, b_1 is the change in the total health services output emanating from employment of an extra unit of the ith human resources for health, and AP_{Li} is the average product of labour. Similarly, the marginal product of health systems' physical capital (MP_K) is

$$MP_K = b_2 \left(\frac{Q}{K_i} \right) = b_2 (AP_{Ki})$$

where K_i is the quantity of the ith category of physical capital used within a given period, b_2 is the change in the total health services output emanating from employment of an extra unit of the ith physical capital, and AP_{K_i} is the average product of capital.

Marginal Rate of Technical Substitution and Elasticity of Substitution

Due to resource constraints in health systems, health decision-makers in developing countries are increasingly considering substitution of health systems' inputs. For example, clinical officers can be substituted for physicians as a way of dealing with deficiencies in numbers of physicians. Indeed, this is already happening in countries like Kenya, Mozambique, Sudan, and Tanzania. Clinical officers usually undergo a three-year training programme in public health, nursing care, and surgical procedures that covers anatomy, orthopaedics, pathology, pharmacology, psychology, and psychiatry. They become skilled and well-rounded medical professionals able to diagnose and treat illness, perform surgery, and educate their communities [11]. Clinical officers cannot be certified by the medical councils of developed countries and thus cannot easily emigrate to seek employment. African countries are also substituting certified nursing assistants for nurses, pharmaceutical technologists for pharmacists, and laboratory technicians for laboratory technologists among others.

The slope of each isoquant ($-\partial CO/\partial DO$) indicates the substitution levels (trade off) of clinical officers for physicians when output is held constant. The slope of an isoquant decreases in absolute terms as we move downwards along the isoquant showing the increasing difficulty of substituting clinical officers for physicians. The rate at which a health DMU can substitute one health system input for another and still produce the same level of total health services output is known as the marginal rate of technical substitution (MRTS) [9]. The MRTS between two inputs such as physicians and clinical officers is equal to the negative ratio of their marginal products. Thus,

$$MRTS_{CO,DO} = -\left(\partial CO/\partial DO\right) = \frac{\partial Q/\partial CO}{\partial Q/\partial DO} = \left(MP_{CO}/MP_{DO}\right)$$

where ∂ stands for change in the concerned variable; $MP_{CO} = \partial Q/\partial CO$ is the marginal product of clinical officers' time (which means the change in health services output resulting from a very small change in this input while keeping all other inputs constant); $MP_{DO} = \partial Q/\partial DO$ is the marginal product of physicians' time (which means the change in health services output resulting from a very small change in this input while keeping all other inputs constant).

The weakness of MRTS as a measure of the degree of substitutability of health systems' inputs is its dependence on the units in which the inputs are measured. A better measure of the ease of substitution is elasticity of substitution (σ), which is the percentage change in the ratio of clinical officers to physicians divided by the percentage change in the rate of technical substitution [9]. Thus,

$$\sigma = \frac{percentage\ change\ in\ \partial CO/\partial DO}{percentage\ change\ in\ \dfrac{\partial Q/\partial CO}{\partial Q/\partial DO}}.$$

Elasticity of substitution is a pure number that is independent of the units used to measure clinical officers or physicians since both the numerator and denominator are measured in the same units [10]. A diminishing rate of technical substitution indicates that as a DMU increases the level of input 1 (for example clinical officers) and adjusts input 2 (for example physicians) so as to stay on the same isoquant, the technical rate of substitution declines. A diminishing technical rate of substitution indicates how the ratio of marginal product, which is the slope of the isoquant, changes as a DMU increases the level of one factor and reduces the level of the other factor so as to stay on the same isoquant [8]. How many physicians would be freed by increasing the number of clinical officers without affecting the quantity (and quality) of health services produced? Marginal rate of technical substitution can also be obtained by estimating a Cobb-Douglas production function using regression analysis as follows:

$$MP_{L,K} = \frac{\partial Q/\partial L}{\partial Q/\partial K} = \frac{b_1(Q/L)}{b_2(Q/K)} = \left(\frac{b_1}{b_2}\right) x \left(\frac{K}{L}\right).$$

Factor Intensity

The factor intensity of any production process (method or activity) is measured by the slope of the line through the origin representing the particular process [10]. Figure 4.9 shows the factor intensity of the ratio of clinical officers to physicians.

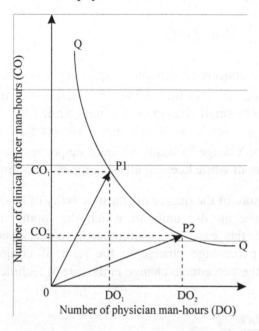

Figure 4.9   Health system factor/input intensity

It reveals that:

$$\frac{CO_1}{DO_1} \succ \frac{CO_2}{DO_2}.$$

The upper part of isoquant (Q) contains the more clinical officer-intensive production processes, while the lower part of the isoquant includes the more physician-intensive processes. The results of a regression analysis of a Cobb-Douglas production function indicate that the factor intensity equals b_1/b_2. For example, if $b_1 = 1.036$ and $b_2 = 3.270$, then $1.036/3.270 = 0.31682$. The higher this ratio, the more clinical-officer intensive the method of production and the lower the ratio, the more physician-intensive the method.

EFFICIENCY OF PRODUCTION

Efficiency of production refers to the ability of a health system's DMU to generate maximum health services output from a given set of inputs. For example, the expanded programme on immunisation (EPI) of a particular African country combines community health nurses (L) and cold-chain management (K) to fully immunise a child against all vaccine-preventable diseases at point P (Figure 4.10). The technical inefficiency of this DMU could be represented by the distance QP, which is the amount by which all the health system's inputs (L and K in this case) could be proportionately reduced without reducing output (i.e., the number of children immunised). Efficiency of production is usually expressed in percentage terms by the ratio *QP/0P*, which represents the percentage by which all inputs could be reduced. The technical efficiency (TE) of a DMU is usually measured by the ratio $TE_1=0Q/0P=1-(QP/0P)$.

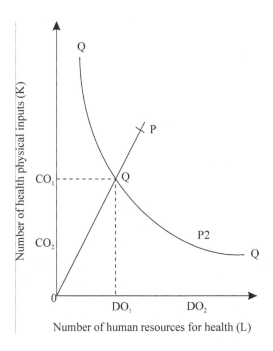

Figure 4.10   Technical efficiency or efficiency of production

Technical efficiency will take a value between zero and one and hence provides an indicator of the degree of technical inefficiency of a DMU. A value of one indicates that the DMU is fully technically efficient; for example, at point Q which lies on the efficiency isoquant [12]. Efficiency of production can be estimated through either mathematical programming such as data envelopment analysis (discussed later) or regression analysis. In a Cobb-Douglas production function, efficiency in organisation of a health system's inputs is measured by the intercept b_0. A more efficient DMU will have a larger b_0 than a less efficient one.

Returns to Scale

Since all variables vary in the long run, a health system DMU must also consider the best way to increase health service output. One strategy to achieve such a goal would be to change the scale of the DMU's operation by increasing all of the health system's inputs proportionately. For example, if it takes one health promotion officer working with one bicycle in rural Africa to deliver education on healthy lifestyle topics such as personal hygiene, balanced diet, use of condoms, family planning, avoidance of substance abuse, and behavioural change to 200 households in a month, how will output be affected if a health promotion programme (a DMU) uses two such officers and two bicycles? There are three possible outcomes [10].

First, the output could increase by a larger proportion than each of the health system's inputs. Thus, doubling of all the health system's inputs could more than double the health service outputs; in this case the number of households reached with knowledge on healthy lifestyles. This situation is termed as increasing returns to scale (IRS). Also referred to as economies of scale, IRS may result from technical or managerial indivisibilities or a combination of both types of the health system's inputs such as organ transplant units, magnetic resonance imaging units, hospital buildings, and greater specialisation (for instance subdivision of tasks as the human resources for health and health technologies increase).

Second, doubling of the health system's inputs may lead to an increase in health service output by a smaller proportion than each of the health system's inputs. This is a case of decreasing returns to scale (DRS), which might result from an expansion of a health system's DMU (i.e., a health facility or programme) that makes it difficult to coordinate tasks, supervise work, obtain and disseminate information, or maintain good communication between management and health workers. Such a situation could also be brought about by limitations affecting the population in the catchment area whose health requires a preventive programme or is to be addressed by the health facility. Third, doubling of all the health system's inputs could double the outputs. In other words, the health services output might increase by exactly the same proportion as the health system's inputs. This is a case of constant returns to scale (CRS). In such a situation, the size of a DMU has no effect on the productivity of its factors.

Returns to scale describes how health services output(s) changes when all of a health system's inputs are varied in equal proportions. Returns to scale can remain constant, it can increase, or it may decrease depending on whether outputs increase in equal proportion to, more than, or less than inputs respectively. The occurrence of increasing returns to scale, decreasing returns to scale, or constant returns to scale in a DMU is an empirical issue that can be ascertained by estimating the elasticity of a health system's output. Thus,

> Output elasticity is defined as the percentage change in (a health service) output resulting from 1% increase in all the health system's inputs. If output elasticity exceeds 1, there are increasing returns to scale; if it equals 1, there are constant returns to scale; and if it is less than 1, there are decreasing returns to scale. [9, p. 209]

For illustration, let us assume that a health promotion programme uses health promotion officers and bicycles to reach and educate households in rural Africa on disease prevention and healthy lifestyles. The quantities of both output and inputs are summarised in Table 4.4. In a real situation, such data can be obtained from any of the sources such as (*a*) time series studies on the volumes of health systems' inputs over various periods in the past and the health services outputs during each period, (*b*) cross-sectional studies showing the inputs and outputs of various DMUs of the health promotion industry at a given time such as one month or one year, and (*c*) technical information supplied by health promotion officers (including information obtained by experiments or the daily work experience in the technical health-promotion process).

Table 4.4   Production function of a health promotion programme

No. of households educated (Q)	Log of households educated (log Q)	Health promotion officers (HPO)	Log of health promotion officers (log HPO)	Bicycles (BIKE)	Log of bicycles (log BIKE)
100	4.60517	4	1.38629	2	0.693147
300	5.703782	6	1.79176	3	1.098612
550	6.309918	8	2.07944	4	1.386294
850	6.745236	10	2.30259	5	1.609438
1,200	7.090077	12	2.48491	6	1.791759
1,600	7.377759	15	2.70805	7	1.94591
2,000	7.600902	19	2.94444	8	2.079442
2,350	7.762171	25	3.21888	9	2.197225
2,500	7.824046	33	3.49651	10	2.302585
2,500	7.824046	40	3.68888	11	2.397895

In order to estimate the output elasticity of the health promotion programme, we can estimate the following exponential functional (Cobb-Douglas) form of the production function:

$$Q = \alpha^{\beta 0} HPO^{\beta 1} BIKE^{\beta 2} e^{\varepsilon}$$

where Q is the total number of households reached with health education on disease prevention and healthy lifestyles, HPO is the number of health promotion officers, BIKE is the number of bicycles for transportation in the programme, α is the intercept term, and β_1 and β_2 are coefficients. Taking the logarithms of Q, HPO, and BIKE we obtain the following double-log equation:

$$\ln Q = \beta_0 + \beta_1 \ln HPO + \beta_2 \ln BIKE + \varepsilon$$

where "$\ln Q$" refers to the natural logarithm of Q. In a double-log equation, an individual regression coefficient, for example β_1, can be interpreted as an elasticity because

$$\beta_1 = \Delta(\ln Q)/\Delta(\ln HPO) \approx \frac{\Delta Q/Q}{\Delta HPO/HPO} = \eta_{Q,HPO} \,.$$

The way to interpret coefficient β_1 in a double-log equation is that if HPO changes by one per cent while BIKE is held constant, then Q will change by β_1 per cent. In a Cobb-Douglas production function, output elasticity equals the sum of the exponents (i.e., $\beta_1 + \beta_2$). Thus, if the sum of the exponents exceeds 1, increasing returns to scale are indicated; if it equals 1, constant returns to scale prevail; and if it is less than 1, decreasing returns to scale are indicated [8-10].

Using SPSS statistical software [13], we regressed $\log Q$ on $\log HPO$ and $\log BIKE$ to obtain the following regression coefficients: $\log Q$=3.866-1.036 $\log HPO$+3.270 $\log BIKE$ as shown in (Table 4.5). Since the sum of β (-1.036) and λ (3.270) of 2.2337 is greater than 1, increasing returns to scale are indicated in this hypothetical health promotion programme.

Table 4.5   Regression results

	B	Std. Error	t	Significance level
(Constant)	3.866	.095	40.778	.000
Log HPO	-1.036	.167	-6.215	.000
Log BIKE	3.270	.224	14.589	.000

Note: Dependent variable is log Q

PRODUCTION FUNCTION OF A MULTIPLE OUTPUT HEALTH SYSTEM DECISION-MAKING UNIT

In a realistic situation, most health system DMUs generate more than one product. For example, an expanded immunisation programme might provide immunisation against diseases such as polio, diphtheria, tuberculosis, whooping cough, measles, tetanus, and hepatitis B. Similarly, a district hospital could provide various types of preventive health services such as antenatal or postnatal care, family planning, child growth monitoring, immunisation, and health promotion outreach among others. A health centre too may provide multiple health services. There is need, therefore, to extend the analysis from the reality of single-product or single-service DMUs to that of multiple product or service DMUs (firms). For the sake of simplicity, we will assume that a health DMU employs human resources for health (L) and health technology (K) to produce the two products of preventive (Q_P) and curative (Q_C) services. The production functions of the two health services can be expressed as follows: $Q_P = f_1(L,K)$; $Q_C = f_2(L,K)$. Figure 4.11 is the Edgeworth box used to illustrate production efficiency.

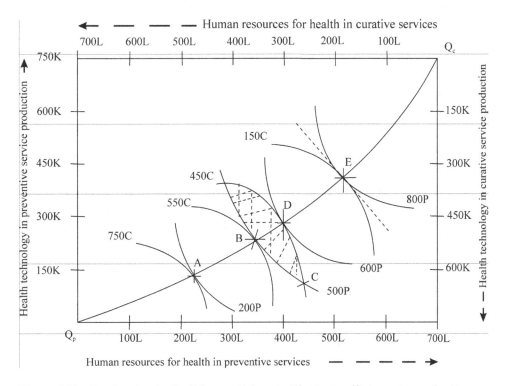

Figure 4.11   Production in the Edgeworth box to illustrate efficiency in production

Some 700 human resources for health hours and 750 health technology hours are available for the production process. The origin for preventive health services (P) is Q_P, while the origin for curative health services is Q_C. The points in the Edgeworth box represent every possible combination of human resources for health and health technology required to produce preventive and curative health services. For instance, point C represents the input of 438 human resources for health hours and 102 health technology hours to produce preventive health services. Point C also represents the health system's input of 254 human resources for health hours and 660 health technology hours to produce curative health services.

Various production isoquants in the Edgeworth box depict the levels of health service outputs produced with various combinations of health system inputs. An individual isoquant represents the total production of a health service that can be obtained without distinguishing the DMU that produced it. There are four isoquants representing 200, 500, 600, and 800 units of preventive health services outputs. The isoquants increase in output as one moves from the lower left to the upper right side because one or both of the health system's inputs increases as well. The Edgeworth box also has four isoquants showing 150, 450, 550, and 750 units of curative health services outputs. These isoquants depict an increase in output as one moves from the upper right to the lower left side, again because one or both health system's inputs is increasing. For example, isoquant 200P represents all combinations of human resources for health and health technology for producing 200 units of preventive health services, whilst isoquant 450C shows all combinations of human resources for health and health technology for producing 450 units of curative health services. It is clear that Point C simultaneously depicts 500 units of preventive and 450 units of curative health services.

Input Efficiency

How can a health system's inputs be combined efficiently? We need to search for combinations of human resources for health and health technology that can be used to produce each of the two health services outputs efficiently. A specific allocation of a health system's inputs to the production process is technically efficient if increasing the output of one health service does not lead to a decrease in the output of another service.

Figure 4.11 illustrates that inputs that are allocated inefficiently will generate more of one or both health services if reallocated. For example, input allocation at point C is technically inefficient because any combination of the health system's inputs in the shaded area generates more of both preventive and curative health services. As one moves from C to B by reallocating some human resources for health from production of preventive to curative health services and some health technology from production of curative to preventive health services, a DMU produces the same volume of preventive health services (500 units) but a larger volume of curative health services (550 units up from 450 units).

Production Contract Curve

The production contract curve represents all the technically efficient combinations of a health system's inputs. For example, points A, B, D, and E in Figure 4.11 are efficient allocations since they all lie on the production contract curve that connects Q_P and Q_C. It is important to note that in an Edgeworth production box with two fixed inputs of a health system and two health services, efficient use of inputs occurs when the isoquants of the two health services are tangent. All the points that are off the production contract curve, such as C, are technically inefficient since human resources for health and health technology can be reallocated to increase the output of at least one of the health services.

Production Possibilities Frontier

The production possibilities frontier (PPF) or product transformation curve shows the alternative combinations of two health services, for example preventive and curative services, that can be produced when all the available health system's inputs such as human resources for health and physical capital are utilised efficiently (Figure 4.12). The curve sets the boundary between attainable and unattainable levels of health services production given the available health system's inputs and technology.

The production possibilities frontier curve in Figure 4.12 is derived from the production contract curve in the Edgeworth box in Figure 4.11. The labelling of the production possibilities frontier corresponds to the points on the health services production contract curve. Point Q_P depicts one extreme in which only preventive services are produced and Point Q_C shows the other extreme in which only curative health services are produced. Points *A, B, D,* and *E* correspond to the four other labelled points from the Edgeworth box production contract curve. Every point on both the contract curve and the production possibilities frontier describes an efficiently produced level of both preventive and curative services.

All points (such as C) that lie inside the production possibilities frontier are off the contract curve in the Edgeworth box and indicate inefficient allocation of a health system's inputs. The production possibilities frontier is downward-sloping because the production of more preventive health services requires health policy makers to reallocate a health system's inputs from production of curative services, which in turn lowers the level of curative health services. This is a real challenge in sub-Saharan African countries where most of the human resources (specialists, general physicians, and nurses) and other health systems' inputs are allocated to hospital-based curative services rather than the more cost-effective preventive health services.

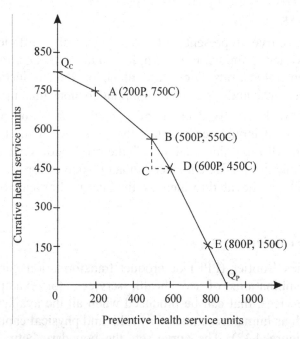

Figure 4.12   Health service production possibilities frontier

Marginal Rate of Transformation

The slope of the PPF at any point yields the marginal rate of transformation (MRT) between curative and preventive health services at that point. The PPF is concave or bowed out, which means that its slope becomes steeper as preventive health services increase. The MRT measures the level of curative health services that must be given up to produce one additional unit of preventive health services (as health systems' inputs are shifted from production of one service to the other). For example, if MRT was 2, which means that giving up one unit of curative services will allow a DMU to produce two units of preventive health services, it would make economic sense to reduce production of curative services by one unit so as to produce two extra units of preventive services. The marginal rate of transformation (the slope of the PPF) is presented as [9]:

$$-\frac{\partial Q_C}{\partial Q_P} = \frac{MP_{L,c}}{MP_{L,P}} = \frac{MP_{K,P}}{MP_{K,C}}$$

Calculation of MRT is illustrated in Table 4.6. For example, the MRT of the technically efficient point B can be derived as follows:

$$MP_{L,P} = \frac{(500-200)}{(340-223)} = \left(\frac{300}{117}\right) = 2.56$$

$$MP_{K,P} = \frac{(500-200)}{(240-132)} = \left(\frac{300}{108}\right) = 2.78$$

$$MP_{L,C} = \frac{(550-750)}{(368-479)} = \left(\frac{-200}{-111}\right) = 1.81$$

$$MP_{K,C} = \frac{(550-750)}{(514-621)} = \left(\frac{-200}{-107}\right) = 1.880$$

$$MRT_{C,P} = \frac{1.81}{2.56} = \frac{1.880}{2.78}$$

Table 4.6   Derivation of the production possibility curve

Technically efficient points	Preventive (T)	HRH-P (U)	HTL-P (V)	MP(HRH-P) (X)	MP(HTL-P) (Y)	MRTS (Z) = (X/Y)	MRPT
A	200	223	132	0.90	1.52	0.592	
B	500	340	240	2.56	2.78	0.920	-1.50
D	600	403	282	1.60	2.38	0.671	-1.00
E	800	516	420	1.76	1.45	1.217	-0.67
	Curative (T)	HRH-C (U)	HTL-C (V)	MP(HRHC) (X)	MP(HTLC) (Y)	MRTS (Z) = (X/Y)	
A	750	479	621	1.57	1.21	1.297	
B	550	368	514	1.81	1.880	0.961	
D	450	301	467	1.49	2.115	0.703	
E	150	186	337	2.62	2.307	1.134	

COST OF HEALTH SERVICES

Health systems decision-making units (DMU) may be categorised according to their legal structure or proprietorship or ownership as public/government or private or they can also be distinguished on the basis of the type of market structure in which they operate [14,15]. Market structure refers to the characteristics of output markets that influence the behaviour of DMUs including the number of DMUs in the market, their size, and the type of health services produced. The categorisation of DMUs by the type of market that they operate in is based on the output markets that influence the pricing and output behaviour of DMUs and which is in turn used to analyse the economic decisions that they make.

The primary objective of private-for-profit DMUs is to maximise profits or the difference between total revenue and total costs. The primary objective of public and private-not-for-profit DMUs is to produce maximum health services at the minimum cost possible; otherwise, wastage of scarce health systems resources would be immoral and unethical. The total economic costs of production are the full opportunity costs (the value of the most desirable alternative given up when choosing an option) of all resources used in the production of the DMU's health service outputs. This includes both explicit costs (expenditure of money to buy health service-producing inputs) and implicit costs (opportunity costs of using resources already owned by a DMU). For example, the cost of providing organ transplant services is the value of maternal and child health services (assuming this is the most valuable alternative use) that could have been provided with the health workforce, medical equipment, pharmaceuticals, and non-pharmaceutical supplies used currently in provision of organ transplant services. The opportunity costs and the DMU's production function determine the cost of producing a given health service.

Short-Run Total Cost Functions

The decision by a DMU concerning the type of health service to produce and the production technology to be used in producing this service depends partly on the time dimension of the decision [14,15]. Economists distinguish between long-run and short-run decisions. A long-run decision is a planning decision that applies where all health systems inputs are variable including the amount of physical capital inputs employed by a DMU. On the other hand, a short-run decision is a constrained decision since the amount of at least one of the health system inputs (such as production technology and physical capital) employed by the firm is fixed. A DMU's cost function portrays various relationships between the cost of health systems inputs and rate of output of health services. The production function of a DMU and the prices it pays for health system inputs determine its cost functions, which could be short-run or long-run [9]. In a nutshell, cost function is the minimum cost of producing a specific level of health service output.

The short-run cost function is the minimum cost of producing a given level of health service output by varying only the health system's variable inputs [8]. Conversely, long-run cost function depicts the minimum cost of producing a specific level of health service output by adjusting all the health systems inputs. According to Koutsoyiannis [10], a DMU's total cost is a multivariable function both in the short-run and the long-run (i.e., it is determined by many factors). Symbolically, a DMU's short-run cost function can be expressed as follows:

$$TC_{SR} = f\left(Q, T, w_f, \overline{K}\right).$$

The long-run cost function of a DMU can be expressed as

$$TC_{LR} = f\left(Q, T, w_f\right),$$

where TC_{SR} is the short-run total cost; TC_{LR} is the long-run total cost; Q is the health service output; T is the healthcare technology; w_f is a vector of health system factor/input prices; and $\overline{K}$ refers to the fixed health system inputs. Any change in T, w_f, and $\overline{K}$ results in a shift in the cost curve of a DMU hence the name shift factors. Changes in health service output levels result only in movements along the cost curve.

Total economic cost (TC) is the sum of total fixed costs (TFC) and total variable costs (TVC) and is represented as $TC = TFC + TVC$. Table 4.7 shows the short-run costs of Kathera Health Centre, which provides outpatient treatment services. In Table 4.7 total cost in Column D is derived by adding TFC in Column B and TVC in Column C at each health service output.

Total fixed costs refer to the total costs incurred by the DMU for fixed health system inputs in a given time period [9]. Thus, TFC refers to any costs that, in the short-run, do not vary with the level of a health service output (e.g., salaries of hospital director or superintendent, hospital matron, hospital human resource manager, hospital and health centre buildings; and medical equipment/technologies among others).

Table 4.7   Short-run costs for Kathera Health Centre in Kathera dollars (K$)

Number of patients treated per day (A)	Total fixed cost (B)	Total variable cost (C)	Total cost (D=B+C)
0	1,500,000	0	1,500,000
1	1,500,000	200,000	1,700,000
2	1,500,000	333,333	1,833,333
3	1,500,000	433,333	1,933,333
4	1,500,000	500,000	2,000,000
5	1,500,000	600,000	2,100,000
6	1,500,000	733,333	2,233,333
7	1,500,000	1,000,000	2,500,000
8	1,500,000	1,666,667	3,166,667
9	1,500,000	3,000,000	4,500,000
10	1,500,000	5,666,667	7,166,667

The total cost function for Kathera Health Centre is shown in Figure 4.13. Therefore, the total cost of producing a specific level of health service output is derived by multiplying the optimal quantity of each health system input used by their respective input prices and then summing up all these costs. The fixed cost function of the DMU can be depicted graphically by a horizontal straight line at all levels of health service output. In this hypothetical health centre, the total fixed cost remains as K$1.5 million irrespective of whether the health centre attends to zero or ten patients.

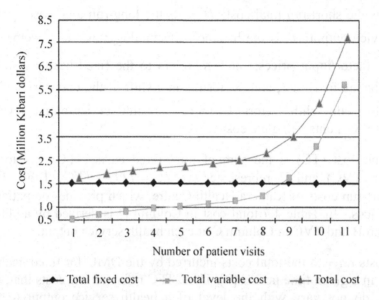

Figure 4.13   Fixed, variable, and total cost of Kathera Health Centre

Total variable costs are the total costs incurred by the DMU for variable health systems inputs per time period. Variable costs include payments for medicines, non-pharmaceutical supplies, human resources for health (such as physicians, nurses, radiologists, laboratory technologists/technicians, health promotion officers, and community health workers), fuel, and capital inputs preventive maintenance among others. Total variable costs rise as the DMU's health service output rate rises since higher output rates require higher variable health system input rates that entail larger variable costs. For example, the larger the number of patients treated at Kathera Health Centre, the larger the quantity of medicines that must be used and the higher the total cost of the medicines.

The total variable cost schedule for Kathera Health Centre is shown in Table 4.7. The total variable costs are zero when health service output is zero, but they rise as output rises. Figure 4.13 shows the corresponding total variable cost function. Up to a health service output rate of seven patient visits per day, the rate of TVC increase is declining (because DMU uses limited amounts of variable health system inputs with the fixed inputs) but beyond that output level the rate of TVC increase is rising. Thus, the TVC function follows the law of diminishing marginal returns. Please note that the TC function and the TVC function of Kathera Health Centre have the same shape since they change by only a constant amount, which is the TFC.

The TC, TFC, and TVC functions of Kathera Health Centre (or any other health system DMU) show the minimum total, fixed, and variable costs of the DMU incurred in producing various levels of health service output in the short run. Thus, cost functions show the minimum costs of producing various levels of health service output on the assumption that the health system DMU uses the optimal or least-cost health system input combinations to produce each level of health service output.

Short-Run per Unit Cost Functions

Average fixed, average variable, average total, and marginal cost functions of a health system DMU can be derived from the total fixed, total variable, and total cost functions. Average fixed cost (AFC) is obtained by dividing a health centre's total fixed cost (TFC) by its level of health service output (Q) (that is $AFC = TFC/Q$). Table 4.8 shows the derivation of average fixed cost for Kathera Health Centre.

The fixed cost per unit of health service will fall as output increases because total fixed costs are spread over a larger output. For example, the AFC of treating one patient in Kathera Health Centre is K$1.5 million while the AFC of treating ten patients is K$0.15 million. Why is AFC behaving this way? This is because the total fixed cost is held constant in the short run, and thus AFC decreases as the rate of health centre output increases. This means that, as shown in Figure 4.14, AFC declines continuously because total fixed costs are spread over more and more units of health service output as the health centre's health service output expands.

Table 4.8   Derivation of average fixed cost for Kathera Health Centre

Number of patients treated per day (A)	Total fixed cost (B)	Average fixed cost (C=B/A)
1	1,500,000	1,500,000
2	1,500,000	750,000
3	1,500,000	500,000
4	1,500,000	375,000
5	1,500,000	300,000
6	1,500,000	250,000
7	1,500,000	214,286
8	1,500,000	187,500
9	1,500,000	166,667
10	1,500,000	150,000

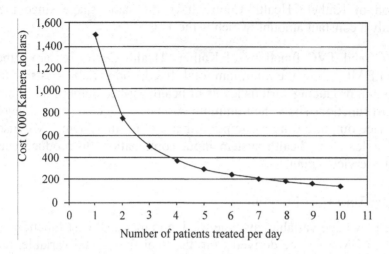

Figure 4.14   Average fixed cost for Kathera Health Centre

Average variable cost (AVC) equals total variable cost (TVC) divided by the level of health service output (Q) of a health centre (i.e., $AVC=TVC/Q=ATC-AVC$). Table 4.9 presents a numerical derivation of average variable cost. The average variable cost per patient treated decreases from K$2,000 for patient 1 to a minimum of K$1,200 for the fifth patient and then starts increasing. Figure 4.15 depicts the U-shaped AVC curve of Kathera Health Centre.

Table 4.9   Derivation of average variable cost for Kathera Health Centre

Number of patients treated per day (A)	Total variable cost (B)	Average variable cost (C=B/A)
1	2,000	2,000
2	3,333	1,667
3	4,333	1,444
4	5,000	1,250
5	6,000	1,200
6	7,333	1,222
7	10,000	1,429
8	16,667	2,083
9	30,000	3,333
10	56,667	5,667

Why does the AVC curve assume this shape? To answer this question, let us assume that human resources for health (HRH) is the only variable health system input for Kathera Health Centre. The TVC for any health service output level (Q) equals the wage rate w (which is assumed to be fixed) times the quantity of HRH used.

Therefore,

$$AVC = \frac{TVC}{Q} = \frac{w(HRH)}{Q} = \frac{w}{Q/HRH} = \frac{w}{AP_{HRH}} \; .$$

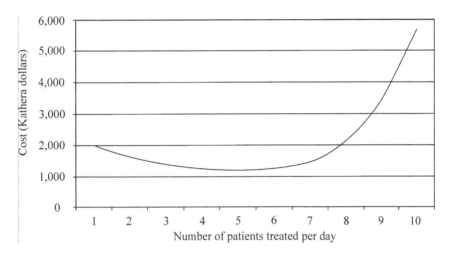

Figure 4.15   Average variable cost for Kathera Health Centre

According to production theory, the average physical product of HRH (AP_{HRH} or Q/HRH) usually rises first, reaches a maximum, and then falls. It then follows that the AVC curve first falls, reaches a minimum, and then rises as shown in Figure 4.15. Average total cost (ATC) is obtained by dividing the health centre's total cost (TC) by its level of health service output (Q); that is, $ATC = TC/Q = AFC + AVC$. Table 4.10 shows the numerical derivation of ATC for Kathera Health Centre. The ATC decreases from K\$ 1.502 million for the first patient treated to K\$ 0.156 million for the tenth patient treated.

As portrayed in Figure 4.16, the ATC curve is also U-shaped like the AVC curve. The ATC curve continues to fall after the AVC curve begins to rise as long as the decline in AFC exceeds the rise in AVC. Once again, the declining ATC is attributed to spreading of the fixed costs over greater quantities of health service output and, at low quantities, the result of increasing marginal productivity.

Marginal cost (MC) is the change in total variable costs (TVC) or the change in total costs (TC) that results from expanding (or reducing) health service output by one unit (i.e., $MC = \partial TVC/\partial Q = \partial TC/\partial Q$); where ∂ means "change in" and Q is the health service output. Marginal cost can be calculated from either the total variable cost (column B) or the total cost (column C) as shown in Table 4.11.

Table 4.10 Derivation of average total cost of Kathera Health Centre

Number of patients treated per day (A)	Total cost (B)	Average total cost (C=B/A)
1	1,502,000	1,502,000
2	1,503,333	751,667
3	1,504,333	501,444
4	1,505,000	376,250
5	1,506,000	301,200
6	1,507,333	251,222
7	1,510,000	215,714
8	1,516,667	189,583
9	1,530,000	170,000
10	1,556,667	155,667

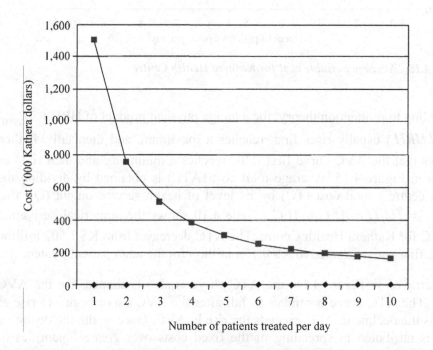

Figure 4.16   Average total cost of Kathera Health Centre

For example, the marginal cost of increasing health centre output from 3 to 4 patients is obtained as follows:

$$MC = \partial TVC/\partial Q = (5{,}000 - 4{,}333)/(4-3) = K\$667 \quad \text{or}$$

$$MC = \partial TC/\partial Q = (1{,}505{,}000 - 1{,}504{,}333)/(4-3) = K\$667.$$

The marginal cost decreases from K\$2,000 for the first patient to a minimum of K\$667 for the fourth patient and thereafter increases sharply to a maximum of K\$26,667 for the tenth patient treated. The marginal cost of treating the tenth patient is 4.7 times the average variable cost of treating the same patient (i.e., $26667/5667$). For this reason economists advise that health policy makers should base their decisions on the marginal cost instead of average costs. As shown in Figure 4.17, the Kathera Health Centre marginal cost curve reaches its minimum before the AVC curve and intersects the AVC curve from below at its lowest point.

Why does the marginal cost curve have a U-shape? It is important to remember that:

$$MC = \frac{\partial TVC}{\partial Q} = \frac{\partial(w \times HRH)}{\partial Q} = \frac{w(\partial HRH)}{\partial Q} = \frac{w}{\partial Q/\partial HRH} = \frac{w}{MP_{HRH}}.$$

According to production theory, the marginal product of HRH (MP_{HRH} or $\partial Q/\partial HRH$) increases, attains a maximum, and then declines with increases in health service output. It follows that the marginal cost normally decreases, reaches a minimum, and then increases. Therefore, the rising portion of the marginal cost curve reflects the operation of the law of diminishing returns. It is important to note that marginal cost equals average cost when the latter is at a minimum [9].

Table 4.11   Derivation of marginal cost of Kathera Health Centre

Number of patients treated per day (A)	Total variable cost (B)	Total cost (C)	Marginal cost (D)
1	2,000	1,502,000	2,000
2	3,333	1,503,333	1,333
3	4,333	1,504,333	1,000
4	5,000	1,505,000	667
5	6,000	1,506,000	1,000
6	7,333	1,507,333	1,333
7	10,000	1,510,000	2,667
8	16,667	1,516,667	6,667
9	30,000	1,530,000	13,333
10	56,667	1,556,667	26,667

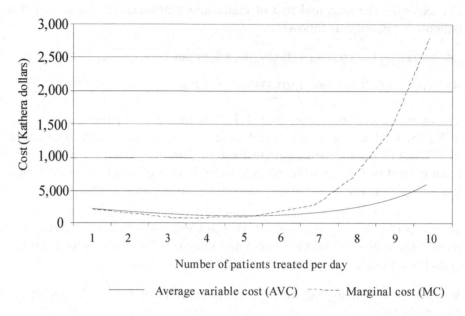

Figure 4.17   Average and marginal costs of Kathera Health Centre

Long-run per Unit Cost Functions

Long-run refers to the period during which all health systems inputs are variable including the amount of physical capital inputs employed by a DMU. All DMU costs are variable in the long run. In the health sector, the long-run period may range from weeks to years. For example, acquisition of clinical equipment may take only a few days, whilst construction of a new health centre or hospital may take one or more years. Thus, in the long run a health system DMU can produce more health services output by adjusting all its inputs, including plant size. The long-run average cost function shows the minimum cost per unit of producing each health service output level when any desired scale of DMU can be built.

Let us assume that it is possible for a health system DMU to construct four alternative scales of a health centre. The short-run average cost function for each scale of the health centre is represented by $S_1 S_1'$, $S_2 S_2'$, $S_3 S_3'$, and $S_4 S_4'$, from the smallest to the largest respectively (Figure 4.18). Which scale would be the most preferred? The choice will depend on the long-run health service output rate that health policy makers want produced since the DMU will want to produce this output rate at a minimum average cost. For example, if the national health policy makers plan to provide a health service quantity of $0Q_1$, then the most appropriate health centre scale would be $S_1 S_1'$. In Figure 4.18, the long-run average cost (LRAC) function is the solid part of the short-run average cost functions, $S_1 ABCDS_4'$.

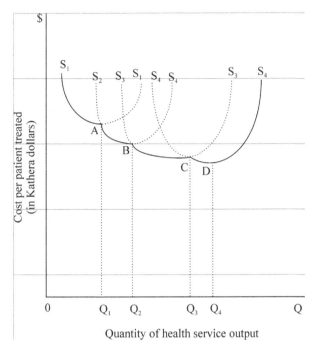

Figure 4.18   Kathera Health Centre long-run average costs as an
envelop of short-run average total cost curves

The broken-line segments of the short-run functions are not included since they are not the lowest average costs. In the long-run, the LRAC of health service production is less than or equal to the short-run average cost (SRAC) of production [14,15]. Figure 4.19 presents the LRAC function, which portrays the minimum long-run cost per unit of producing each output level as the envelop of SRAC functions. The LRAC function is tangent to each of the SRAC functions at the output where the scale of a health centre corresponding to the SRAC function is optimal [9]. Figure 4.20 shows the long-run total cost (LTC) curve derived from the health system DMU's expansion path and shows the minimum long-run total costs of producing various levels of health service output [15].

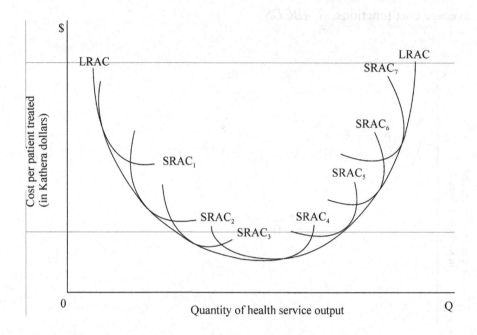

Figure 4.19   Kathera Health Centre long-run average cost function

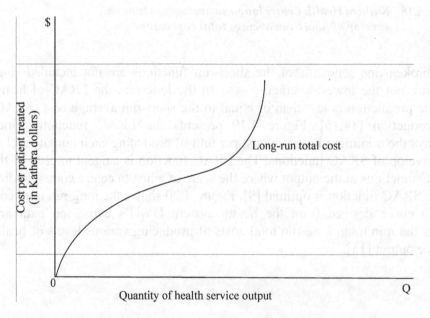

Figure 4.20   Kathera Health Centre total cost function

Figure 4.21 shows the long-run marginal cost function describing the relationship between health service output and the cost resulting from the production of the last unit of output if Kathera Health Centre has time to make the optimal changes in the quantities of all inputs used. Of course, the long-run marginal cost must be less than long-run average cost when the latter is decreasing, equal to long-run average cost when the latter is at minimum, and greater than long-run average cost when the latter is decreasing. When the DMU has built the optimal scale of plant for producing a given level of output, then LRMC will be equal to SRMC at that output [9].

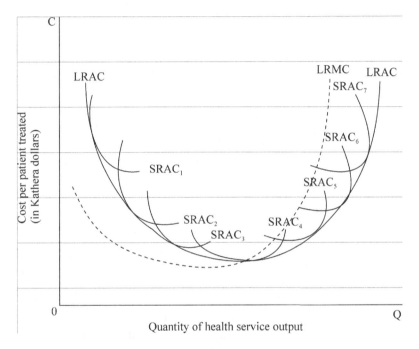

Figure 4.21   Kathera Health Centre long-run marginal cost (LMC) function

Challenges in Measuring Efficiency of Health Facilities

O'Neill and Largey [16] argue that the objective functions of health service practitioners (and health facilities) may differ but they include developing innovative techniques, being at the forefront of chosen specialties, playing a greater role in administration, showing a greater degree of responsiveness to non-medical expectations of clients, maximising user fee revenues/ professional incomes, cost-containment, and nature and amount of work among others. According to Evans [17], the process of training and socialisation, the regulation of practice conduct by professional bodies, and public expectations all tend to discourage pure profit-seeking behaviour but encourage substitution or addition of objectives based on professional self-image or perceptions of patient interests. O'Neill and Largey [16, p.50] also posit that "...the difficulties associated with defining and measuring output, accounting for casemix and the heterogeneous nature of inputs make the concept of a production frontier, i.e., defining the maximum output that can be obtained from a given amount and combination of input, fuzzy".

The output of health facilities (health centres and hospitals) is not homogeneous [18] and thus it is important to reflect their multiproduct nature in cost function analyses. Evans [17] argues that the measurement of cost per unit of output in terms of per diems or total costs per separation is misleading for several reasons: hospitals are multiproduct firms producing some combination of inpatient care, outpatient services, education, research, and community services; inpatient care itself may vary in terms of diagnostic, therapeutic, and custodial services that it embodies over different types and severity of illnesses; and the outcomes of treatment may vary with the quality of care provided.

Utilisation of health facility services is not exogenous. Instead, health facility management in liaison with medical staff influence the need for admission and length of stay and can, in addition, influence costs per day or admission [17]. According to Finkler [18, p. 287], "within the hospital industry, the evidence is conflicting as to whether the long run average cost (LRAC) curve is L- or U-shaped". He argues that econometric techniques are unable to distinguish between diseconomies due to size and those due to inefficient production of specific products. Therefore, researchers should guard against the temptation of lumping teaching, tertiary, provincial/regional, and district hospitals together in the analysis since mix and quality of their products (services) might differ significantly. Instead, comparisons should be made of health facilities offering the same product line mix or they should adjust for product line mix; for travel, inconvenience, and other costs that change as average DMU size changes; and for other potential reasons for cost differences such as different levels of quality.

CONCEPTS OF EFFICIENCY MEASUREMENT

This section focuses on the measurement of productive efficiency. According to Professor Farrell [19], the pioneer of efficiency measurement, the total economic efficiency of a health system consists of technical efficiency (the ability of a DMU to obtain maximum health services output from the available set of the health system's inputs) and allocative efficiency (the ability of a DMU to use the health system's inputs in optimal proportions given their respective prices).

Input-oriented Efficiency Measures

The input-oriented technical efficiency measures attempt to address the question: "By how much can a DMU's health system's input quantities be proportionately reduced without changing its health services output quantities?" Figure 4.22 is an example of a HIV/AIDS prevention community-based programme that employs physical capital such as bicycles (BIKE) and human resources for health such as community health workers (CHW) to produce a single output (condom distribution, Q) assuming constant returns to scale. Isoquant QQ' represents the various combinations of the health system's inputs of BIKE and CHW that a perfectly efficient community-based programme may use to produce a unit of output.

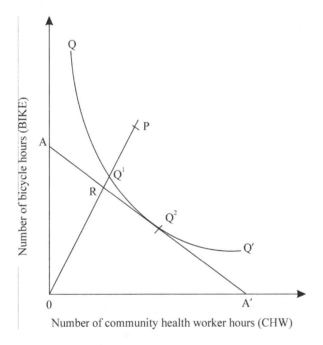

Figure 4.22 Technical efficiency or efficiency of production of a HIV/AIDS prevention community-based programme

A technically inefficient community-based programme (P) is observed to employ a combination of *BIKE* and *CHW* to distribute one condom. An efficient community-based programme (Q) produces the same output as P using only a fraction of the two health system's inputs. The technical inefficiency of the community-based programme P equals the distance $Q^1 P$ (i.e., the volume by which the two inputs could be proportionately reduced without reducing output). The technical efficiency of programme P is $0Q^1/0P$.

Technical efficiency scores take a value between 0 (totally inefficient) and 1 (100% efficient). The information needed for estimation of technical efficiency of community-based condom distribution programmes includes the quantities of each health system's input used by a specific programme in a year and the quantities of condoms distributed by each programme during that period. A programme operating at point Q^1 is 100% technically efficient but not allocatively efficient because the same level of output could be produced at a lower cost at point Q^2.

Following Farrell [19], we define allocative efficiency (AE) as the ability of a DMU to use a health system's inputs in optimal proportions given their respective prices. Allocative efficiency measures the success of a DMU in choosing the optimal set of a health system's inputs. If AA' has a slope equal to the ratio of the prices of BIKE to CHW then Q^2 (and not Q^1) is the optimal method of production. The allocative efficiency of a community-based programme operating at P is equal to $0R/0Q^1$ because RQ^1 depicts the reduction in production costs that would occur if production were to take place at the technically and allocatively efficient point Q^2.

Allocative efficiency scores take a value between 0 (total allocatively inefficient) and 1 (100% allocatively efficient). Thus, to be able to practically measure allocative efficiency we need to collect data on quantities of health system inputs used, average input prices, and health services outputs produced by each community-based programme. For example, to estimate the allocative efficiency of community-based HIV/AIDS prevention programme, one would require information on the total number of community health worker hours in a year, total number of bicycle hours in a year, average hourly remuneration of a community health worker, and average price of hiring a bicycle for each community-based programme in the country.

The overall efficiency, total economic efficiency (EE), or cost efficiency of the community-based programme, P, is defined as the ratio $0R/0P$; where the distance RP indicates the scope for cost reduction. The product (or multiplication) of technical and allocative efficiency scores provides the overall economic efficiency; that is,

$$EE_I = TE_I \times AE_I = \left(0Q^1/0P\right) \times \left(0R/0Q^1\right) = \left(0R/0P\right) \text{ [12]}.$$

Overall efficiency can take only values between 0 and 1 (or 0 and 100%). A DMU will only be economically or cost efficient if it is both technically and allocatively efficient [12, 19]. If the community-based programme moved from point Q^1 to Q^2, its economic or cost efficiency would increase by $(0P-0R)/0P$. This would constitute an improvement in technical efficiency measured by the distance $(0P - 0Q^1)/0P$ and in allocative efficiency measured by the distance $(0Q^1 - 0R)/0Q^1$.

Output-oriented Efficiency Measures

Output-oriented efficiency measures attempt to address the question: "By how much can the quantities of a DMU's health services output be proportionately expanded without altering the quantities of the health system's inputs used?" Figure 4.23 shows a community-based condom distribution programme that employs community health workers' time (X) to distribute condoms (Y) among a target population. It depicts scenarios that assume constant returns to scale (CRS) and variable returns to scale (VRS) technology. Under CRS, Farrell's [19] input-oriented technical efficiency measure of an inefficient programme operating at P would be equal to AB'/AP and the output-oriented measure of technical efficiency would be CP/CE. The input- and output-oriented measures would yield the same efficiency score in a CRS scenario.

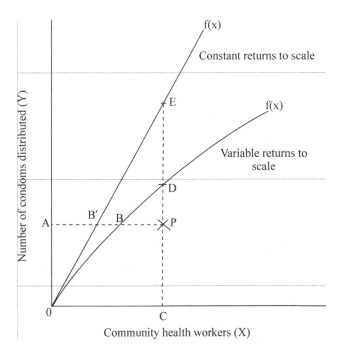

Figure 4.23   Output-oriented technical efficiency measure of a community-based condom distribution programme

Under variable returns to scale, Farrell's input-oriented technical efficiency measure of an inefficient programme operating at P would be equal to AB/AP and the output-oriented measure of technical efficiency would be CP/CD. The input- and output-oriented measures would lead to different efficiency scores under a VRS scenario (either increasing or decreasing) [12]. Figure 4.24 shows four community health centres (A, B, C, D) that use a single input (x_1), such as community health nurses, to produce curative services (y_1) and preventive health services (y_2).

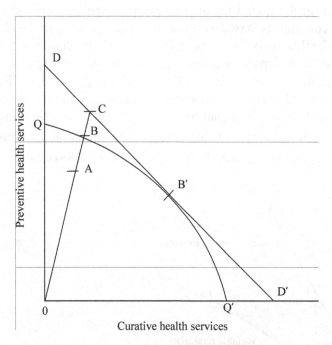

Figure 4.24 Community health centre output-oriented technical and allocative efficiencies

The line QQ' is the unit production possibility frontier and point A, which lies below the frontier, corresponds to an inefficient community health centre. The two health services outputs could be increased by the distance AB with the existing health system's input endowment. Thus, output-oriented technical efficiency is measured by the ratio (TE_O): $0A/0B$. If we have the wage rate of a community health nurse we can draw an iso-revenue line DD' and define allocative efficiency (AO_O) as $0B/0C$. The overall economic efficiency (EE_O) is equal to $TE_O \times AE_O = (0A/0C) = (0A/0B) \times (0B/0C)$.

According to Farrell [19, p. 255], the aforementioned measures of efficiency assume that the efficient production function (i.e., the standard of perfect efficiency) against which to compare the observed performance of health systems' DMUs is known. He indicates that there are two possible candidates: a theoretical function specified by engineers and an empirical function based on the best results observed in practice. The health services' production process is too complex for engineers or technicians to come up with an accurate theoretical standard of perfect efficiency. The pragmatic approach, as Farrell observes, is to compare observed performance with the best actually achieved levels than with some unattainable level.

METHODS OF MEASURING EFFICIENCY

The two main approaches that have been used to quantify technical efficiency, allocative efficiency, and total economic efficiency scores of DMUs are mathematical programming [20] and stochastic frontier regression analysis [21]. The focus of this book is to demonstrate application of the data envelopment approach (DEA) in Africa. Data envelopment is a linear programming technique for measuring the relative performance of health systems' DMUs (hospitals, health centres, dispensaries and programmes) that usually employ multiple inputs to produce multiple health services. In such a scenario, a realistic efficiency measure would have to be defined as [20]:

$$\text{Efficiency} = \frac{\text{weighted sum of inputs}}{\text{weighted sum of inputs}}$$

Charnes, Cooper, and Rhodes [20] propose that the efficiency (E) of a target DMU j_0 can be obtained by solving the following fractional linear programming model:

$$\text{Maximise } E_{j_0} = \frac{\sum_{r=1}^{t} u_r y_{rj_0}}{\sum_{i=1}^{m} v_i x_{ij_0}}$$

Subject to

$$\frac{\sum_{r=1}^{t} u_r y_{rj_0}}{\sum_{i=1}^{m} v_i x_{ij_0}} \leq 1, \; j = 1,...,n,$$

$$u_r, v_i \geq \varepsilon, \forall r \text{ and } i,$$

where y_{rj} = quantity of health services output r from health system DMU j; x_{ij} = quantity of health systems' input i from health system DMU j; u_r = the weight given to output r; v_i = the weight given to input i, and n = the number of DMUs.

The unknown weights u_r and v_i are chosen by the DEA in a manner that maximises the efficiency of the j_0 decision-making unit. The estimated efficiency score for any DMU has an upper boundary of 1 (the efficiency score cannot exceed 1 or 100%). The DEA software solves the above-mentioned model for as many times as is necessary for the size of the population or size of the sample of DMUs.

Measuring Technical Efficiency

Example 1: Technical efficiency of a single input and single health services output under constant returns to scale

Table 4.12 contains data on the number of nurses and total maternal and child health visits at 11 health centres in Kenya. The performance ratio of "number of maternal and child health visits per nurse" in column C indicates that Kaviani is the most efficient health centre in providing maternal and child health services since it has the highest number of patients (2,604) for each nurse employed. In contrast, Isinya is the least efficient among the health centres with only 141 maternal and child health cases per nurse employed.

As shown in column D, the efficiency of each of the 11 health centres relative to Kaviani can be determined by dividing the ratio of maternal and child health visits per nurse for each health centre by the ratio for Kaviani. Multiplying each of the health centre's relative efficiency scores in column D by 100 indicates that Kaviani is 100% efficient while Kitengela is only 6% efficient. In this case, Kaviani is an example of a centre with the best performance that all other health centres should strive to emulate. Kaviani could serve as a reference health centre when setting targets for improving the performance of other health centres. For instance, in order to equal Kaviani's performance, Kitengela could be given the target of increasing its maternal and child health visits from 2,089 to 36,460. Its output to input ratio would then be $36,460/2,089 = 2,604$, to make it 100% efficient.

Table 4.12 Health centre performance

Decision-making unit	Input: nurses (A)	Output: maternal and child health visits per year (B)	Output/input: maternal and child health visits per nurse C = (B/A)	Relative efficiency D = (C/2604)
Athi-River	4	7,129	1,782	0.68
Bissel	3	3,611	1,204	0.46
Githunguri	11	7,365	670	0.26
Isinya	9	1,267	141	0.05
Karuri	25	25,782	1,031	0.40
Kasigau	3	6,164	2,055	0.79
Kaviani	4	10,417	2,604	1.00
Kigumo	12	10,599	883	0.34
Kihara	10	3,311	331	0.13
Kitengela	14	2,089	149	0.06
Lari	12	7,812	651	0.25

Example 2:   Technical efficiency of a single input and two health services outputs under constant returns to scale

Let us extend the example above by assuming that the 11 health centres employ nurses to produce the two health services outputs of maternal and child health visits and curative outpatient health care. Our task is to assess how efficiently the health centres use their single input of nurses to produce the two health services outputs. The input and output data for this situation are presented in Table 4.13.

Columns D and E are obtained by dividing the health centres' health services outputs by their respective inputs. The higher the ratio of output to input, the more efficient a health centre is in producing the output. The health centre with the highest ratio of curative service visits per nurse is Bissel and is therefore regarded as the most efficient in attending to patients for these services. However, Kaviani has the highest ratio of maternal and child health visits per nurse implying that it is the most efficient in providing these services. Which measure do we use to measure efficiency in this situation? We have to employ an efficiency frontier graph generated using Banxia Frontier Analyst software [22]. It plots curative services visits per nurse against maternal and child health visits per nurse for all the 11 health centres (Figure 4.25).

Table 4.13 Input and output data for selected health centres in Kenya

Decision-making unit (DMU)	Nurses (A)	Curative service visits (B)	Maternal and child health (MCH) visits (C)	Curative service visits per nurse D = (B/A)	MCH visits per nurse E = (C/A)	Relative efficiency in production of curative visits F = (D/3336)	Relative efficiency in production of MCH visits G = (E/2604)
Athi-River	4	10,077	7,129	2,519	1,782	0.76	0.68
Bissel	3	10,009	3,611	3,336	1,204	1.00	0.46
Githunguri	11	17,949	7,365	1,632	670	0.49	0.26
Isinya	9	4,824	1,267	536	141	0.16	0.05
Karuri	25	14,691	25,782	588	1,031	0.18	0.40
Kasigau	3	7,183	6,164	2,394	2,055	0.72	0.79
Kaviani	4	9,294	10,417	2,324	2,604	0.70	1.00
Kigumo	12	33,004	10,599	2,750	883	0.82	0.34
Kihara	10	22,357	3,311	2,236	331	0.67	0.13
Kitengela	14	19,110	2,089	1,365	149	0.41	0.06
Lari	12	30,889	7,812	2,574	651	0.77	0.25

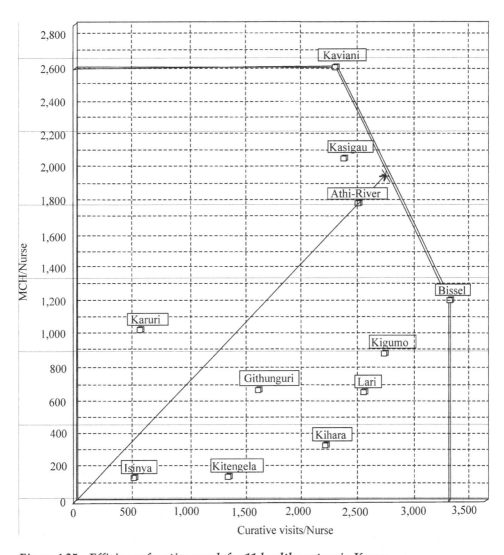

Figure 4.25 ***Efficiency frontier graph for 11 health centres in Kenya***

Figure 4.25 depicts Bissel and Kaviani as the most efficient health centres. We can construct the efficiency frontier by drawing a line between Bissel and Kaviani and straight lines from Bissel to the Y axis and from Kaviani to the X axis. The efficiency frontier is a fundamental concept of DEA. This frontier envelops all the nine inefficient health centres within it and vividly depicts the relative efficiency of each health centre. The health centres on the frontier are 100% relatively efficient (i.e., Bissel and Kaviani) while those below the frontier are inefficient and have a score of less than 100%. The inefficient health centres can become efficient by increasing their health services outputs by equal proportions while keeping their health systems' inputs constant.

Alternatively, they can be made efficient by reducing inputs while keeping outputs constant.

The two-dimensional efficiency frontier graph is useful only when dealing with two health services outputs and one input or with one output and two inputs. When confronted with scenarios involving two or more health service outputs or two or more inputs, an analyst has to resort to the use of DEA software such as Banxia Frontier Analyst (available for sale) or DEAP Version 2.1 (available for free) [23]. The constant returns to scale technical efficiency for each DMU can be obtained by solving the following input-oriented linear programme [24]:

$$TE_{jo} = \max_{u_r v_j} \sum_{r=1}^{N} u_r y_{rjo}$$

Subject to:

$$\sum_r u_r y_{rj} - \sum_i v_i x_{ij} \leq 0; \forall j$$

$$\sum_i v_i x_{ij} = 1$$

$$u_r, \ v_i \ \geq 0; \forall r, \ \forall i.$$

where TE_{j_0} is the technical efficiency score of DMU j_0, u_r is a vector of output weights to be determined by the solution to the linear programming problem, v_i is a vector of input weights to be determined by the solution to the linear programming problem, y_{rj_0} is the observed amount of output r for DMU j_0, x_{ij} is the observed amount of input i for DMU j.

Variable returns to scale technical efficiency (VRSTE) can be obtained by solving the following input-oriented linear programme [24]:

$$TE_{j_0} = \max_{u_r v_i} \sum_{r=1}^{N} u_r y_{rj_0} + u_0$$

Subject to:

$$\sum_r u_r y_{rj} - \sum_i v_i x_{ij} \ + \ u_0 \ \leq 0; \ \forall j$$

$$\sum_i v_i x_{ij} = 1$$

$$u_r, \ v_i \ \geq 0; \ \ \forall r, \ \forall i.$$

The preceding two examples assume that the health centres in question manifest constant returns to scale. However, this assumption is often not valid for health systems' DMUs. Table 4.14 depicts estimations of constant returns to scale technical efficiency (CRSTE), variable returns to scale technical efficiency (VRSTE), and scale efficiency (SE) scores. Note that $CRSTE = VRSTE \times SE$ and $SE = CRSTE/VRSTE$. The VRSTE scores indicate only the technical inefficiency emanating from non-scale factors. These scores are also referred to as pure technical efficiency.

Table 4.14 also shows three results related to returns to scale. First, Ngewa and Thinu health centres have VRSTE and SE scores of 1 (or 100%), which means that they are both pure technical and scale efficient (they represent the optimal scale within the sample). In this situation, doubling the two health system's inputs of nurses and beds also doubles their two health services outputs (curative outpatient visits and maternal and child health visits). This means that there are no economies or diseconomies of scale.

Second, Nyanche Health Centre has increasing returns to scale (IRS), suggesting that doubling the two inputs would more than double the outputs. Third, the remaining nine health centres excluding Ngewa, Thinu, and Nyanche manifest decreasing returns to scale (DRS) implying that doubling their inputs less than doubles their outputs (suggesting that these centres are too large and are suffering diseconomies of scale). Five health centres, namely, Limuru, Ngewa, Thinu, Nyanche, and Wangige are technically efficient under variable returns to scale but show scale inefficiencies. Limuru and Wangige are generating health services outputs with decreasing returns to scale and are too large to be considered as scale efficient.

What do the efficiency scores mean? Recall that efficiency scores usually vary from 0 to 1. An efficiency score of 1 indicates that a health centre is 100% efficient relative to its peers. Any health centre with an efficiency score of less than 1 is inefficient. For example, the variable returns to scale technical efficiency score for Namanga Health Centre is 0.612 (or 61.2%). This implies that the health centre should be able to reduce the use of all its health system's inputs by 38.8% without reducing its health services output. In addition, since Namanga has a scale efficiency score of 0.857 (or 85.7%), it has the scope to further increase its health services output by 14.3% by reducing the size of its operations. The latter approach is even more pertinent since the health centre is manifesting decreasing returns to scale.

Cost Efficiency and Allocative Efficiency

Assuming that the prices of health systems' inputs for each DMU are known, the cost efficiency score for each observation can be calculated by solving N linear programmes of the following form [25]:

Minimise $\sum_{k=1}^{k} P_{kn} x_{kn}; w_1, ..., w_n \quad x_{1n}, ..., x_{km}$

Subject to:

$$\sum_{j=1}^{N} w_j y_{ij} - y_{in} \geq 0 \quad i = 1, ..., I$$

$$\sum_{j=1}^{N} w_j x_{kj} - x_{kn} \leq 0 \quad k = 1, ..., K$$

$$w_j \geq 0 \quad j = 1, ..., N$$

where N is the number of DMUs in the sample producing I different health systems' outputs with K different health systems' inputs; y_{ij} is the observed amount of output i for the jth DMU; x_{km} is the observed amount of input k from the nth DMU; w_j are weights applied across the N DMUs; and $p_{1n}, ..., p_{kn}$ are the health system's input prices for the K inputs that the nth DMU faces.

Total cost efficiency (CE) or economic efficiency is found by dividing the costs that would be incurred by a DMU if it used the cost minimising level of inputs by the actual costs the DMU faces. Thus, the CE for the nth DMU can be calculated as follows [25]:

$$CE = \sum_{k=1}^{K} P_{kn} x_{kn}^{*} / \sum_{k=1}^{K} P_{kn} x_{kn}$$

If one has already estimated both the technical and allocative efficiency scores, cost efficiency is simply a product of the two. A cost efficiency score would mean that a DMU is cost efficient, while a score of less than 1 would imply existence of cost inefficiencies. Allocative efficiency (AE) is the ratio of the cost efficiency score to the technical efficiency score. It can be obtained using the formula $AE = \sum_{k=1}^{K} P_{kn} x_{kn}^{*} / TE_n \sum_{k=1}^{K} P_{kn} x_{kn}$; where TE_n is the technical efficiency score [27].

Table 4.14 *Estimation of technical and scale efficiency among health centres with multiple inputs and multiple outputs*

DMU	Curative OPD visits	MCH	Nurses	Beds	Constant returns to scale technical efficiency (CRSTE)	Variable returns to scale technical efficiency (VRSTE)	Scale efficiency = CRSTE/VRSTE	Returns to scale
Limuru	21,595	7,002	11	17	0.803	1.000	0.803	DRS
Namanga	8,979	4,432	7	27	0.525	0.612	0.857	DRS
Ndeiya	9,179	2,939	7	18	0.536	0.573	0.936	DRS
Ngewa	18,191	7,421	8	8	1.000	1.000	1.000	-
Ngong	6,206	1,134	12	20	0.212	0.287	0.736	DRS
Nyanche	2,956	2,437	2	10	0.605	1.000	0.605	IRS
O-Rongai	6,608	4,857	10	11	0.312	0.57	0.548	DRS
Sagala	8,581	3,432	4	16	0.878	0.903	0.972	DRS
Simba	7,693	3,206	4	24	0.787	0.809	0.972	DRS
Thinu	7,334	6,157	3	4	1.000	1.000	1.000	-
Wangige	7,743	9,833	13	8	0.799	1.000	0.799	DRS
Wundanyi	12,983	7,224	7	35	0.759	0.987	0.769	DRS
Mean	**9,837**	**5,006**	**7**	**17**	**0.685**	**0.812**	**0.833**	

DEAP version 2.1 software [12] can be used to estimate technical, allocative, and cost efficiencies. Execution of DEAP requires five files (Box 4.1) as contained in the following description:

(1)   The start-up file DEAP.000, which stores key parameter values (you do not need to change these);

(2)   A data file (e.g., eg1-dta.txt) that has to be created by the user. In the example below, I entered the data in Excel as shown in Table 4.15. The names of health centres (DMUs) are in column 1, output (number of outpatient visits) in column 2, first input (number of clinical officers) in column 3, second input (number of nurses) in column 4, third input (number of support staff) in column 5, price of the first input (annual remuneration of clinical officers) in column 6, price of the second input (annual remuneration of nurses) in column 7, and price of the third input (annual remuneration of support staff) in column 8. Information on prices of inputs has been included to facilitate estimation of both allocative and cost efficiencies. I then copied only the data (without the names of the health centres or names of variables), opened Notepad and then the data file eg1.dta provided in DEAP, erased the demonstration data, and pasted my data on Notepad and saved it.

(3)   An instruction file (e.g., eg1-ins.txt). In Notepad I opened the instruction file eg1.ins that comes with the DEAP software and modified it as shown in the list of items for the instruction file eg4.ins. Since in my sample of Zambian health centres I had hypothetical data on 15 health centres, I changed the statistic at the beginning of the third row to 15. Since the data were for only one year, I typed 1 at the beginning of the fourth row. In this hypothetical example I had one output (outpatient visits) and thus I typed 1 at the beginning of the fifth row. Since I had three inputs, I typed 3 at the beginning of the sixth row. Given that I assumed that the health centres strived to minimise their inputs, I typed 0 at the beginning of the seventh row to indicate input orientation. I assumed that some of the health centres would manifest economies or diseconomies of scale; thus I typed 1 at the beginning of row eight to signify variable returns to scale. Lastly, since the objective was to estimate cost efficiency, I typed 1 at the beginning of the ninth row to signify COST-DEA.

(4)   An output file (e.g. eg1-out.txt). This file is created automatically by the programme.

(5)   The executable file DEAP.EXE. This file comes with the programme. Thus, after modifying the instruction file, I went into DEAP and clicked on DEAP.EXE to start the programme. The software prompted me to "Enter instruction filename" to which I typed eg1-ins.txt. After a few seconds I clicked on the output file (eg1-out.txt) to access my output,

which included an efficiency summary (Table 4.16; see also Box 4.1) and a summary of cost minimising input quantities.

Illustrative Interpretation of Efficiency Scores

Table 4.16 presents the DEAP efficiency summary output. Remember that technical efficiency is the ability of a health centre to obtain maximum health services outputs from a given set of inputs. Of the 15 health centres, 12 had a technical efficiency score of 1 implying that they had 100% technical efficiency. The overall sample average technical efficiency score was 0.893 (or 89.3%). However, the average technical efficiency score among the three inefficient health centres was 46.4%. This finding indicates that on average the three inefficient health centres could potentially reduce inputs by 53.6% and still produce their current levels of health services outputs.

Bwacha and Kansuswa health centres were allocatively efficient with a score of 1 (or 100%). Allocative efficiency indicates whether inputs for a given level of output and set of input prices are chosen to minimise the cost of production assuming that the health centre being examined is already fully technically efficient [27]. Allocative efficiency equals cost efficiency divided by technical efficiency. The overall sample average allocative efficiency score was 0.517 (or 51.7%). However the average allocative efficiency score among the 13 inefficient health centres was 0.443 (or 44.3%). These findings confirm that a health centre that is operating using best practices in engineering or technical terms could still be allocatively inefficient if it is not using inputs in proportions that minimise costs given the relative input prices [25].

Finally, recall that cost efficiency is the product of the technical and allocative efficiency scores and that a health centre can attain a score of 100% in cost efficiency only if it has attained 100% scores in both technical and allocative efficiency. As shown in Table 4.16, only Bwacha and Kansuswa health centres were cost efficient since they had efficiency scores of 1. The remaining 13 health centres were cost inefficient with an average cost inefficiency of 35.7%. This implies that, the cost in those inefficient health centres was, on average, 64.3% [= (1-0.35.7) × 100)] higher than would be necessary if they were operating in the best-practice cost efficiency frontier. In other words, the average cost efficiency score of 35.7% for the non-frontier health centres indicates that the excess cost in those health centres is 64.3%.

Table 4.15 Data needs for estimating cost efficiency for selected health centres in Zambia

Health centres	Outpatient visits	Clinical officers	Nurses	Support staff	Annual salary of clinical officers (Kwacha)	Annual salary of nurses (Kwacha)	Annual salary of support staff (Kwacha)
Bwacha	6,500	1	1	2	390,000	245,000	85,000
Chowa	9,334	1	16	3	271,939	256,394	70,000
Mukobeko	9,788	1	5	9	199,868	141,913	95,000
Nakoli	10,000	1	8	2	683,000	440,000	98,000
Butondo	10,623	1	11	2	207,144	204,000	85,000
Chibolya	12,600	5	2	2	460,000	330,000	88,000
Chimwemwe	13,525	1	6	2	682,600	640,253	99,000
Bulangililo	15,820	4	22	4	265,000	251,000	65,000
Kawama	16,241	1	21	3	203,676	199,868	70,000
Kwacha	16,676	1	21	4	201,867	199,868	70,000
Luangwa	19,501	3	17	4	221,867	199,500	75,000
Mindolo	20,092	1	14	2	217,500	189,000	91,000
Ipusukilo	20,679	1	29	8	199,868	199,868	75,000
Kamuchanga	24,410	3	18	7	199,868	179,810	70,000
Kansuswa	27,092	1	8	2	206,332	141,913	70,000

Box 4.1: List of items for the instruction file eg4.ins

eg1.dta   DATA FILE NAME
eg1.out   OUTPUT FILE NAME
15   NUMBER OF FIRMS
1   NUMBER OF TIME PERIODS
1   NUMBER OF OUTPUTS
3   NUMBER OF INPUTS
0   0 = INPUT AND 1 = OUTPUT ORIENTED
1   0 = CRS AND 1 = VRS
1   0 = DEA(MULTI-STAGE),
           1 = COST-DEA,
           2 = MALMQUIST-DEA,
           3 = DEA(1-STAGE),
           4 = DEA(2-STAGE)

Table 4.16 DEAP efficiency summary output

Health centres	Technical efficiency	Allocative efficiency (AE=CE/TE)	Cost efficiency (CE=TE X AE)
Bwacha	1.00	1.00	1.00
Chowa	1.00	0.20	0.20
Mukobeko	1.00	0.391	0.391
Nakoli	1.00	0.419	0.419
Butondo	1.00	0.331	0.331
Chibolya	1.00	0.498	0.498
Chimwemwe	1.00	0.646	0.646
Bulangililo	0.50	0.421	0.211
Kawama	1.00	0.261	0.261
Kwacha	1.00	0.264	0.264
Luangwa	0.50	0.667	0.333
Mindolo	1.00	0.48	0.48
Ipusukilo	1.00	0.229	0.229
Kamuchanga	0.391	0.954	0.373
Kansuswa	1.00	1.00	1.00
Mean	**0.893**	**0.517**	**0.442**

EFFICIENCY CHANGE, TECHNICAL CHANGE AND PRODUCTION GROWTH

Invention is the creation of new production techniques and processes and also new products such as computers that can be developed into usable processes and products through innovation [26]. Investment in new health technologies may improve productivity of DMUs, lower production costs and prices to clients, and provide clients with improved health services [27, 28]. Innovation is the practical refinement and development of an original invention into a usable production technique (process innovation) or product (product innovation) [26]. According to Todaro [29], innovation may also involve introduction of new social and management methods such as total quality management, human resources motivation, decentralisation, and contracting commensurate with modern ways of conducting economic activities. Innovation can contribute to faster growth of health services production. Investment in research and development is critical for invention and innovation.

Technology is the result of the application of scientific and technical knowledge to improve health services and production processes [26]. Technological progress is "increased application of new scientific knowledge in form of inventions and innovations with regard to both physical and human capital" [19, p.766]. Thus, technological change – the advance of technology – often takes the form of new methods of producing existing health commodities (products and services) and new techniques of organisation, marketing, distribution, and management.

Technological progress may take a number of forms [29] such as labour- or capital-augmenting technical progress or labour- or capital-saving technological progress. Labour-augmenting technical progress raises the productivity of an existing quantity of human resources for health through, for example, basic and post-basic education, on-the-job training programmes, access to educational materials on the Internet, and active participation in professional associations. Labour-saving technological progress refers to the generation of higher levels of health services outputs using an unchanged quantity of labour inputs as a result of some invention (such as the computer, magnetic resonance imaging, or laser surgical methods) or an innovation (such as telemedicine or decentralisation of authority, responsibility, and financial resources to health districts) [29]. Capital-augmenting technical progress raises the productivity of capital by innovation and invention. Capital-saving technological progress results from some health invention or innovation that facilitates the generation of higher levels of health services outputs using the same quantity of capital inputs [29, 30].

African countries, with partner support, have since the early 1980s been implementing various forms of health sector reforms such as cost containment, cost recovery, social health insurance, decentralisation, service integration, privatisation, contracting, resource allocation and management, and provider payment mechanisms with a view to increasing the total health systems' factor productivity. Health decision-makers, both policy makers and managers, are interested in knowing the extent to which health services productivity has increased over time in response to various health sector reforms and new techniques. According to Mansfield [9], if the production function were readily observable, a comparison of the production function at two different times would provide the health decision-maker with a simple measure of the effect of technological change during an intervening period. Since production functions are not readily observable, a better measure of the rate of technological change is total factor productivity (TFP) that relates changes in outputs to changes in all health systems' inputs. Thus, if a health system DMU uses multiple inputs to produce one output then the total factor productivity would be [9]:

$$TFP = \frac{Q}{\alpha_1 X_1 + \alpha_2 X_2 + ... + \alpha_n X_n}$$

where Q is the quantity of health services, X_1 is the quantity of the first health system input used, X_2 is the quantity of the second health system input used, X_n is the quantity of the nth health system input used, α_1 is the price of the first input, α_2 is the price of the second input, and α_n is the price of the nth input in some base period.

To calculate the changes in total factor productivity for a health system DMU over a period of time, health system managers must obtain data on the quantity of health services outputs and inputs during that period. In addition, they have to obtain base-year health systems' input prices to be used for all years and not just the base year. Table 4.17 shows quantities of health systems' output and inputs for the hypothetical Njuri-Ncheke Health Centre during 2000 and 2007.

Table 4.17 Health systems' inputs and outputs for the Njuri-Ncheke Health Centre
for 2000 and 2007

	Quantity in 2000	Quantity in 2007	Year 2000 prices (shillings)
Output			
Health services	2,000,000	2,866,764	–
Inputs			
Clinical officers	8	8	30,000
Nurses	19	19	24,000
Allied health personnel	10	10	18,000
Administrative staff	15	15	12,000
Medicines	918,000	682,600	0.05
Supplies	650,000	640,253	0.005

If we insert the data into the formula above, we find that the total factor productivity for 2000 was:

$$TFP_{2000} = \frac{2,000,000}{30,000(8) + 24,000(19) + 18,000(10) + 12,000(12) + 0.05(918,000) + 0.005(650,000)} = 1.81$$

The total factor productivity for 2007 was:

$$TFP_{2007} = \frac{2,866,764}{30,000(8) + 24,000(19) + 18,000(10) + 12,000(12) + 0.05(682,600) + 0.005(640,253)} = 2.62$$

From 2000 to 2007, total productivity increased by 44.89% [(2.62-1.81)/1.18)]. Note that in order to hold the health centre's prices constant, input prices for year 2000 were used even for year 2007. When confronted with a multiple-output and multiple-input situation and the absence of input prices, one has to resort to the use of indices such as the Malmquist total factor productivity index to measure changes in total health services outputs relative to health systems' inputs over time [31].

Malmquist Total Factor Productivity Index

The Malmquist index can be decomposed into the product of a pure efficiency change component, a scale efficiency component, and a technological change component. It does not require assumptions on profit, revenue, or cost minimisation nor on input and output prices. Instead, estimation of the Malmquist index requires only the quantities of health services outputs and inputs for a set of DMUs during a period of two or more years. Following Fare et al. [32] to define the output-oriented Malmquist index of productivity change for Afroland health centres, we assume that for each time period t = 1,...,T the health service production technology, S^t, models the transformation of n health systems' inputs $x^t \in \Re^N_+$ (i.e., doctors, nurses, laboratory technicians, support staff, medicines, and medical equipment) into m health services outputs $y^t \in \Re^M_+$ (e.g., curative outpatient visits, antenatal visits, child delivery, immunised children, and community outreach visits). The technology consists of a set of all feasible input and output vectors; that is, $S^t = \{(x^t, y^t) : x^t can produce y^t\}$.

The Malmquist index calls for definition of distance functions with respect to two different time periods, for example $D^t_0(x^{t+1}, y^{t+1})$, which measures the maximum proportional change in health services outputs required to make (x^{t+1}, y^{t+1}) feasible in relation to technology at t and $D^t_0(x^t, y^t)$, which measures the maximum proportional change in health services output needed to make (x^t, y^t) feasible in relation to the technology at $t+1$.

Caves et al. [31] define the Malmquist productivity index (M) as:

$$M_0^t = \frac{D_0^t\left(x^{t+1}, y^{t+1}\right)}{D_0^t\left(x^t, y^t\right)} \quad \text{or} \quad M_0^{t+1} = \frac{D_0^{t+1}\left(x^{t+1}, y^{t+1}\right)}{D_0^{t+1}\left(x^t, y^t\right)}$$

Leveraging the above equation, Fare et al. [32] specified the output-oriented Malmquist productivity change index as the geometric mean of the two productivity indices above and subsequently decomposed it into various sources of productivity change as follows:

$$M_0 = \left(x^{t+1}, y^{t+1}, x^t, y^t\right) = \left[\frac{D_0^t\left(x^{t+1}, y^{t+1}\right)}{D_0^t\left(x^t, y^t\right)}\right] \times \left[\frac{D_0^t\left(x^{t+1}, y^{t+1}\right)}{D_0^{t+1}\left(x^{t+1}, y^{t+1}\right)} \times \frac{D_0^t\left(x^t, y^t\right)}{D_0^{t+1}\left(x^t, y^t\right)}\right]$$

$$\text{Efficiency change} = \left[\frac{D_0^t\left(x^{t+1}, y^{t+1}\right)}{D_0^t\left(x^t, y^t\right)}\right]$$

$$\text{Technological change} = \left[\frac{D_0^t\left(x^{t+1}, y^{t+1}\right)}{D_0^{t+1}\left(x^{t+1}, y^{t+1}\right)} \times \frac{D_0^t\left(x^t, y^t\right)}{D_0^{t+1}\left(x^t, y^t\right)}\right]^{1/2}$$

Figure 4.26 illustrates the decomposition of productivity growth for constant returns to scale technology [33]. S^t and S^{t+1} represent the production technologies in periods t and $t+1$. The health system DMU produces at point P in period t and at point Q in period *t+1*.

Using the formula by Fare et al. [32], the decomposition of the Malmquist index (M_0) and its components from Figure 4.17 is given as:

$$M_0\left(x^{t+1}, y^{t+1}, x^t \cdot y^t\right) = \left[\frac{0D}{0F} \times \frac{0B}{0A}\right] \left[\frac{0F}{0E} \times \frac{0C}{0B}\right]^{1/2}$$

The first component of the stated index measures the technical efficiency change relative to a constant returns to scale technology (the change in the distance of observed production from maximum feasible production) between years t and $t+1$. Thus:

$$\text{Constant returns to scale efficiency change} = \left[\frac{0D}{0F} \times \frac{0B}{0A}\right]$$

According to Fare *et al.* [32], constant returns to scale efficiency change is the product of pure efficiency change and scale efficiency change. Pure efficiency change measures pure technical efficiency change relative to a variable returns to scale technology [33]. Thus:

$$\text{Pure efficiency change} = \left[\frac{0D}{0H} \times \frac{0G}{0A} \right]$$

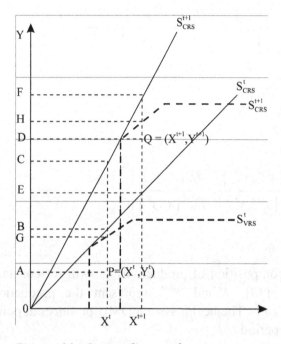

Figure 4.26   Output distance functions

Source: Fulginiti & Perrin [35]

Change in scale efficiency is the change in productivity resulting from a scale or size change that brings a health system's DMU closer to or moves it further from the optimum scale of output as identified by a variable returns to scale technology [33]. Thus:

$$\text{Scale efficiency change} = \left[\frac{0H}{0F} \times \frac{0G}{0B} \right]$$

As indicated in the equation below, technical change is the geometric mean of the shift in technology evaluated at x^{t+1} and the shift in technology evaluated at x^t is as follows [33]:

$$\text{Technical change} = \left[\frac{0F}{0E} \times \frac{0C}{0B} \right]^{\frac{1}{2}}$$

According to Grifell-Tatje and Lovell [34], the Malmquist productivity index attains a value greater than, equal to, or less than unity depending on whether a DMU experiences productivity growth, stagnation, or decline respectively net of the contribution of scale economies between periods t and $t+1$.

The next task is to demonstrate with an example how the Malmquist total factor productivity index is estimated and decomposed using data envelopment analysis. The example uses real data from 10 municipal hospitals in Angola (Table 4.18).

Once again the DEAP version 2.1 software [12] comes in handy in estimating the output-oriented Malmquist total factor productivity index and its component. The execution of DEAP requires five files (Box 4.2) as contained in the following description:

1. The start-up file DEAP.000 which stores key parameter values. You do not need to change these.

2. A data file (e.g. eg4-dta.txt), which you will have to create. In the Angolan example, I entered the data in Excel as shown in Table 4.18. The names of municipal hospitals (DMUs) are in column 1, a numerical code for each hospital is in column 2, the year under consideration (in our case 1 = year 2000, 2 = year 2001, and 3 = year 2002) is in column 3, the first output (number of outpatient visits) is in column 4, the second output (number of admissions) is in column 5, the first input (number of doctors and nurses) is in column 6, and the second input (number of hospital beds) is in column 7. I then copied only the data without the names of the health centres or of the variables, opened Notepad and then the data file provided in DEAP (e.g., 4-dta.txt), erased the demonstration data, and pasted my data on notepad and saved it.

3. An instruction file (such as eg4-ins.txt). In notepad, I opened instruction file eg4-ins.txt, which comes with the DEAP software, and modified it as shown in Box 4.2. Since in my sample of Angolan municipal hospitals I had hypothetical data on 10 hospitals, I changed the statistic at the beginning of the third row to 10. Since the data were for three years, I typed 3 at the beginning of the fourth row. In this example, I had two outputs and thus I typed 2 at the beginning of the fifth row. Given that I had two inputs, I typed 2 at the beginning of the sixth row. I assumed that the hospitals strived to maximise their health services outputs, so I typed 1 at the beginning of the seventh row to indicate output orientation.

Table 4.18 Outputs and inputs in selected municipal hospitals in Angola

Name of hospital	Hospital code	Number of outpatient visits	Number of patients admitted	Number of doctors and nurses	Number of beds
2000 - (Year 1)					
Cajueiros	1	214,753	53,143	664	134
Kilamba Kiaxi	2	131,995	8,971	273	80
Cacuaco	3	24,723	3,876	234	35
Samba	4	15,823	3,590	197	25
Maternidade Caxito	5	192,532	11,858	247	45
Caxito	6	39,711	21,098	318	80
Catete	7	4,238	232	46	36
Ambriz	8	6,798	102	37	23
Muxima	9	2,173	145	127	18
Porto Amboim	10	14,388	993	118	45
2001 - (Year 2)					
Cajueiros	1	244,016	53,143	886	134
Kilamba Kiaxi	2	142,061	10,802	273	80
Cacuaco	3	27,989	5,987	234	35
Samba	4	16,098	3,430	197	25
Maternidade Caxito	5	13,423	2,980	247	45
Caxito	6	42,329	25,023	318	80
Catete	7	5,459	379	47	36
Ambriz	8	62,001	439	37	23
Muxima	9	2,737	302	127	18
Porto Amboim	10	26,486	1,875	118	45
2002 - (Year 3)					
Cajueiros	1	255,084	49,789	886	134
Kilamba Kiaxi	2	135,121	12,490	273	80
Cacuaco	3	35,578	6,732	234	35
Samba	4	16,061	3,004	197	25
Maternidade Caxito	5	17,148	3,781	247	50
Caxito	6	53,421	32,996	318	87
Catete	7	7,242	498	47	36
Ambriz	8	10,108	623	37	23
Muxima	9	3,595	803	127	18
Porto Amboim	10	22,578	1385	118	45

Since the Malmquist index is usually estimated under constant returns to scale, I typed 0 at the beginning of row eight to signify variable returns to scale. Lastly, since the objective was to estimate the Malmquist index, I typed 2 at the beginning of the ninth row to signify Malmquist DEA.

4. An output file (e.g. eg4-out.txt). This file is automatically created by the programme.

5. The executable file DEAP.EXE. This file comes with the programme. After modifying the instruction file, I went into DEAP and clicked on DEAP.EXE to start the programme. The software prompted me to "Enter instruction filename" to which I typed eg4-ins.txt. After a few seconds I

clicked on the output file (eg4-out.txt) to access my output, which included the Malmquist index summary of annual means (Table 4.19) and a Malmquist index summary of firm/DMU means (Table 4.20).

```
Box 4.2:    Instruction file called eg4-ins.txt

eg4-dta.txt   DATA FILE NAME
eg4-out.txt   OUTPUT FILE NAME
10        NUMBER OF FIRMS
3         NUMBER OF TIME PERIODS
2         NUMBER OF OUTPUTS
2         NUMBER OF INPUTS
1         0 = INPUT AND 1 = OUTPUT ORIENTED
0         0 = CRS AND 1 = VRS
2         0 = DEA(MULTI-STAGE),
          1 = COST-DEA,
          2 = MALMQUIST-DEA,
          3 = DEA(1-STAGE),
          4 = DEA(2-STAGE)
```

In Table 4.19, the last row and the last column show that on average the municipal hospitals' health services productivity increased by 34.3% over the three-year period. The growth was largely due to improvement in efficiency. Whereas efficiency improved by 41.4%, on average, technology regressed by 5% per annum.

Table 4.19 Malmquist index summary of annual means (output oriented)

Year	Efficiency change (A = C × D)	Technical change (B)	Pure efficiency change (C)	Scale efficiency change (D = A/C)	Total factor productivity change (E = B × C × D) or (E = A × B)
2001	1.477	1.044	1.000	1.477	1.542
2003	1.353	0.865	1.000	1.353	1.170
Mean	1.414	0.950	1.000	1.414	1.343

Productivity Growth

To trace the source of inefficiency, we need to scrutinise the results in Table 4.20 containing a summary of the average annual values of the Malmquist productivity index and its constituent components for each municipal hospital. Seven of the 10 hospitals registered improvements in productivity since they had Malmquist indices greater than 1 including Maternidade Caxito (380.7%),

Samba (75.9%), Cajueiros (62.1%), Kilamba Kiaxi (54.7%), Cacuaco (47.5%), Caxito (39.0%), and Porto Amboim (6.2%).

Table 4.20 Malmquist index summary of firm (DMU) means

Decision-making units	Efficiency change (A = C × D)	Technical change (B)	Pure efficiency change (C)	Scale efficiency change (D = A/C)	Total factor productivity change (E = B × C × D) or (E = A × B)
1 = Cajueiros	1.238	1.309	1.000	1.238	1.621
2 = Kilamba Kiaxi	1.679	0.922	1.000	1.679	1.547
3 = Cacuaco	1.137	1.297	1.000	1.137	1.475
4 = Samba	1.360	1.294	1.000	1.360	1.759
5 = Maternidade Caxito	4.181	1.150	1.000	4.181	4.807
6 = Caxito	1.109	1.253	1.000	1.109	1.390
7 = Catete	1.282	0.758	1.000	1.282	0.972
8 = Ambriz	0.956	0.574	1.000	0.956	0.548
9 = Muxima	1.000	0.777	1.000	1.000	0.777
10 = Porto Amboim	1.750	0.607	1.000	1.750	1.062
Mean	1.414	0.950	1.000	1.414	1.343

Note: All Malmquist index averages are geometric means

In five of the seven hospitals, productivity growth was caused both by improvements in efficiency change (movements of the hospitals towards the frontier) and technical change (movements of the best practices frontier). However, Kilamba Kiaxi and Porto Amboim hospitals experienced technical regress.

Three (30%) of the municipal hospitals had Malmquist indices of less than 1 signifying deterioration in performance over time. Ambriz, Muxima, and Catete experienced total factor productivity regress of 45.2%, 22.3%, and 2.8% respectively. In Catete and Muxima deterioration in productivity was caused by technological regress. In Ambriz Hospital, however, productivity decline resulted from both efficiency and technological deterioration.

Pure Efficiency Change

Recall that the first component of Malmquist productivity index (MPI) provides a measure of the contribution, to productivity change, of a change in technical efficiency between periods t and $t+1$. Efficiency change = pure efficiency change × scale efficiency change. As indicated in Table 4.20 the average pure efficiency change (column C) was equal to 1 in all the hospitals, which means that the relative technical efficiency of all the hospitals remained the same between years 2000 and 2002.

Scale Efficiency Change

The scale efficiency change index attains a value greater than, equal to, or less than one if the scale of a DMU's production contributes positively, not at all, or negatively to productivity change [34]. With the exception of Amriz and Muxima, all the other hospitals had a scale efficiency change value of greater than one, which means that the scale of production of these hospitals contributed positively to productivity change. Ambriz registered a scale efficiency change score of 0.956 implying that the scale of production on average reduced the hospital's efficiency change slightly by 4.4%. Maxima had a scale efficiency score of 1 indicating that its scale of production did not affect its efficiency change. The average scale efficiency change score for the entire sample was 1.414 suggesting that, on average, the scale of production improved efficiency change by 41.4%.

Technical Change

The technical change component of MPI provides a measure of the contribution to productivity change of whatever change occurs between periods t (2000 in our example) and $t+1$ (2001 and 2002 in our example). Five (50%) of the hospitals experienced technical progress, none experienced technical stagnation, and five experienced technical regress. The average technical change score was 0.950 indicating a 5% technical regression.

ADVANTAGES AND LIMITATIONS OF DEA

The key advantages of DEA are that (*a*) it can handle multiple health service inputs and outputs and requires information only on quantities of outputs and inputs for estimation of technical efficiency; (b) it can decompose economic efficiency into pure technical efficiency, scale efficiency, and allocative efficiency; and (*c*) it identifies well-performing peer DMUs whose practice can be emulated by the inefficient DMUs [12, 19].

The main limitations of DEA are that (*a*) it is deterministic rather than statistical; (*b*) it measures efficiency relative to best practice within a particular sample, which makes it impossible to meaningfully compare different studies; and (*c*) its scores are sensitive to input and output specification and size of the sample. The first limitation is usually ameliorated by employing a two-stage procedure; that is, estimating efficiency scores using DEA and then regressing those scores against various climatic, topographic, demographic, socio-economic, and governance factors [12, 19].

ACKNOWLEDGEMENTS

This chapter has benefited greatly from the work of HR Varian, E Mansfield, A Koutsoyiannis, M Todaro, MJ Farrell, R Fare, S Grosskopf, M Norris M, Z Zhang, and T Coelli among others. The author's contribution has been to adapt the production theory to the health sector and to illustrate estimation of various theoretical concepts with data from Africa.

REFERENCES

1. World Health Organization. *Basic documents*. Geneva: World Health Organization; 2005.

2. Culyer AJ. The morality of efficiency in health care — some uncomfortable implications. *Health Economics* 1992;1:7–18.

3. Kirigia JM, editor. *Economic evaluation of public health problems in sub-Saharan Africa*. Nairobi: University of Nairobi Press; 2009.

4. Kirigia JM, Saidou BP. Kirigia JM, Barry SP. Health challenges in Africa and the way forward. *International Archives of Medicine* 2008;1:27. Available at: http://www.intarchmed.com/content/1/1/27.

5. Culyer AJ. *The economics of health*. Aldershot: Edward Elgar; 1991.

6. Mooney GH. *Economics, medicine and health care*. London: Harvester Wheatsheaf; 1986.

7. Kirigia JM, Sambo LG, Anikpo E, Karisa E, Mwabu G. Health economics: potential applications in HIV/AIDS control in Africa. *African Journal of Health Sciences* 2005; 12(1–2):1–12.

8. Varian HR. *Intermediate microeconomics: a modern approach*. New Delhi: W.W. Norton and Company; 2006.

9. Mansfield E. *Managerial economics: theory, applications and cases*. London: W.W. Norton and Company; 1990.

10. Koutsoyiannis A. *Modern microeconomics*. London: MacMillan Education; 1979.

11. AMREF. Webpage. Nairobi; 2010. [http://www.amref.org/what-we-do/train-health-workers/clinical-officers/]

12. Coelli TJ. *A guide to DEAP version 2.1: a data envelopment analysis (computer) program*, Centre for Efficiency and Productivity Analysis Working Paper 96/08. Department of Econometrics, University of New England; Armidale, NSW Australia; 1996.

13. SPSS Inc. *Statistical Package for Social Scientists*. Chicago: SPSS; 2009. http://www.spss.com/products/

14. Brickley JA, Smith CW, Zimmerman JL. *Managerial economics and organizational architecture*. Boston: McGraw-Hill-Irwin; 2007.

15. Salvatore D. *Managerial economics: principles and worldwide applications*. Oxford: Oxford University Press; 2008.

16. O'Neill C, Largey A. Issues in cost function specification for neonatal care: the Fordham case. *Journal of Public Health Medicine* 1997;19(1):50-54.

17. Evans RG. *Strained mercy: the economics of Canadian health care*. Toronto: Butterworths; 1984.

18. Finkler SA. On the shape of the hospital industry long run average cost curve. *Health Services Research* 1979;4(4):281-289.

19. Farrell MJ. The measurement of productivity efficiency. *Journal of the Royal Statistical Society* 1957;120(3):253–290.

20. Charnes A, Cooper WW, Rhodes E. Measuring the efficiency of decision-making units. *European Journal of Operational Research* 1978;2(6):429–444.

21. Evans DB, Tandon A, Murray CJL, Lauer JA. Comparative efficiency of national health systems: cross national econometric analysis. *BMJ* 2001;323:307-310.

22. Banxia Holdings. *Banxia efficiency analysis software*. Kendal: 2000–2008. www.banxia.com/frontier/index.html.

23. Coelli TJ. *DEAP [computer program]. version 2.1*. Centre for Efficiency and Productivity Analysis. University of Queensland. Brisbane, Australia; 1996. http://www.uq.edu.au/economics/cepa/coelli.htm

24. Boussofiane A, Dyson RG, Thanassoulis E. Applied data envelopment analysis. *European Journal of Operational Research* 1991;52(1):1–15.

25. Commonwealth of Australia. *Data envelopment analysis: a technique for measuring the efficiency of government service delivery*. Melbourne, Australia; 1997.

26. Pass C, Lowes B, Davies L. *Collins internet-linked dictionary of economics*. Glasgow: HarperCollins; 2005.

27. Kirigia JM, Seddoh A, Gwatwiri D, Kainyu LH, Seddoh J. Determinants, opportunities, challenges and the way forward for countries in the WHO African Region. *BMC Public Health* 2005;5:137. Available at: [http://www.biomedcentral.com/1471–2458/5/137].

28. Kirigia JM, Wambebe C. Status of resources for health research in ten African countries. *BMC Health Services Research* 2006; 6:135. Available at: http//:www.biomedcentral.com/1472-6963/6/135.

29. Todaro MP. *Economic development*. New York: Addison Wesley Longman; 2000.

30. Jhingan ML. *The economics of development and planning*. New Delhi: Vikas; 1982.

31. Caves DW, Christensen LR, Diewert WE. The economic theory of index numbers and the measurement of input, output, and productivity. *Econometrica* 1982;50(6):1393–1414.

32. Fare R, Grosskopf S, Norris M, Zhang Z. Productivity growth, technical progress, and efficiency change in industrialized countries. *The American Economic Review* 1994;84(1):66–83.

33. Fulginiti LE, Perrin RK. LDC agriculture: nonparametric Malmquist productivity indexes. *Journal of Development Economics* 1997;53:373–390.

34. Grifell-Tajte E, Lovell CAK. The sources of productivity change in Spanish banking. *European Journal of Operational Research* 1997;98(2):364–380.

Part II

Application of Data Envelopment
Analysis in Health Systems in Africa

Learning Objectives

By the end of Part 2 you should be well-acquainted with the following applications of DEA:

1. Measurement of technical and scale efficiency of hospitals and health centres in Africa;

2. Measurement of allocative and cost efficiency of health centres in Africa;

3. Measurement and decomposition of productivity growth among national health systems, hospitals, and health centres in Africa using Malmquist total factor productivity index;

4. Interpretation of technical, scale, allocative, and cost efficiency scores and of Malmquist productivity index results.

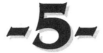

Technical Efficiency of Public Hospitals and Health Centres in Ghana*

*Daniel Osei, Sellasie d'Almeida, Melvin O. George,
Joses M. Kirigia, Ayayi O. Mensah and Lenity H. Kainyu*

ABSTRACT

The Government of Ghana has been implementing various health sector reforms (e.g., user fees in public health facilities, decentralisation, and sector-wide approaches to donor coordination) in a bid to improve efficiency in health care. However, to date, except for the pilot study reported in this paper no attempt has been made to make an estimate of the efficiency of hospitals and/or health centres in Ghana. The objectives of this study, based on data collected in 2000, were (*a*) to estimate the relative technical efficiency (TE) and scale efficiency (SE) of a sample of public hospitals and health centres in Ghana; and (*b*) to demonstrate policy implications for health sector policy makers.

The Data envelopment analysis (DEA) approach was used to estimate the efficiency of 17 district hospitals and 17 health centres. This was an exploratory study. Eight (47%) hospitals were technically inefficient with an average TE score of 61% and a standard deviation (STD) of 12%. Ten (59%) hospitals were scale inefficient manifesting an average SE of 81% (STD = 25%). Out of the 17 health centres, 3 (18%) were technically inefficient with a mean TE score of 49% (STD=27%). Eight health centres (47%) were scale inefficient with an average SE score of 84% (STD = 16%).

* The original article appeared in *Cost Effectiveness and Resource Allocation* 2005;3(9):1-3. Reproduced with the permission of BioMed Central Ltd.

This pilot study demonstrated to policy makers the versatility of DEA in measuring inefficiencies among individual facilities and inputs. There is need for the Planning and Budgeting Unit of the Ghana Health Services to continually monitor the productivity growth, allocative efficiency, and technical efficiency of all its health facilities (hospitals and health centres) during the implementation of health sector reforms.

BACKGROUND

The strategic health objectives of Vision 2020 in Ghana envisage a significant reduction in the rates of infant, child, and maternal mortality; effective control of the risk factors that expose individuals to major communicable diseases; increased access to health services, especially in rural areas; establishment of a health system effectively reoriented towards delivery of public health services; and effective and efficient management of the health system [1].

The Ministry of Health, following the thrust of Vision 2020, developed its current policy and strategy guidelines in 1995 in the Medium-Term Health Strategy (MTHS) document [2]. The five main objectives of the MTHS are improving access to health services; improving quality of care; improving efficiency; fostering partnership between private and public health service-providers; and improving financing of health services.

Subsequently, the first [3] and second [4] Health Sector Five-Year Programme of Work were developed to enable the country attain the MTHS objectives. One of the five underlying objectives of the two programmes of work is "improved efficiency in health services delivery". Furthermore, the Ghana Poverty Reduction Strategy 2002-2004 [5] also highlights "enhancing efficiency in health service delivery" as one of the three priority health sector-related interventions. Thus, efficiency concerns are deeply embedded in the national Vision 2020, national poverty reduction strategy, health policy, and programme of work.

In a bid to improve the efficiency of health services delivery, the Ministry of Health is implementing the following health sector reforms: separation of functions between the Ministry of Health (policy formulation, planning, donor coordination, and resource mobilisation) and the Ghana Health Services (responsible for service delivery); autonomy of tertiary hospitals; decentralised planning and budgeting systems, strengthening of financial management and performance monitoring system, and investing in overall management development capacity within the sector; sector-wide approach (SWAP); and strengthening of existing regulatory bodies and laws [6,7].

Since 1978, data envelopment analysis (DEA) has been extensively used in the Americas [8-10], Western Europe [11-17], and Asia [18, 19] to shed light on the efficiency of various aspects of national health systems. In Africa, the application of DEA in the health sector has been quite limited. So far, the approach has been applied to health facilities in only three countries, that is, South Africa [20-22], Kenya [23, 24], and Zambia [25]. Yet, assessment of efficiency ought to be more prevalent in low-income countries like Ghana in order to optimise health benefits from the available meagre health sector resources.

In Ghana, prior to the current study, no attempt had been made to estimate the efficiency of healthcare facilities using either parametric (econometric) or non-parametric methods. The Planning Unit in the Ministry of Health (with support from the World Health Organization) decided to undertake a limited pilot study to demonstrate to policy makers the potential usefulness of DEA in the pursuit of health sector efficiency objectives. Once policy makers were adequately sensitised, hopefully, a national efficiency study would be conducted among all health centres and district, regional, and tertiary hospitals. The objectives of the exploratory study reported in this paper were (*a*) to estimate the relative technical efficiency of a sample of public hospitals and health centres in Ghana; and (*b*) to demonstrate policy implications for health sector policy makers.

METHODS

Study Area

Ghana is situated on the west coast of Africa. It is divided into ten administrative regions (i.e., Upper East, Upper West, Northern, Brong Ahafo, Ashanti, Volta, Eastern, Greater Accra, Central, and Western) and 110 districts. The organisation of health services more or less mimics the country's administrative structure. The country's health services are organised at the following levels [2]:

1. *Community:* Delivered through outreach programmes, resident or itinerant herbalists, traditional birth attendants, and/or retail drug peddlers.

2. *Sub-district:* A health centre services a geographical area with a population of 15,000 to 30,000. It provides basic curative care, disease prevention services, and maternity services (primary healthcare). A health centre constitutes an essential component of the close-to-client health services.

3. *District:* A district hospital provides support to sub-districts in disease prevention and control, health promotion, and public health education; referral outpatient and inpatient care, training and supervision of health centres; maternity services, especially the management of complications and emergencies; and surgical contraception.

4. *Regional:* A regional hospital provides specialised clinical and diagnostic care; management of high-risk pregnancies and complications of pregnancy; technical and logistical backup for epidemiological surveillance; and research and training.

5. *Tertiary:* At the apex of the referral system, there are two government-owned teaching hospitals that offer specialised services, undertake research, and provide undergraduate and postgraduate training in health and allied areas.

6. *National (*i.e., Ministry of Health headquarters): The national level is responsible for the development of national health policy and for providing strategic direction for service delivery as well as coordination and monitoring.

Ghana's population of 19.7 million is served by a total of 2,189 health facilities of which 952 are government owned, 181 are owned by religious organisations, 75 are quasi-government, and 980 belong to the private sector. Out of the total number of health facilities, there are 2 teaching hospitals, 9 regional hospitals, 91 district hospitals, 124 other hospitals, 558 health centres, 1,085 clinics, and 320 maternity homes. All these health facilities are serviced by 1,294 doctors, 29 dentists, 207 pharmacists, and 326 medical assistants along with other paramedical and support staff [7]. The country spends a total of US$ 252 million (4.2% of the GDP of US$ 6 billion) annually on health. About 53.5% of this expenditure is incurred by the government and 46.5% by the households through out-of-pocket expenses. The total per capita expenditure on health at an average exchange rate is US$ 11 [26].

The life expectancy at birth in Ghana is 57.4 years. The infant and under-five-years mortality rates per 1,000 live births are 57 and 97 respectively [26]. The probability of dying between ages 15 and 59 years is 303 per 1,000 live births. The maternal mortality is 214 per 100,000 live births. Nearly 72% of the population has access to improved sanitation, while 73% has access to an improved water supply source [27]. The question is whether the people of Ghana are deriving maximum healthcare benefits from the aforementioned investments in the health sector especially from hospitals and health centres which consume over 75% of both the recurrent and capital budgets of the Ministry of Health. The next sub-section presents a DEA conceptual framework which is used to shed light on this issue.

DEA Conceptual Framework

In the production process, hospitals and health centres turn inputs (factors of production) into outputs (health services). We can divide the inputs into the broad categories of labour, materials, and capital each of which will often include more narrow sub-divisions. Labour inputs include skilled health personnel (doctors, nurses, paramedics, support staff) and unskilled workers (drivers, watchmen, gardeners, ward attendants, cooks, etc.) as well as the entrepreneurial efforts of managers of health facilities. Materials include pharmaceuticals, non-pharmaceutical supplies, and any other goods that health facilities require to produce healthcare. Capital includes buildings, medical equipment, vehicles, and beds.

The relationship between inputs and the production process and the resulting outputs is described in Figure 5.1. It is clear that hospitals and health centres employ multiple inputs to produce multiple outputs. We used the DEA approach since it allows the measurement of relative efficiency when decision-making units (in this case hospitals/health centres) have multiple inputs and multiple outputs.

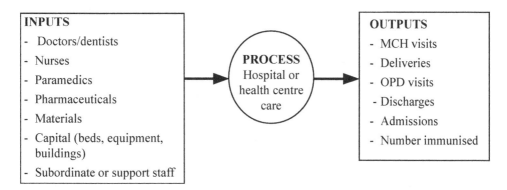

Figure 5.1   Relationship between inputs and the production process and resulting outputs

Data envelopment analysis is a linear programming methodology for evaluating relative efficiency of each production unit among a set of fairly homogeneous decision-making units (DMUs), for example, district hospitals or health centres. It sketches a production possibilities frontier (data envelop or efficient frontier) using combinations of inputs and outputs from best performing health facilities. Health facilities that compose the "best practice frontier" are assigned an efficiency score of one (or 100%) and are deemed technically efficient compared to their peers. The efficiency of the health facilities below the efficiency frontier is measured in terms of their distance from the frontier. The inefficient health facilities are assigned a score between one and zero. The larger the score the more efficient a health facility is. Since hospitals and health centres employ multiple inputs to produce multiple outputs, their individual technical efficiency can be defined as [28]:

$$\text{Technical efficiency score} = \frac{\text{weighted sum of outputs}}{\text{weighted sum of inputs}}$$

The technically inefficient health facility uses more weighted inputs per weighted output or produce less weighted output per weighted input than those health facilities on the "best practice frontier". Algebraically, the technical efficiency score of each hospital and health centre in the sample were obtained by solving the models (1) and (2) in Figure 5.2 [29].

Model 1	DEA weights model, input-oriented, CRS	Model 2	DEA weights model, input-oriented, VRS

$$\text{Eff} = \underset{u_r, v_i}{\text{Max}} \sum_r u_r y_{rj_0}$$

s.t.

$$\sum_r u_r y_{rj} - \sum_i v_i x_{ij} \leq 0; \; \forall j$$

$$\sum_i v_i x_{ij_0} = 1$$

$$u_r, v_i \geq 0; \forall r, \forall i.$$

$$\text{Eff} = \underset{u_r, v_i}{\text{Max}} \sum_r u_r y_{rj_0} + u_0$$

s.t.

$$\sum_r u_r y_{rj} - \sum_i v_i x_{ij} + u_0 \leq 0 \quad ; \forall j$$

$$\sum_i v_i x_{ij_0} = 1$$

$$u_r, v_i \geq 0 \quad ; \forall r, \forall i.$$

Figure 5.2   DEA Models

Where:

y_{rj} = the amount of output r produced by a hospital or health centre j,

x_{ij} = the amount of input i used by a hospital or health centre j

u_r = the weight given to output r, ($r =1,..., t$ and t is the number of outputs)

v_i = the weight given to input i, ($I =1, ..., m$ and m is the number of inputs)

n = the number of hospitals or health centres

j_0 = the hospital or health centre under assessment

We need to explain what we mean by constant returns to scale and variable returns to scale. Returns to scale refers to the changes in output as all inputs change by the same proportion. For instance, suppose that for a specific hospital (or health centre) j we start from an initial level of inputs (doctors = D, other technical staff = T, subordinate staff = S, beds = B) and output (Q):

$$Q_O = f(D, T, S, B)$$

and increase all the factors by the same proportion ϕ, we will obviously obtain a new level of output Q^* that is higher than the original level Q_0. Thus:

$$Q^* = f(\phi D, \phi T, \phi S, \phi B).$$

If Q^* increases (*a*) by the same proportion, ϕ, as the inputs we say that there are constant returns to scale (CRS); (*b*) less than proportionally with the increase in inputs we have decreasing returns to scale (DRS); and (*c*) more than proportionally with the increase in the inputs we have increasing returns to scale (IRS). Those hospitals and health centres manifesting CRS are said to be operating at their most productive scale sizes. In order to operate at the most productive scale size, a health facility displaying DRS should scale down both outputs and inputs. If a health facility is exhibiting IRS, it should expand both outputs and inputs in order to become scale efficient [8]. We have illustrated below how DEA works using hypothetical hospitals.

Let us assume that a hypothetical country called Nkrumah has 9 district hospitals. Each hospital produces two outputs: outpatient department visits (OPVisits) and inpatient admissions (Admissions) from a single input of technical staff. The number of staff employed, OPVisits, Admissions, ratio of OPVisits to staff, and ratio of Admissions to staff are contained in Table 5.1.

Table 5.1 Illustration of DEA analysis using a hypothetical example of nine hospitals

DMUs	OPVisits (A)	Admissions (B)	Staff (C)	OP visits/staff D=(A/C)	Admissions/staff E=(B/C)
Anim	7,020	5,451	102	69	53
Akoa	20,566	7,610	92	224	83
Addai	25,200	7,148	143	176	50
Mensa	33,568	7,958	96	350	83
Kofi	17,406	2,429	95	183	26
Gyau	10,573	8,094	117	90	69
Anani	10,500	8,944	115	91	78
Amoi	20,421	10,969	117	175	94
Asamoa	20,647	8,619	46	449	187

The efficiency of each hospital in producing the two outputs was estimated by dividing each of their outputs by their input and determining which hospital had the highest ratios. The results are contained in the last two columns of Table 5.1. The higher the ratio of an output to input the more efficient a hospital is in producing that output. In this example, Asamoa hospital had the highest number of OPVisits (449) and Admissions (187) for each member of technical staff employed. By plotting OPVisits/staff against Admissions/staff for the nine hospitals we derive the production possibilities frontier graph contained in Figure 5.3.

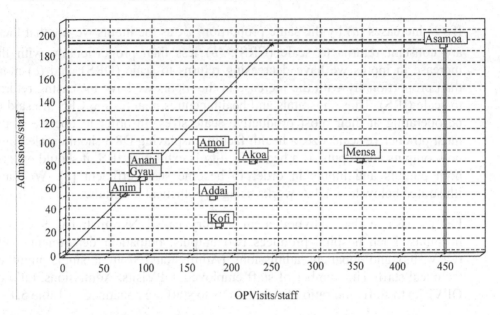

Figure 5.3   Production possibilities frontier graph

Figure 5.3 shows the efficiency frontier, which is the fundamental concept of DEA. The straight lines from Asamoa hospital to the Y-axis (labelled Admissions/staff) and from Asamoa to the X-axis (labelled Opvisits/staff) represent the efficient frontier. The efficiency frontier, derived from the most efficient hospital (Asamoa hospital in our example) in the dataset/sample, represents a standard of technically best performance that can be achieved from available input and technology endowment. Consequently, it is used as a threshold against which to measure the performance of all other hospitals.

The efficiency frontier "envelops" the inefficient hospitals within it and clearly shows the relative efficiency of each hospital. A hospital like Asamoa, which is located on the frontier, is considered 100% technically efficient. Any hospital, like Mensa, Amoi, Akoa, Anani, Kofi, Addai, Gyau, and Anim that is below the production possibilities frontier is relatively less efficient and is given a technical efficiency rating of less than 100%.

Anim hospital, for instance, could become efficient if it increased its outputs in the same proportions while holding its input constant; that is, assuming an output-oriented model/situation. Instead, it could become efficient by reducing its input while keeping its outputs the same; that is, assuming an input-oriented scenario. Its technical efficiency is calculated by the ratio of its distance from the origin over the distance from the origin to the point of intersection on the production possibilities frontier or the efficiency frontier. This gives Anim hospital a technical efficiency score of 28.52%. Likewise, Mensa hospital is 77.90% as efficient as Asamoa hospital (the best practice hospital), Amoi hospital is 50.04%, Akoa hospital is 49.80%, Anani hospital is 41.51%, Kofi hospital is 40.82%, Addai hospital is 39.26%, and Gyau hospital is 36.92%. These scores were estimated assuming constant returns to scale (CRS).

However, health services production processes often are not linear and thus it may be more appropriate to assume variable returns to scale (VRS). Thus, we estimated the DEA model assuming VRS and the efficiency scores for various hospitals were as follows: Asamoa = 100%, Amoi = 100%, Mensa = 100%, Akoa = 50%, Anani = 48.54%, Kofi = 48.42%, Anim = 45.10%, Addai = 44.49%, and Gyau = 39.32%. This finding implies that if Akoa, Anani, Kofi, Anim, Addai, and Gyau hospitals were to operate efficiently, they are capable of producing their current output levels with 50%, 51.5%, 51.58%, 54.9%, 55.51%, and 60.68% less inputs respectively than they are currently using. Whereas in the CRS model only Asamoa hospital had a 100% efficiency score, in the VRS model three hospitals (Asamoa, Amoi, and Mensa) achieved a pure technical efficiency score of 100%.

The impact of hospital scale/size on their technical efficiency was evaluated using a three-step process. First, the model was estimated assuming CRS. Second, the model was run assuming VRS. Third, scale efficiency was obtained by dividing each hospital's CRS technical efficiency score by its VRS technical efficiency score. Akoa and Asamoa hospitals have a scale efficiency score of 100% implying they had an optimal size. Gyau scored 94%, Addai scored 88%, Anani scored 86%, Kofi scored 84%, Mensa scored 78%, Anim scored 63%, and Amoi scored 50%. These seven hospitals were scale inefficient since they were not operating at their most productive size for their observed input mix. It is important to mention that DEA is only an exploratory tool for efficiency measurement and indicates directions for further investigations into how to improve/enhance efficiency.

Input and output orientation

In the hospital analysis, the input orientation assumed that these facilities had limited control over the volume of their outputs. There was no linkage between staff earnings and output; thus, there was no incentive for inducing demand for health services. Otherwise, in Ghana hospital management has got greater control over the use of inputs. Thus, an input-oriented DEA model was used for hospital analysis.

On the other hand, output orientation was assumed for health centres. The management of health centres has no control over inputs, especially its staffing. However, given their primary healthcare orientation with a strong bias towards health promotion and disease prevention, they can influence a great number of people seeking, for example, antenatal and postnatal care, family planning services, birthing services, immunisations, and health education through their public health outreach work among communities. Thus, the output-oriented DEA model was used for the health centre analysis.

Strengths and weaknesses of DEA

We chose to employ the DEA approach to estimate technical efficiency of individual hospitals and health centres because of its unique strengths such as: (*a*) it can handle multiple input and multiple output models/scenarios typical of hospitals and health centres; (*b*) it does not require an assumption of a functional form relating inputs to outputs (as regression methods do); (*c*) health facilities are directly compared against a peer or combination of peers; (*d*) inputs and outputs can be in very different units; and (*e*) it does not require information on prices of inputs and outputs [22,30].

Even though we chose to use DEA, we were fully aware that it has two main limitations. Firstly, it attributes any deviation from the "best practice frontier" to inefficiency while some could be due to statistical noise (such as epidemics or measurement errors). Secondly, given that DEA is a deterministic or nonparametric technique, it is difficult to conduct statistical tests of hypotheses concerning the inefficiency and the structure of the production function [22,31,32].

Variables

The hospital DEA model had a total of seven variables including three outputs and four inputs. The three outputs for each individual hospital were the number of maternal and child care visits (i.e., antenatal care, postnatal care, family planning, tetanus toxoid, child immunisation, and growth monitoring); the number of child deliveries; and the number of patients discharged (not including deaths). The four inputs were number of medical officers; number of technical officers (including medical assistants, nurses, and paramedical staff); number of support or subordinate staff (including orderlies, ward assistants, cleaners, drivers, gardeners, watchmen, etc.); and number of hospital beds.

On the other hand, the health centre DEA model was estimated with a total of six variables including four outputs and two inputs. The four outputs for each individual health centre were number of child deliveries; number of fully-immunised children under the age of 5 years; number of other maternal (i.e., antenatal care, postnatal care, and family planning services) and childcare (nutritional/child growth monitoring) visits; and number of outpatient curative visits. The two inputs were number of technical staff (including medical assistants, nurses, and paramedical staff); and number of support or subordinate staff (including cleaners, drivers, gardeners, watchmen, and others). The choice of inputs and outputs for the DEA analysis was guided, in part, by the previous DEA healthcare studies in the African Region and availability of data.

Data

The data used in this study are for year 2000. In order to have a feel of the usefulness of DEA in the measurement of technical efficiency of hospitals and health centres, the policy makers instructed the Planning and Budget Unit (PBU) to draw a pilot sample of 21 hospitals and 21 health centres. The PBU decided to use simple random sampling technique to draw the two samples. Data were collected from a random sample of 21 public health centres using a WHO African regional office efficiency questionnaire for primary healthcare facilities [32]. However, information on health personnel in four health centres was missing; thus, they were left out of the analysis. Data were also collected from a random sample of 21 district hospitals. However, information on inputs and outputs from only 17 hospitals was included in the analysis. Data on hospitals were collected using a WHO/AFRO efficiency questionnaire for hospitals [33]. The data were analysed using the DEAP software developed by Professor Tim Coelli [31].

RESULTS

Hospital Analysis

In year 2000, all 17 hospitals in the sample produced a total of 200,589 maternal and child health (MCH) visits, 24,152 deliveries, and 69,361 discharges. Those outputs were produced employing a total of 55 medical officers/dentists, 1,345 technical staff, 721 subordinate staff, and 1,543 beds. Table 5.2 presents the means and standard deviations for input and output variables of the 17 district hospitals.

Table 5.2   Means and standard deviations for public hospital inputs and outputs

Variable	Mean	Standard deviation
Outputs		
Maternal and child healthcare visits	11,799	9,516
Deliveries	1,421	1,186
Inpatient discharges	4,080	2,274
Inputs		
Doctors/dentists	3	3
Technical staff (including nurses)	79	34
Subordinate staff	42	27
Beds	91	43

The VRS model technical and scale efficiency scores for individual hospitals are contained in Table 5.3. Of the 17 hospitals, 9 (53%) were technically efficient since they had a relative technical efficiency (TE) score of 100%. The remaining 8 (47%) had a TE score of less than 100%, which means that they were technically inefficient. The TE score among the latter facilities ranged from 74% in Atua hospital to 43% in Winneba hospital. This finding implies that Atua and Winneba hospitals could potentially reduce their current input endowments by 26% and 57% while leaving their output levels unchanged. The average TE score among the inefficient hospitals was 61% (standard deviation=12%), which means that these hospitals could, on average, produce their current levels of output with 39% less inputs than they were currently using.

Seven (41%) of the hospitals had a scale efficiency (SE) of 100%, which means that they had the most productive size for that particular input-output mix. The remaining 10 (59%) hospitals had a SE of less than 100% and as such they were scale inefficient. The average SE among the inefficient hospitals was 81% (standard deviation = 25%), meaning that, on average, the scale inefficient hospitals could reduce their size by 19% without affecting their current output levels. All the seven scale-efficient hospitals displayed constant returns to scale (CRS) implying that they were operating at their most productive scale sizes. Eight of the 10 scale-inefficient hospitals had increasing returns to scale (IRS) while one of the hospitals revealed decreasing returns to scale (DRS). In order to operate at the most productive scale size (MPSS), a hospital exhibiting DRS should scale down both its outputs and inputs. Similarly, if a hospital is displaying IRS, it should expand both its outputs and inputs.

Table 5.3   *Technical and scale efficiency scores for district hospitals*

DMU (Hospital)	Technical efficiency (%)	Scale efficiency (%)
Swendru	100.0	100.0
Half Asin	100.0	100.0
Turkwa	100.0	100.0
Kwesiminstmu	100.0	100.0
Yendi	100.0	100.0
Takoradi	100.0	100.0
St Francis Xavier	100.0	100.0
West End	100.0	91.6
Walewale	100.0	43.9
Atua	74.4	99.8
Tetteh Quarshie	73.6	99.9
Cape Coast	68.6	93.2
Akuse	66.3	43.9
Axim	57.4	50.9
Suhum	56.5	98.0
Akim	46.0	99.6
Winneba	42.7	93.9

Health Centre Analysis

The total output of all health centres in the sample combined was as follows: 67,739 MCH visits; 4,541 deliveries; 28,909 fully immunised children; and 81,665 outpatient curative visits. The total input endowment of all health centres consisted of 181 technical staff and 87 subordinate staff. Table 5.4 presents the means and standard deviations for input and output variables of 17 health centres.

Table 5.4   Means and standard deviations for public health centre inputs and outputs

Variable	Mean	Standard deviation
Outputs		
Maternal and child healthcare visits	3,985	2,579
Deliveries	267	207
Fully-immunised children	1,701	1,526
OPD curative visits	4,804	5,475
Inputs		
Medical assistants/nurses/other technical staff	11	5
Subordinate staff	5	3

The VRS technical and scale efficiency scores for individual health centres are given in Table 5.5. Out of the 17 health centres, 14 (82%) were technically efficient since they had a relative technical efficiency (TE) score of 100%. The remaining 3 (18%) had a TE score of less than 100% and thus were deemed to be technically inefficient. The TE score among the latter facilities varied from about 80% at Daboase and 42% at Tikobo to 27% at the Abomoso health centre. This means that Daboase, Tikobo, and Abomoso could potentially produce 20%, 58%, and 73% more outputs respectively using their current input endowment if they were to operate efficiently.

On the other hand, 9 (53%) of the health centres were scale efficient because they had a relative scale efficiency (SE) score of 100%. The remaining 8 health centres (47%) had an SE of less than 100% and as such were scale inefficient. The average SE among the inefficient health centres was 84% (standard deviation = 16%). This implies that, on average, the scale inefficient health centres could produce their current output levels with 17% less capacity than they were actually using. All the 9 scale-efficient health centres exhibited constant returns to scale (CRS). Except for Abomoso, all the other 7 scale-inefficient health centres manifested decreasing returns to scale (DRS).

*Table 5.5   Technical and scale efficiency scores for public health
centres*

DMU (Health centres)	Technical efficiency (%)	Scale efficiency (%)
Diare	100.0	100.0
Nafong	100.0	100.0
Anyingse	100.0	100.0
Anyinam	100.0	100.0
Akroso	100.0	100.0
Elubo	100.0	100.0
Adisadel	100.0	100.0
Nkwanyawum	100.0	100.0
Adukrom	100.0	100.0
Osino	100.0	98.3
Fanti Nyankomasia	100.0	90.1
Okrakwadwo	100.0	88.7
Ewim	100.0	69.5
Savelugu	100.0	67.6
Daboase	79.7	58.5
Tikobo	42.0	96.6
Abomoso	26.6	99.9

DISCUSSION

Hospital Analysis

Forty-seven per cent of the hospitals in the sample were technically inefficient and 59% were scale inefficient. A similar study among 55 public hospitals in Kwazulu-Natal Province in South Africa found 40% of the hospitals to be technically inefficient and 42% to be scale inefficient [20,22]. Another DEA analysis of 54 public hospitals in Kenya revealed that 26% of them were technically inefficient while about 30% were scale inefficient [23]. Masiye *et al.* [25] undertook DEA among 20 hospitals in Zambia and found 75% of them to be technically inefficient. Thus, the available evidence indicates that although there is significant technical inefficiency among health facilities in Ghana, Kenya, South Africa, and Zambia the magnitude of inefficiency does vary.

Table 5.6 shows the total output increases and/or input reductions needed to make inefficient district public hospitals efficient. The inefficient hospitals could be technically efficient if they were to increase their output levels by 25% more MCH visits, 12% more deliveries, and 1% more discharges while holding their current input endowment constant. Alternatively, the inefficient hospitals could become technically efficient if they were to reduce their current number of medical officers/dentists by 44%, technical staff by 22%, subordinate staff by 28%, and beds by 29% while holding the output constant.

Table 5.6   Total output increases and/or input reductions needed to make inefficient district public hospitals efficient

Variable	Radial movement (A)	Slack movement (B)	Total value (C=A+B)
Outputs			
Maternal and child healthcare visits	0	50,845	50,845
Deliveries	0	2,865	2,865
Inpatient discharges	0	808	808
Inputs			
Doctors/dentists	13	11	24
Technical staff (including nurses)	292	0	292
Subordinate staff	173	27	200
Beds	397	51	448

Policy implications for hospitals

As regards the excess resources which were wasted and not utilised in the production of hospital outputs, decision-makers in the Ghana Ministry of Health have a number of policy options available to them. These are as follows:

1.   Do nothing and continue with the wasteful situation as it exists. However, judging from the strategic and policy documents produced by the Ministry of Health, it is clear that this option is considered unacceptable by its policy makers.

2.   Option related to excess medical officers/dentists and other technical staff; in our opinion, given the need for strengthening health services at sub-district and community levels, it would not be rational to offer any category of technical staff the option of early retirement. Instead, excess medical officers/dentists and other technical staff should be transferred to health centres to provide primary healthcare. We believe that this would increase health coverage and quality of service provided at sub-district and community levels.

3.   Options related to excess subordinate staff include (*a*) offering employees early retirement with severance pay plans (i.e., voluntary retirement); (*b*) forced retrenchment with severance package; and (*c*) transfer of excess labour force to under-staffed primary healthcare facilities.

4.   Options related to excess beds and space include (*a*) convert the space occupied by excess beds to provide outpatients secondary prevention services; (*b*) rent excess beds and space to private medical practitioners if there is a demand for them; and (*c*) sell excess beds and the space they occupy and use the money thus realised to improve the quality of hospital care.

5. Closure of some hospitals; holding equity and political concerns constant, in principle, health policy makers could opt to close down those hospitals with efficiency score below a certain threshold. However, in reality, members of parliament representing the concerned constituencies might be opposed to such an option due to potential political fallout.

6. Conversion of specific hospitals into health centres; this option would entail downsizing both the services provided and staff composition and their numbers. If this option were to be pursued, there would be need for working out details of the conversion process.

Implementation of any of the aforementioned options will need to be preceded by more detailed studies into the determinants of inefficiencies.

Health Centre Analysis

In the Ghana pilot study reported in the paper, 18% of the health centres were technically inefficient and 47% were scale inefficient. A DEA study of 155 primary healthcare clinics in Kwazulu-Natal Province in South Africa found 70% of them to be technically inefficient while 84% manifested some scale inefficiency [21]. A similar study of 32 public health centres in Kenya revealed that 56% of them were technically inefficient while 41% were scale inefficient [24].

Table 5.7 presents the total output increases and/or input reductions needed to make inefficient public health centres efficient. In order to become efficient, health centres will need to expand (*a*) maternal and child health visits by 9%; (*b*) deliveries by 11%; (*c*) fully-immunised children by 9%; and (*d*) outpatient curative visits by 6%. If the excess inputs in district hospitals were to be transferred to primary healthcare facilities, health centres would potentially be able to increase their outputs by even larger magnitudes than those indicated above.

Table 5.7   *Total output increases and/or input reductions needed to make inefficient public health centres efficient*

Variable	Radial Movement (A)	Slack movement (B)	Total movement (C=A+B)
Outputs			
Maternal and child healthcare visits	5,306	1,100	6,406
Deliveries	507	0	507
Fully-immunised children	2,645	74	2,719
OPD curative visits	3,451	1,564	5,015
Inputs			
Medical Assistants/nurses/ other technical staff	0	7	7
Subordinate staff	0	1	1

Policy implications for health centres

Health centres provide affordable promotive, preventive, and basic curative care in localities inhabited mainly by the poor. Their location makes them critically important in the ongoing efforts to scale up pro-poor cost-effective public health interventions geared at achieving the health-related Millennium Development Goals [34] and New Partnership for Africa's Development (NEPAD) health targets [35]. Thus, the importance of these close-to-client health facilities in all efforts to reduce the burden of disease and improve health conditions, especially in rural areas, cannot be overemphasised.

Health promotion strategies and methods may be crucial in inducing the necessary demand for services mentioned above in order to reduce technical inefficiencies in health centres [36]. Health promotion uses approaches/methods such as advocacy (including lobbying); health education; communication for behavioural change; social marketing; social mobilisation; information, education, and communication (IEC); legislation; and economic and environmental policies to reduce health risks involving health as well as non-health sectors (e.g., agriculture, education, housing, sanitation, trade, transport, and water) [37,38].

Given their strategic position amongst communities and closeness to actual and potential clients, health centres make a vital contribution to the development, implementation, monitoring, and evaluation of health-promoting initiatives. For example, through the combined use of the aforementioned health promotion strategies and approaches, health centre personnel (with some additional basic health-promotion training) can proactively motivate and persuade households to (*a*) support pregnant women to seek antenatal care, give birth under the care of skilled birth attendants, and seek postnatal care; (*b*) get their children immunised against vaccine-preventable diseases; and (*c*) take their children to outpatient departments for integrated management of childhood illnesses (IMCI).

Apart from health promotion, once the Ghana National Health Insurance (GNHI) programme is fully implemented up to the community level, demand for health services is bound to increase due to reduction in financial barriers. The GNHI consists of Social Health Insurance Schemes (District Mutual Health Insurance Schemes and Private Mutual Health Insurance Schemes) and Private Commercial Health Insurance Schemes [39, 40].

Limitations of the Study

It could be argued that the objective function of health facilities is to maximise health gains from available resources. The ideal output indicator would be the one that captures in a sensitive, valid, reliable, and culturally acceptable manner changes in both the quantity and quality of the lives of those who interact with hospitals and health centres [20]. However, given the unavailability of data on either disability-adjusted life expectancy (DALE) [41] or quality-adjusted life years (QALY) [42,43] gained due to care in each of the facilities in the data set, we opted to use proxies that had been used in similar studies in the past [20-24].

It may be argued that there may be variation in the quality of care provided by different health facilities (for instance, facilities offering higher quality of care may require more personnel time and other inputs than those offering low quality of care). Given the fact that all the hospitals studied were district-level public hospitals designed and resourced to provide a fairly similar level and mix of care, it is unlikely that there would be any significant variance in the quality of care across these facilities. The health centres studied were also fairly homogeneous in size and mix of services provided [2]. The analysis assumed that the case mix of a specific hospital and its efficiency reference set (ERS) hospitals was similar. We were not able to verify whether that assumption was plausible. However, due to the fact that the study hospitals were all non-specialist first referral-level hospitals, the above assumption was most likely to hold.

Drugs were largely supplied from the Central Medical Stores. However, some health facilities often used their cost-sharing funds to make supplementary acquisitions as and when needed. Unfortunately, data on drug expenditure were not forthcoming in most of the questionnaires; thus, it was decided to drop this variable from the analysis altogether. Lastly, since the sample for health centres constituted only 3.7% of the total number of public health centres and hospitals formed about 22% of the public district hospitals, the results cannot be generalised to the entire population of health centres and hospitals in Ghana.

Suggestions for further research

In the light of the challenges of health financing, equity, and efficiency (both allocative and technical) confronting the public health sector, there is an urgent need for (*a*) conducting technical and allocative efficiency studies in all the public, private-for-profit, and religious mission hospitals and health centres with a view to identifying inefficiencies in individual health facilities and their inputs; and (*b*) conducting Malmquist productivity index analysis to monitor and evaluate the effects of different healthcare reforms on productivity growth, technical progress, and efficiency change in health facilities over time [44].

CONCLUSIONS

Various governments in Africa have embarked on health sector reforms to improve the performance of their national health systems. Monitoring and evaluating the effects of those reforms on productivity growth, technical progress, and efficiency change of fixed health facilities that consume the majority of the recurrent and development budgets of ministries of health is of paramount importance. Our study tried to contribute to establishing baseline technical and scale efficiency information that could be used in monitoring the efficiency effects of future policy changes. We have also briefly described how health promotion strategies and methods could be used to reduce inefficiencies in health centres.

Competing Interests

The author(s) declare that they have no competing interests.

Authors' Contributions

DO, SD and MOG collected the data and participated in analysis and drafting of sections of the document. OM, LHK and DG participated in drafting sections of the manuscript. JMK did literature review and participated in the development of the conceptual framework, data analysis, and writing of sections of the document. All the authors read and approved the final manuscript.

ACKNOWLEDGEMENT

We are grateful to the Ministry of Health, Ghana, and the Ghana Health Services for authorising and facilitating the study. We are indebted to the two anonymous peer reviewers for their constructive comments and suggestions that helped to improve the quality of our manuscript. A.S. Kochar provided commendable editorial support. We owe profound gratitude to Sabbaoth El Mekodeshkum for multifaceted support, without which the manuscript would never have been completed.

Any mistakes remaining in the paper are those of the authors and should not be attributed to any of the persons acknowledged. The article contains the views of the authors only and does not represent the opinions, decisions or stated policies of either the Ghana Ministry of Health, the Ghana Health Services, the Kenyatta University, or the World Health Organization.

REFERENCES

1. Republic of Ghana. *The Ghana Vision 2020*. Accra: Republic of Ghana; 1999.

2. Republic of Ghana, Ministry of Health. *Medium-term health strategy towards Vision 2020*. Accra: Republic of Ghana; 1999.

3. Republic of Ghana, Ministry of Health: *Health sector 5-year programme of work 1997-2001*. Accra: Republic of Ghana; 1999.

4. Republic of Ghana, Ministry of Health: *Health sector 5-year programme of work 2002-2006*. Accra; 2001.

5. Republic of Ghana, Ministry of Health. Ghana Poverty Reduction Strategy 2002-2004: An agenda for growth and prosperity. Accra: Republic of Ghana; 2002.

6. Republic of Ghana, Ministry of Health. *Institutional reform in the health sector*. Accra: Republic of Ghana; 1999.

7. World Health Organization Regional Office for Africa. *WHO Country cooperation strategy: Ghana*. Brazzaville: World Health Organization; 2002.

8. Chattopadhy S, Ray CS. Technical, scale, and size efficiency in nursing home care: a nonparametric analysis of Connecticut homes. *Health Economics* 1996;5:363-373.

9. Shroff HFE, Gulledge TR, Haynes KE, Oneill MK. Siting efficiency of long-term healthcare facilities. *Socio-economic Planning Science* 1998;32(1): 25-43.

10. White KR, Fache RN, Ozcan YA. Church ownership and hospital efficiency. *Hospital and Health Services Administration* 1996;41(3):297-310.

11. Hollingsworth B, Parkin D. The efficiency of the delivery of neonatal care in the UK. *Journal of Public Health Medicine* 2001;23(1):47-50.

12. Jacobs R. Alternative methods to examine hospital efficiency: data envelopment analysis and stochastic frontier analysis. *Health Care Management Science* 2001;4:103-115.

13. Ersoy K, Kavuncubasi S, Ozcan YA, Harris II JM. Technical efficiencies of Turkish hospitals: DEA approach. *Journal of Medical Systems* 1997;21(2):67-74.

14. Zavras AI, Tsakos G, Economou C, Kyriopoulos J. Using DEA to evaluate efficiency and formulate policy within a Greek national primary healthcare network. *Journal of Medical Systems* 2002;26(4):285-292.

15. Linna M, Nordblad A, Koivu M. Technical and cost-efficiency of oral health care provision in Finnish health centers. *Social Science and Medicine* 2002;56:343-353.

16. Salinas-Jimenez J, Smith P. Data envelopment analysis applied to quality in primary health care. *Annals of Operational Research* 1996;67:141-161.

17. Giuffrida A, Gravelle H. Measuring performance in primary care: econometric analysis and DEA. *Applied Economics* 2001;33:163-175.

18. Chang H. Determinants of hospital efficiency: the case of central government-owned hospitals in Taiwan. *Omega International Journal of Management Science* 1998;26(2):307-317.

19. Wan TTH, Hsu N, Feng R, Ma A, Pan S, Chou M. Technical efficiency of nursing units in a tertiary care hospital in Taiwan. *Journal of Medical Systems* 2002;26(1):21-27.

20. Kirigia JM, Lambo E, Sambo LG. Are public hospitals in Kwazulu-Natal Province of South Africa technically efficient? *African Journal of Health Sciences* 2000;7(3-4):25-32.

21. Kirigia JM, Sambo LG, Scheel H. Technical efficiency of public clinics in Kwazulu-Natal Province of South Africa. *East African Medical Journal* 2001;78(3 Suppl):S1-S13.

22. Zere EA, Addison T, McIntyre D. Hospital efficiency in sub-Saharan Africa: evidence from South Africa. *South African Journal of Economics* 2000;69(2):336-358.

23. Kirigia JM, Emrouznejad A, Sambo LG. Measurement of technical efficiency of public hospitals in Kenya: using data envelopment analysis. *Journal of Medical Systems* 2002;26(1):39-45.

24. Kirigia JM, Emrouznejad A, Sambo LG, Munguti N, Liambila W. Using data envelopment analysis to measure the technical efficiency of public health centers in Kenya. *Journal of Medical Systems* 2004;28(2):155-166.

25. Masiye F, Ndulo M, Roos P, Odegaard K. A comparative analysis of hospitals in Zambia: a pilot study on efficiency measurement and monitoring. In:Seshamani V, Mwikisa CN, Odegaard K, editors . *Zambia's health reforms: selected papers 1995-2000*. Lund: Swedish Institute for Health Economics and University of Zambia, Department of Economics; 2002. p 95-107.

26. World Health Organization. *The world health report 2002*. Geneva: World Health Organization; 2002.

27. United Nations Development Programme. *Human development report 2003: Millennium Development Goals: a compact among nations to end human poverty*. New York: Oxford University Press; 2003.

28 Charnes A, Cooper WW, Rhodes E. Measuring efficiency of decision-making units. *European Journal of Operational Research* 1978;2(6):429-444.

29. Emrouznejad A. Ali Emrouznejad's Data Envelopment Analysis HomePage 1995-2001,www.DEAzone.com.

30. Commonwealth of Australia. *Data envelopment analysis: a technique for measuring the efficiency of government service delivery*. Melbourne: Commonwealth of Australia; 1997.

31. Coelli TJ. *A guide to DEAP version 2.1: a data envelopment analysis (computer) program*, Centre for Productivity and Efficiency Analysis (CEPA) Working Paper *96/08*. Department of Econometrics, University of New England, Armidale, NSW Australia; 1996.

32. World Health Organization Regional Office for Africa. *Primary health care facility economic efficiency analysis data collection instrument*. Brazzaville: World Health Organization; 2000.

33. World Health Organization Regional Office for Africa. *Hospitals economic efficiency analysis data collection instrument*. Brazzaville: World Health Organization; 2000.

34. United Nations Organization. *Millennium Development Goals (MDG)*. New York: United Nations; 2000.

35. New Partnership for Africa's Development (NEPAD). *Human development programme: NEPAD health strategy*. Pretoria: NEPAD; 2001.

36. World Health Organization. *Ottawa charter for health promotion*. First International Conference on Health Promotion; 21 November 1986; Ottawa. Geneva: World Health Organization; 1986. WHO/HPR/HEP/95.1.

37. Egger G, Spark R, Lawson J. *Health promotion strategies and methods*. Sydney: McGraw-Hill; 1990.

38. World Health Organization Regional Office for Africa. *Health promotion: a strategy for the African Region*. Harare: World Health Organization; 2001.

39. Republic of Ghana, Ministry of Health. *National health insurance policy framework*. Accra: Republic of Ghana; 2004.

40. International Labour Organization. *Improving social protection for the poor: health insurance in Ghana*. Geneva: International Labour Organization; 2005.

41. World Health Organization. *The world health report 2000 –health systems: improving performance*. Geneva: World Health Organization; 2000.

42. Kirigia JM. Health impacts of epidemiological environment change: measurement issues. *Environment and Development Economics* 1996;1(3):359-367.

43. Kirigia JM. Cost-utility analysis of schistosomiasis intervention strategies in Kenya. *Environment and Development Economics* 1998;3:319-346.

44. Fare R, Grosskopf S, Norris M, Zhang Z. Productivity growth, technical progress, and efficiency change in industrialized countries. *The American Economic Review* 1994;84(1):66-83.

-6-

Measurement of Technical Efficiency of Public Hospitals in Kenya: Using Data Envelopment Analysis*

Joses M. Kirigia, Ali Emrouznejad and Luis G. Sambo

ABSTRACT

In sub-Saharan Africa (SSA), there is a huge knowledge gap of health facilities' performance. The objective of this study was to measure relative technical efficiencies of 54 public hospitals in Kenya using the data envelopment analysis (DEA) technique. Fourteen (26%) of the public hospitals were found to be technically inefficient. The study singled out the inefficient hospitals and provided the magnitudes of specific input reductions or output increases needed to attain technical efficiency.

Keywords: DEA, hospital efficiency, and health efficiency

INTRODUCTION

Without a wider use of economics in healthcare inefficiencies will abound and decisions will be made less explicitly and hence less rationally than is desirable: we will go on spending large sums to save life in one way when similar lives in greater numbers could be saved in another way. The price of inefficiency, inexplicitness and irrationality in health care is paid in death and sickness. Gavin H. Mooney [1,p.55]

In sub-Saharan Africa (SSA) public hospitals absorb about 45%-69% of current government health sector expenditure [2-5]. For example, in the 1998/99 fiscal year, Kenya's Ministry of Health spent US$90,795,433 (75.1%) on curative care at the tertiary, provincial, district, and sub-district hospitals [6]. However, although fixed health facilities (hospitals and health centres)

---

* The original article appeared in *Journal of Medical Systems* 2002;26(1):39-45. Reproduced with the permission of Plenum Publishing Corporation.

constitute an important component of health systems in SSA, there is a huge knowledge gap of the performance of individual health facilities. Two DEA studies conducted in South Africa have demonstrated that public healthcare facilities are not maximising healthcare outcomes from the available resource endowments [7].

Inefficiency is akin to a torn rice sack: if the holes are not identified and sealed/mended, it would be impossible to fill the sack. Likewise, unless inefficiencies are identified and eliminated, resources will keep on leaking out of the healthcare system and thus reducing the extent to which health systems are able to achieve goals of health status improvement, responsiveness to client's rational expectations, and fairness in healthcare financing [8]. Inefficiency signifies denying additional citizens the opportunities to realise health improvements at zero extra cost. This is what makes inefficiency both immoral and unethical. The objectives of this study were (*a*) to measure individual hospital's technical and scale efficiency with a view to identifying the inefficient ones and the magnitudes of input reductions needed to make them efficient and (*b*) to make the policy implications of the results explicit for policy makers and hospital managers.

DATA

Input data for individual hospitals were obtained from the published recurrent expenditure estimates [6]. Output data were obtained from the Health Information System [9] office of the Ministry of Health (MoH). Hospitals were assumed to use mainly eleven inputs as follows: medical officers/ pharmacists/dentists, clinical officers, nurses (including enrolled, registered, and community nurses), administrative staff, technicians / technologists, other staff, subordinate staff, pharmaceuticals, non-pharmaceutical supplies, maintenance of equipment, vehicles, and buildings, and food and rations.

The way the Health Information System data are summarised suggests that hospitals produce eight distinct intermediate outputs from the inputs as follows: outpatient department casualty visits, special clinic visits, MCH/FP visits, dental care visits, general medical admissions, paediatric admissions, maternity admissions, and amenity ward admissions. Input and output data were available for 54 district level hospitals. These constituted 55% of all district level public hospitals.

DEA CONCEPTUAL FRAMEWORK

Charness, Cooper, and Rhodes [10] suggested a comprehensive index that incorporates multiple output and input variables to measure technical efficiency (TE) of a decision-making unit (DMU) relative to a group of DMUs. The index is in the form of an output-to-input ratio with a "virtual" input (output) representing the weighted sum of all inputs (outputs) [11]. It is computed by solving two fractional programming models under the assumption of constant returns to scale (CRS in Model 1) and variable returns to scale (VRS in Model 2) as shown in Figure 6.1.

Model 1	DEA weights model, input-oriented, CRS	Model 2	DEA weights model, input-oriented, VRS

$$\text{Eff} = \underset{u_r, v_i}{\text{Max}} \sum_r u_r y_{rj_0}$$

s.t.

$$\sum_r u_r y_{rj} - \sum_i v_i x_{ij} \leq 0; \forall j$$

$$\sum_i v_i x_{ij_0} = 1$$

$$u_r, v_i \geq 0; \forall r, \forall i.$$

$$\text{Eff} = \underset{u_r, v_i}{\text{Max}} \sum_r u_r y_{rj_0} + u_0$$

s.t.

$$\sum_r u_r y_{rj} - \sum_i v_i x_{ij} + u_0 \leq 0 \quad ; \forall j$$

$$\sum_i v_i x_{ij_0} = 1$$

$$u_r, v_i \geq 0 \quad ; \forall r, \forall i.$$

Figure 6.1   DEA models

Where:

y_{rj} = the amount of output r produced by hospital j,

x_{ij} = the amount of input i used by hospital j,

u_r = the weight given to output r, ($r = 1,...,t$ and t is the number of outputs)

v_i = the weight given to input i, ($I = 1, ..., m$ and m is the number of inputs)

n = the number of hospitals,

j_0 = the hospital under assessment

From Model 2 it is possible to derive scale efficiency, that is, whether a hospital is operating on an optimal scale of production or not. Note that [12] scale efficiency score = CRS TE score ÷ VRS TE score.

RESULTS AND DISCUSSION

Table 6.1 presents means and standard deviations for input and output variables of 54 district hospitals.

Table 6.1   Means and standard deviations for public hospitals inputs and outputs

Category of variable	Mean	Standard deviation
Doctors/pharmacists/dentists	4	5
Clinical officers	9	7
Nurses	99	64
Administrative staff	26	25
Technicians & technologists	33	31
Other technical staff	17	17
Subordinate staff	55	51
Drugs (in Ksh)	196,218	74,479
Non-pharmaceutical supplies (in Ksh)	5,664	6,531
Maintenance (in Ksh)	9,752	9,948
Food rations (in Ksh)	100,536	88,760
Beds	183	164
OPD casual visits	35,419	23,244
Special care visits	5,829	8,545
MCH-FP visits	20,935	12,865
Dental care visits	1,108	2,062
Inpatient Department General Admissions	3,839	11,644
Paediatrics Ward Admissions	1,376	1,716
Maternity Ward Admissions	1,391	1,502

Technical and scale efficiency scores for individual hospitals can be found in Table 6.2. It is important to recall that efficiency scores range from 0 (totally inefficient) to 1 (100% TE). Out of 54 district hospitals included in the analysis, 40 (74%) were technically efficient, whilst the remaining 14 (26%) were technically inefficient. Among the inefficient hospitals, 2 (14%) had a TE score of 51-60%, 2 (14%) scored 61-70%, 2 (14%) scored 71-80%, 2 (14%) scored 81-90%, and 6 (43%) scored 91-99%. The inefficient hospitals had an average TE score of 84% and a standard deviation of 15.5%. This implies that, on average, these hospitals could reduce their utilisation of all inputs by about 16% without reducing output.

On the other hand, out of the 54 hospitals analysed, 1 (1.9%) had a scale efficiency score of 61-70%, 2 (3.7%) scored 71-80%, 3 (5.6%) scored 81-90%, 10 (20.4%) scored 91-99%, and 38 (70.5%) scored about 100%. Sixteen (29.6%) of the hospitals were scale inefficient; meaning their scale efficiency score was less than unity. The average scale efficiency score in the whole sample was 90% (with a standard deviation of 9.7) implying that there is room to increase total output by about 10%. Data envelopment analysis has demonstrated that 26% of the hospitals are run inefficiently and need to either reduce their inputs or increase their outputs in order to become efficient. Total input reductions and/or output increases needed to make inefficient public hospitals efficient are presented in Table 6.3.

Table 6.2   Technical and scale efficiency scores for public hospitals

DMU (Hospitals)	Technical efficiency	Scale efficiency	DMU (Hospitals)	Technical efficiency	Scale efficiency
Gatundu	100	100	Nanyuki	100	100
Tambach	100	100	Chuka	100	100
Nandi Hills	100	100	Bungoma	100	100
Ngao	100	78	Mt. Elgon	100	100
Tigoni	100	100	Gilgil Mental	100	100
Kapkatet	100	100	Busia	100	100
Karatina	100	100	Homa Bay	100	98
Makueni	100	100	Nyahururu	100	100
Ishiara	100	100	Maralal	100	100
Port Reitz	100	100	Kisii Central	100	100
Kathiani	100	100	Moyale	100	100
Miathene	100	100	Muranga	100	100
Kangundo	100	100	Kapsabet	100	93
Bondo	100	100	Narok	99	97
Makindu	100	100	Musambweni	97	100
Naivasha	100	100	Moi (Voi)	97	95
Molo	100	100	Kinango	97	86
Webuye	100	100	Mandera	95	96
Transmara	100	100	Ol Kalou	94	97
Elburgon	100	100	Kwale	89	91
Kilifi	100	100	Iten	86	87
Malindi	100	100	Taveta	80	97
Marsabit	100	100	Loitokitok	77	97
Meru	100	100	Lodwar	70	92
Mathare	100	100	Old Nyanza	69	76
Mbagathi	100	100	Hola	58	85
Thika	100	100	Lamu	54	64

The presence of inefficiencies indicates that a hospital has excess inputs or insufficient outputs compared to those hospitals on the efficient frontier. With regard to hospitals with excess inputs, the MoH policy makers could:

1.   Transfer excess doctors, clinical officers, nurses, technicians/technologists and other technical staff to health centres and dispensaries. This would strengthen these primary healthcare (PHC) facilities remarkably. Given the enormity of resources invested in the production of these cadres of staff, it would not be prudent to offer them early retirement options.

2.   Use the excess expenditure on pharmaceuticals, non-pharmaceutical supplies, maintenance, and food to improve technical and perceived quality of services in PHC facilities.

3.   Send the excess administrative and subordinate staff on early retirement. The saving could be used to improve remuneration for the remaining staff.

Alternatively, the MoH could embark on a campaign to boost demand for underutilised essential curative, promotive, and preventive services such as MCH/FP, sexually transmitted diseases care, and voluntary testing and counseling for HIV/AIDS among others. Such campaigns should be preceded by demand analyses to facilitate identification of variables amenable to policy instruments. Table 6.4 provides the magnitudes by which specific inputs per inefficient hospital ought to be reduced. Armed with this information, the policy makers and healthcare managers could proactively improve efficiency in delivery of health services.

Table 6.3 *Total input reductions and/or output increases needed to make inefficient public hospitals efficient*

Variable	Value
Inputs	
Doctors/pharmacists/dentists	26
Clinical officers	55
Nurses	741
Administrative staff	168
Technicians and technologists	402
Other technical staff	134
Subordinate staff	319
Drugs (in Ksh)	68,1148
Non-pharmaceutical supplies (in Ksh)	21,084
Maintenance (in Ksh)	53,368
Food and rations (in Ksh)	501,987
Beds	530
Outputs	
OPD casual visits	122,495
Special care visits	9,347
MCH-FP visits	38,609
Dental care visits	4,423
Inpatient Department general admissions	66,117
Paediatrics Ward admissions	2,999
Maternity Ward admissions	974

Table 6.4   Input reductions and/or output increases needed to make individual inefficient public hospitals efficient

Hospitals

	Narok	Musambweni	Moi Voi	Kinango	Mandera	Ol Kalou	Kwale	Iten	Taveta	Loitokitok	Lodwar	Old Nyanza	Hola	Lamu
Inputs														
Doctors/pharmacists/dentists	1	2	0	0	2	0	0	1	1	4	2	6	4	3
Clinical officers	4	2	4	0	8	0	0	1	1	5	10	6	7	7
Nurses	10	19	137	30	126	89	4	18	56	12	78	70	51	41
Administrative staff	11	0	0	3	25	11	11	10	15	11	23	17	13	18
Technicians and technologists	29	30	29	1	12	8	17	51	71	17	54	25	35	23
Other technical staff	9	0	10	2	23	1	6	4	26	10	8	14	11	10
Subordinate staff	6	33	12	12	34	35	10	5	23	27	39	26	28	29
Drugs (in Ksh)	2,657	12,584	52,283	53,672	18,228	49,561	54,629	42,823	67,571	52,625	56,612	55,577	74,143	88,183
Non-pharmaceutical supplies (in Ksh)	24	108	297	3,997	2,859	1,169	1,155	511	623	703	2,297	1,513	2,675	3,153
Maintenance (in Ksh)	2,125	3614	12,803	4,025	234	391	2,382	583	7,279	1,390	1,553	2,471	5,350	9,168
Food and rations (in Ksh)	405	16,263	50,484	1,762	60,093	4,134	5,263	45,777	12,959	16,584	155,407	44,820	59,321	28,715
Beds	4	3	3	4	33	30	6	57	72	65	65	57	82	49
Outputs														
OPD casual visits	26,730	0	11,405	13,106	0	21,073	0	0	0	0	32,302	9,402	7,181	1,296
Special care visits	0	432	0	668	3,073	0	3,75	1,347	824	1,162	0	0	1,466	0
MCH-FP visits	0	919	2,660	10,21	14,049	0	2,091	5,051	644	0	0	7,248	0	4,926
Dental care visits	0	0	0	575	679	166	230	0	372	0	0	1,440	758	203
Inpatient department general admissions	29,288	10,162	0	704	306	427	525	7,440	3,268	13,667	330	0	0	0
Paediatrics ward admissions	1,359	0	0	257	157	130	0	954	0	124	18	0	0	0
Maternity ward admissions	321	0	0	454	211	0	337	0	93	0	596	680	235	47

CONCLUSIONS

A few studies have attempted to analyse TE of health facilities in SSA using DEA methodology. Recently two studies [7,13] on South African public hospitals and clinics identified substantive input reductions needed to improve their efficiency. The study reported in this paper is the first attempt in Kenya to estimate TE of hospitals using DEA methodology. Seventy-four per cent of the hospitals had a TE rating of 100% implying that they are operating relatively efficiently compared to their peers. These hospitals are using less input to produce more output compared to their inefficient peers. On average, inefficient hospitals utilised larger numbers of inputs. Even with their excess inputs, however, inefficient hospitals produced less output than their relatively efficient counterparts.

In conclusion, the study has demonstrated that DEA not only helps health policy makers and managers to answer the question: "How well are the public hospitals performing?" but also "By how much could their performance be improved?" We recommend (a) further analyses of the best-performing hospitals and their operating practices with a view to establishing a guide to "best practice" for others to emulate; (b) replication among PHC facilities; (c) similar analyses (using routinely collected data) throughout SSA; (d) strengthening of SSA Ministries of Health personnel capacity for undertaking efficiency analyses; and (e) cultivation of a culture of evidence-based decision-making.

REFERENCES

1. Mooney GH. *Economics, medicine and health care.* New York: Harvester Wheatsheaf; 1986.

2. Mills A. The economics of hospitals in developing countries: part I:expenditure patterns. *Health Policy and Planning* 1990;5(2):107-117.

3. Mills A. The economics of hospitals in developing countries: part II: costs and sources of income. *Health Policy and Planning* 1990;5(3):203-218.

4. Mills A, Kapalamula J, Chisimbi S. The cost of the district hospital: a case study in Malawi. *Bulletin of the World Health Organization* 1993;71(3-4):329-339.

5. Kirigia JM, Fox-Rushby J, Mills A. A cost analysis of Kilifi and Malindi public hospitals in Kenya. *African Journal of Health Sciences* 1998; 5(2):79-84.

6. Kenya Government. *Recurrent expenditures.* Nairobi: Kenya Government; 1998.

7. Kirigia JM, Sambo LG, Lambo E. Are public hospitals in Kwazulu-Natal Province of South Africa technically efficient? *African Journal of Health Sciences* 2000;7(3-4):25-32.

8. World Health Organization. *The world health report 2000 - health systems: improving performance.* Geneva: World Health Organization; 2000.

9. Kenya Government Ministry of Health. *Health information system: hospital statistics.* Nairobi: Kenya Government; 2000.

10. Charnes A, Cooper WW, Rhodes E. Measuring the efficiency of decision making units. *European Journal of Operational Research* 1978;2(6):429-444.

11. Banks DA. Cost and access among non-profit hospitals in jurisdictions with and without public hospitals. *Applied Economics* 1996;28(7):875-881.

12. Coelli T: *A guide to DEAP version 2.1: a data envelopment analysis [computer] program,* Centre for Efficiency and Productivity Analysis (CEPA) Working Paper 96/08, Department of Econometrics, University of New England; Armidale, NSW Australia; 1996.

13. Kirigia JM, Sambo LG, Scheel H. Technical efficiency of public clinics in Kwazulu-Natal Province of South Africa. *East African Medical Journal* 2001;78(3 Suppl):S1-S13.

-7-

Using Data Envelopment Analysis to Measure the Technical Efficiency of Public Health Centres in Kenya*

Joses M. Kirigia, Ali Emrouznejad,
Luis G. Sambo, Nzoya Munguti and William Liambila

ABSTRACT

Data envelopment analysis has been widely used to analyse the efficiency of the health sector in developed countries since 1978 while in Africa only a few studies have attempted to apply DEA in the health organisations. In this paper, we measure technical efficiency of public health centres in Kenya. Our finding suggests that 44% of public health centres are inefficient. Therefore, the objectives of this study are to determine the degree of technical efficiency of individual primary healthcare facilities in Kenya; to recommend the performance targets for inefficient facilities; to estimate the magnitudes of excess inputs; and to recommend what should be done with those excess inputs. The authors believe that these kinds of studies should be undertaken in other countries in the World Health Organization (WHO) African Region with a view to empowering Ministries of Health to play their stewardship role more effectively.

INTRODUCTION

The Kenyan government, over time, has undertaken six types of reforms to eliminate inefficiencies and inequities, namely, harmonisation and decentralisation of healthcare delivery system; expansion of preventive health services including family planning services; introduction of medical insurance scheme for certain categories of employees; selective integration of traditional medicine with modern medicine; and introduction of user-charges in

---

* The original article appeared in *Journal of Medical Systems 2004;28(2):155-166.* Reproduced with the permission of Plenum Publishing Corporation.

government health facilities [1]. There is evidence that the introduction of user fees led to significant reduction in inpatient and outpatient services utilisation at public hospitals and health centres [2,3]. A recent study found that 30% of the public district level hospitals in Kenya were technically inefficient [4]. Given lack of baseline study on the technical efficiency of individual health facilities prior to the introduction of reforms, it is difficult to tell whether there was an improvement in their performance.

This study was motivated by several considerations. First, a substantial proportion of the recurrent budget of the Ministry of Health (MoH) is spent on rural health services (RHS), and thus, it is vital to ensure maximum returns. For example, the net expenditure estimate of the MoH for the financial year 1999/2000 amounted to Kenya shillings (Ksh) 9,265,023,800 [5]. Rural health services accounted for 14.5% (Ksh 1,338,311,880) of that total expenditure. Rural health services consist of health centres and dispensaries (which absorbed Ksh.1,199,699,220); and rural health training and demonstration centres (which absorbed Ksh 138,611,880) [6].

Second, RHS are labour intensive, and thus, it is important to ensure that human resources for health are used efficiently. For instance, 54.3% of the total RHS expenditure in the financial year 1999/2000 was spent on human resources. It consisted of personal emoluments, house allowances, other personal allowances, medical allowances, and leave expenses. Thus, it is important to know how efficiently human resources are being used to optimise RHS contributions to improving the health status of communities, responsiveness to communities' rational expectations, and fairness in financing of care [7]; the trio being the goals of health systems.

Third, efficiency concerns cut across all functions of health systems. Those functions include delivery of personal and non-personal health services; healthcare financing, that is, collecting/raising, pooling, and allocating the revenues to purchase those services; investing in people, buildings, and equipment; and acting as the overall stewards of the resources, powers, and expectations entrusted to them [7]. Availability of information on efficiency of individual health centres would serve to empower the MoH to play its stewardship role more effectively.

Fourth, about 80% of the Kenyan population lives in rural areas. Health needs (preventive, promotive, and curative) of the majority of those people are met by the health centres and dispensaries. Those two levels of health facilities, due to their relatively close proximity to those with unmet healthcare needs, are a critical aspect of both district health services and primary health care. In 1989, there were 2,393 health facilities in Kenya and 1571 of them were government health facilities [8]. Constituting 88.4% of the latter were health centres and dispensaries. Thus, their sheer numbers merit close performance scrutiny to ensure that healthcare delivery is maximised.

Fifth, to date no study in Kenya has attempted to estimate either technical or allocative efficiency of individual health centres. Thus, there was need for such a study to bridge that knowledge/information gap. Sixth, this pioneering application of the data envelopment analysis (DEA) methodology would hopefully motivate health system researchers to replicate the methodology among non-governmental organisations (NGOs) hospitals, health centres, and dispensaries. Such information, used in tandem with the available technical efficiency information on public health facilities, would obviously inform public-private mix debate, and hence guide the MoH in identifying the NGO health facilities that should be subcontracted to provide care efficiently. Indeed, this health sector application may stimulate the application of DEA into other sectors (e.g., education, agriculture, industry, commerce, etc.) in the African Region.

Seventh, the information generated by the current study could constitute good baseline data against which to evaluate the impact of various health sector reforms on health centres' technical efficiency over time. This study identifies the health facilities with "best practice". In future, more detailed studies could examine and document their operating practices to establish a guide to "best practice" for inefficient health centres to emulate.

Eighth, the market for health care in Kenya, like most of the other developing countries, has failed (for various reasons) and it cannot be relied upon to ensure efficient allocation of scarce healthcare resources. Instead, in the case of public health facilities, the government will have to intervene to ensure efficiency in the use of resources. On the other hand, in the non-governmental sector, the management of NGO facilities will have to implement interventions that would ensure efficient use of NGO resources. Thus, both the Government and NGOs require information on the extent of technical efficiency in individual health facilities and inputs and what can be done to optimise their efficiency.

Ninth, this study not only identifies the technical performance of each health centre in the sample, but also the magnitudes of inefficiencies in the use of each input among the inefficient health facilities. Such information would be useful to the policy makers and district health services managers in their effort of designing appropriate policy and managerial interventions for ensuring efficient use of healthcare-producing resources.

Finally, given that the technical efficiency of public hospitals has already been undertaken [4], the researchers found it is necessary to replicate the study among health centres. It is expected that evidence from the current study would guide interventions geared at reallocating excess resources from inefficient hospitals to health centres. This would obviate allocation of more resources to health centres that are already inefficient.

MATERIALS AND METHODS

Data

The total number of public health centres in Kenya is approximately 350 [8]. The current study was carried out in a selection of 32 health centres, that is, 9.1% of the public health centres. Two of the authors visited each of the health facilities in the sample and reviewed their input and output records. Inputs are resources used by health centres to produce outputs (i.e., products or services). Health centres were assumed to utilise the eleven inputs of clinical officers, nurses, physiotherapists, occupational therapists, laboratory technologists, laboratory technicians, administrative and general staff, dental technologists, public health officers, beds, and non-wage recurrent expenditures. The latter is a composite of expenditures on utilities (postal and telegrams, telephone, electricity, water and conservancy, and fuel/gas expenses); drugs; oxygen; dressings and non-pharmaceutical items; patients' food; consumable stores; staff uniforms and clothing; stationery; printing of medical records; non-residential rents and rates; plant and equipment; maintenance of plant, machinery and equipment; and maintenance of buildings and stations.

The records kept at health centres suggest that they produce ten intermediate outputs including diarrhoeal visits, malaria visits, sexually transmitted infections (STI) visits, urinary tract infection visits, intestinal worm visits, antenatal care visits, immunisation visits, family planning visits, and other general outpatient visits.

DEA ANALYTICAL FRAMEWORK

This study chose to use DEA [9] instead of regression methods to estimate technical and scale efficiency for the following reasons: DEA can handle multiple input and multiple output models; it does not require an assumption of a functional form relating inputs to outputs; decision-making units (health centres) are directly compared against a peer or combination of peers; and inputs and outputs can have very different units of measurement [10].

The DEA has been used a lot in developed countries, and to a lesser extent in a few developing countries to analyse efficiency of health facilities. Ersoy et al [11] estimated technical efficiencies of Turkish hospitals using the DEA approach. Parkin and Hollingsworth [12] and Hollingsworth and Parkin [13] used DEA to measure production efficiency of acute hospitals in Scotland. Thanassoulis *et al.* [14] explored output quality targets in the provision of perinatal care in England using DEA. Kooreman [15] used DEA to analyse efficiency of nursing-home care in the Netherlands. Majumdar [16] used DEA to assess efficiency capabilities of firms within the Indian pharmaceutical industry. Ozcan and Bannick [17] utilised DEA to evaluate the trends in department-of-defense hospital efficiency. Ozcan *et al.* [18] assessed efficiency of psychiatric hospitals through DEA. Huang [19] applied DEA in measuring the relative performance of Florida general hospitals. Huang [20] used DEA to evaluate the efficiency of rural primary care programmes in North Carolina, USA.

In Africa, only a few studies have attempted to apply DEA in the health sector. Kirigia *et al.* [21] used DEA to investigate the technical efficiencies among 155 primary healthcare clinics in Kwazulu-Natal Province of South Africa. Kirigia *et al.* [4] measured relative technical efficiencies of 54 district level public hospitals in Kenya. Eyob [22] examined the technical efficiency of 86 public sector hospitals in Eastern, Northern and Western Cape Provinces of South Africa. Kirigia, Sambo and Lambo [23] employed DEA to find out what portion of 55 public hospitals of Kwazulu/Natal Province of South Africa were operating efficiently and for those inefficient hospitals what inputs and outputs contribute most to inefficiency.

According to Emrouznejad [24], DEA is a novel approach to relative efficiency measurement where there are multiple inputs and outputs that are incommensurate. In that kind of scenario, efficiency is equal to the weighted sum of outputs divided by the weighted sum of inputs. Algebraically, Bousssofiane *et al.* [25] expresses the DEA model as a fractional linear program of the following form:

$$TE_0 = Max \frac{\sum_r U_r y_{rj_0}}{\sum_i V_i x_{ij_0}}$$

s.t.

$$\frac{\sum_r U_r y_{rj}}{\sum_i V_i x_{ij}} \leq 1 \; ; \forall j$$

$$U_r \, , V_i \; \geq \varepsilon \; ; \forall r, \forall i$$

Figure 7.1   DEA ratio model

where: TE_0 is the technical efficiency score for decision-making unit j_0; U_r = the weight given to output r, ($r = 1,...,t$ and t is the number of outputs); V_i = the weight given to input i, ($I = 1,...,m$ and m is the number of inputs); n = the number of health centres; t = the number of outputs; m = the number of inputs;

ε = a small positive number; Y_{rj} = amount of output r produced by health centre j; x_{ij} = amount of input i used by health centres j; and j_0 = the health centres under assessment. To ensure analytic tractability to linear programming methods this model can be converted into the following linear programme:

CRS model	VRS model
Min ϕ	Min ϕ
s.t.	s.t.
$\sum_j \lambda_j x_{ij} + S_i^+ = \phi x_{ij_0} \quad \forall i$	$\sum_j \lambda_j x_{ij} + S_i^+ = \phi x_{ij_0} \quad \forall i$
$\sum_j \lambda_j y_{rj} - S_r^- = y_{rj_0} \quad \forall r$	$\sum_j \lambda_j y_{rj} - S_r^- = y_{rj_0} \quad \forall r$
	$\sum_j \lambda_j = 1$
$S_i^+, S_r^- \geq 0 \quad \forall i, \forall r$	
	$S_i^+, S_r^- \geq 0 \quad \forall i, \forall r$
$\lambda_j \geq 0 \quad \forall j.$	$\lambda_j \geq 0 \quad \forall j.$

Figure 7.2   Input-oriented DEA model

where λ_j are dual variables, that is, the shadow prices related to the constraints limiting the efficiency of each DMU to be no greater than 1. Where a constraint is binding, a shadow price will be normally positive and when the constraint is non-binding the shadow price will be zero. In the solution to the primal model, therefore, a binding constraint implies that the corresponding DMU has an efficiency of 1 and there will be a positive shadow price or dual variable. Hence, positive shadow prices in the primal or positive values for the λ_j in the dual correspond to and identify the peer group for any inefficient unit. S_r and S_i are slack variables; if DMU j_0 is efficient, the slacks will be equal to 0 and the efficiency measure Z_0 will be equal to 1. Otherwise, if j_0 is inefficient Z_0 will be less than 1 and some slacks may be positive. Scale efficiency is equal to constant returns to scale technical score divided by variable returns to scale technical score [10]. The data analysis procedure is similar to that explained in Kirigia *et al.* [21].

RESULTS

A further statistical analysis has been taken into consideration. The correlation study has revealed that some inputs/outputs can be redundant or be grouped together in association with using DEA. Therefore, the inputs and outputs selected for DEA analysis are presented in Table 7.1 which contains the means and standard deviations for input and output variables of the 32 health centres.

Table 7.1   Means and standard deviations for efficient and inefficient health centres

	Inefficient Health Centres		Efficient Health Centres	
	Mean	Stdev	Mean	Stdev
Inputs*				
Input 1	5.6	4.2	7.2	4.2
Input 2	0.5	0.6	0.5	0.5
Input 3	0.8	0.7	1.4	1.0
Input 4	3.9	2.1	5.0	1.6
Input 5	462,146.1	294,060.9	615,688.3	301,191.9
Input 6	5.3	3.6	13.6	10.1
Outputs**				
Output 1	14,806.2	9,506.8	5,665.7	2,767.8
Output 2	5,176.6	4,885.1	2,462.8	1,350.4
Output 3	8,909.5	8,324.7	3,931.2	2,078.4
Output 4	5,757.7	5,060.0	1,866.6	991.2

* Inputs

Input 1:   Clinical officers + nurses
Input 2:   Physiotherapist + occupational therapist + public health officer + dental technologist
Input 3:   Laboratory technician + Laboratory technologist
Input 4:   Administrative staff
Input 5:   Non-wage expenditures
Input 6:   Number of beds

** Outputs

Output 1:   Diarrhoeal + malaria + STI + urinary tract infections + intestinal worms + respiratory disease visits
Output 2:   Antenatal + family planning visits
Output 3:   Immunisations
Output 4:   Other general outpatient visits

Technical and scale efficiency scores for individual health centres can be found in Table 7.2. It is vital to remember that efficiency scores range from 0 (totally inefficient) to 1 (100% TE). Out of the 32 health centres included in the analysis, 14 (44%) were technically efficient whereas the remaining 18 (56%) were technically inefficient. Among the inefficient health centres, 2 (13%) had TE score of less than 50%, 9 centres (28%) scored between 51-74%, and 6 centres (19%) scored 75-99%. The inefficient health centres had an average TE score of 65% and a standard deviation of 22%. This implies that on average they could reduce their utilisation of all inputs by about 35% without reducing output.

Table 7.2   Technical and scale efficiency scores for health centres

Health Centre	Technical Efficiency Score	Scale Efficiency	Health Centre	Technical Efficiency Score	Scale Efficiency
Athi-River	1.00	1.00	Mitaboni	0.74	0.97
Bissel	0.96	0.96	Mpinzinyi	0.78	1.00
Enkorika	1.00	1.00	Muthetheni	0.88	0.88
Githunguri	0.26	0.59	Mwala	0.53	0.88
Isinya	1.00	1.00	Mwatate	0.61	0.61
Karuri	0.56	0.78	Namanga	1.00	1.00
Kasigau	0.64	0.64	Ndeiya	0.89	0.91
Kaviani	1.00	1.00	Ngewa	0.88	0.99
Kigumo	0.61	0.92	Ngong	1.00	1.00
Kihara	0.60	0.68	Nyanche	1.00	1.00
Kitengela	0.94	0.94	O-Rongai	1.00	1.00
Lari	1.00	1.00	Sagala	1.00	1.00
Limuru	1.00	1.00	Simba	1.00	1.00
Lusigeti	0.39	0.80	Thinu	1.00	1.00
Masii	0.74	0.81	Wangige	0.23	0.49
Mbale	0.46	0.96	Wundanyi	1.00	1.00

On the other hand, out of the 32 health centres analysed 19 (59%) were scale efficient whilst the remaining 13 (41%) were scale inefficient. Out of the inefficient health centres, 4 (13%) had a scale efficiency score less than 50%, 3 (9%) scored 51-75%, and 6 (19%) scored 76-99%. The average scale efficiency score among the inefficient health centres was 70% (with a standard deviation of 19%); implying there is potential for increasing total outputs by about 30% using the existing capacity/size.

DISCUSSION

Data envelopment analysis has demonstrated that 44% of health centres in the sample are operated inefficiently and need to either reduce their inputs or increase their outputs in order to become efficient. Total input reductions and/or output increases needed to make inefficient public health centres efficient are presented in Table 7.3.

Table 7.3   Input reductions and/or output increases needed to make individual inefficient health centres efficient

Inefficient health centre	Inputs[a]						Outputs[b]			
	Input 1	Input 2	Input 3	Input 4	Input 5	Input 6	Output 1	Output 2	Output 3	Output 4
Mpinzinyi	3.8	0.8	1.5	6.1	510,985	3.8	22,129	7,136	20,425	6,351
Nyanche	2.2	0.0	0.0	1.5	493,763	10.4	21,319	1,698	9,770	5,896
Kasigau	1.2	0.0	0.0	0.6	160,068	4.3	2,017	313	420	956
Muthetheni	6.4	1.1	1.1	3.8	537,643	1.1	12,221	2,811	8,108	6,219
Wangige	4.7	1.4	1.9	5.2	285,846	11.3	2,980	488	870	1,080
Isinya	11.8	1.3	1.7	5.2	249,697	3.5	7,617	9,246	12,423	2,167
Mitaboni	1.6	0.0	0.4	2.0	222,258	4.8	3,460	1,315	3,474	543
Simba	2.0	0.0	0.0	2.0	169,861	1.2	3,754	2,416	5,783	835
Enkorika	5.1	0.8	0.8	3.9	625,283	4.3	11,594	4,321	4,882	7,093
Ngong	4.0	0.4	0.4	2.9	212,463	2.2	8,681	1,258	1,339	3,217
Mbale	4.4	0.5	0.5	2.3	444,930	2.6	4,104	1,309	266	1,727
Sagala	3.3	0.0	0.3	1.8	247,081	1.5	5,886	1,600	2,145	3,644
Wundanyi	2.6	0.2	0.2	1.3	149,188	3.7	3,985	1,045	1,481	1,373
O-Rongai	1.0	0.0	0.0	0.6	87,343	0.9	882	413	429	580
Masii	0.8	0.1	0.2	0.6	71,552	0.6	978	610	788	225
Kitengela	0.3	0.0	0.0	0.5	36,009	1.1	494	102	129	98
Athi-River	0.2	0.0	0.0	0.3	29,115	0.2	388	182	384	65
Namanga	0.1	0.0	0.0	0.0	17,214	0.1	135	43	31	20
Total	55.5	6.6	9.0	40.6	4,550,296	57.3	112,624	36,307	73,149	42,090

[a] For definition of inputs see the note on Table 7.1

[b] For definition of outputs see the note on Table 7.1

The presence of inefficiencies indicates that a health centre has excess inputs or insufficient outputs compared to those health centres on the efficient frontier. Table 7.3 also provides the magnitudes by which specific inputs per inefficient health centre ought to be reduced. Equipped with this information, the policy makers and healthcare managers could proactively improve the efficiency in primary healthcare delivery. Concerning health centres with excess inputs, the MoH policy makers should:

1. Transfer excess clinic officers, nurses, laboratory technologists, laboratory technicians, and public health officers to more efficient health centres and dispensaries. That would further enhance the capacity of primary health care sub-sector to respond to people's legitimate expectations.

2. Send excess administrative and general support staff on early retirement. The savings should be used to improve remuneration for the remaining staff.

3. Consider the following options with regard to excess beds: (*a*) transfer them to efficient health centres; (*b*) sell them; or (*c*) enter into a contract with private clinic practitioners to use them at a price, which should not be less than the marginal costs.

4. Use excess non-wage expenditure to (*a*) improve the degree of responsiveness of dispensaries (i.e., lower-level primary healthcare facilities) to patients' legitimate expectations; (*b*) improve quality of services among efficient health centres; and (*c*) support communities to start or sustain systematic risk and resource pooling and cost-sharing mechanisms for protecting beneficiaries against unexpected healthcare costs. The funds could be used to boost the capacity of the existing community-based health insurance schemes. According to Carrin *et al.* [26], the government has four basic functions for enhancing the capacity of Non-Profit Health Insurance Schemes (NPHIS): that of promoter of health insurance, monitor of NPHIS activities, trainer in all dimensions of insurance, and co-financier.

Alternatively, the MoH policy makers could be more proactive in encouraging demand for (*a*) treatment for diarrhoea, malaria, sexually transmitted diseases, urinary tract infections, intestinal worms infestation, and respiratory diseases; and (*b*) consumption of preventive services, including antenatal care, immunisations, and family planning services. Utilisation promotion activities should be guided by demand analyses to facilitate identification of variables amenable to policy instruments. Mwabu *et al.* [27], Jones and Kirigia [28], Kirigia and Muthuri [29], Jones and Kirigia [30], Kirigia and Kainyu [31], and Kirigia *et al.* [4] are a few examples of demand studies geared at modelling consumer health-related choice behaviour in Africa.

SUGGESTIONS FOR FUTURE RESEARCH

1. There is need for undertaking technical (TE) and allocative efficiency (AE) studies among the remaining 318 public health centres, 1,038 dispensaries and 45 health clinics. Allocative efficiency will entail collection of data on prices of various inputs in addition to the data required for TE [8].

2. Approximately 822 (34%) of the total number of health facilities in Kenya are owned by non-governmental organisations (both for-profit and non-profit). These facilities serve a substantial proportion of the Kenya population. The role of the private sector in financing and provision of health care is expected to grow. Given the prominent role of the NGO sector in provision of health care, it will be necessary to undertake TE and AE studies among the 83 non-governmental hospitals, 17 maternity hospitals, 31 nursing homes, 94 health centres, 575 dispensaries and 22 health clinics [8].

3. Future efficiency studies ought to incorporate various environmental factors such as existence of District Health Management Teams (DHMTs), District Health Management Boards (DHMBs), accessibility of each health centre, degree of health-related quality of life, and job satisfaction among human resources in each health centre et cetera.

4. Detailed studies among relatively efficient peer health centres would facilitate identification and dissemination of good operating practices that can lead to improved efficiency not only for relatively inefficient health centres but also for relatively efficient ones.

5. It is vital to undertake health facility efficiency analyses in other countries of the WHO African Region that have not yet undertaken such studies.

CONCLUSION

This study found that 44% of the health centres in the Kenyan sample are technically inefficient. Kirigia *et al.* [4] discovered that 26% of the Kenyan public district hospitals were technically inefficient. Kirigia et al. [21] found 70% of the public health clinics in Kwazulu-Natal Province of South Africa to be technically inefficient. Kirigia et al. [23] unravelled technical inefficiencies in 40% of the public hospitals in Kwazulu-Natal Province of South Africa.

This study has demonstrated that DEA is an essential tool for identifying the most and least efficient health centres and strategies for saving resources/inputs and/or increasing outputs. We concur with Boussifiane *et al.* [25] that DEA can be used in identifying efficient operating practices and efficient strategies, setting targets/benchmarks for relatively inefficient health centres, monitoring effects of health sector reforms on efficiency over time, and resource allocation. There is need to conduct DEA studies in all health facilities across the WHO African Region so as to empower Ministries of Health to adequately perform their stewardship role.

In conclusion, we agree with Mansfield [32, p. 181] that "while the secrets of efficient production are not as complex (or secret) as one might think, the price of efficiency, like that of liberty, is eternal vigilance". Thus, we cannot overemphasise the importance of continued use of DEA (or other approaches) to vigilantly monitor efficiency of all healthcare facilities and programmes in the resource-constrained health sectors of the WHO African Region countries.

ACKNOWLEDGEMENTS

We are grateful to the staff of the 32 health centres for their assistance during the data collection exercise. The data collection exercise was funded by WHO/AFRO. We are indebted to Jehovah Shalom for His multi-faceted support. The views and opinions expressed here are the authors' and should *not* be attributed to either the Ministry of Health of the Republic of Kenya, WHO, or any of the acknowledged.

REFERENCES

1. Mwabu GM. Health care reform in Kenya: a review of the process. *Health Policy* 1995;32:245-255.

2. Mwabu GM, Mwanzia J, Liambila W. User charges in government health facilities in Kenya: effect on attendance and revenue. *Health Policy and Planning* 1995;10(2):164-170.

3. Mwabu GM, Wang'ombe JK. Health service pricing reforms in Kenya. *International Journal of Social Economics* 1997;24(1-3):282-293.

4. Kirigia JM, Emrouznejad A, Sambo LG: Measurement of technical efficiency of public hospitals in Kenya: using data envelopment analysis. *Journal of Medical Systems* 2001;26(1):39-45.

5. Kenya Government Ministry of Health. *Summary of health facilities data.* Nairobi: Kenya Government; 1999.

6. Kenya Government. 1990/2000 estimates of recurrent expenditure of the Government of Kenya for the year ending 30th June, 2000. Nairobi: Kenya Government; 2000.

7. World Health Organization. The World Health Organization 2000: health systems - improving performance. Geneva: World Health Organization; 2000.

8. Kenya Government Ministry of Health: *Summary of health facilities data.* Nairobi: Kenya Government;1989.

9. Charnes A, Cooper WW, Rhodes E. Measuring the efficiency of decision making units. *European Journal of Operational Research* 1978;2(6):429-444.

10. Coelli T. A *guide to DEAP version 2.1: a data envelopment analysis (computer) program*, Centre for Efficiency and Productivity Analysis (CEPA) Working Paper 96/08. Department of Econometrics, University of New England; Armidale, NSW Australia; 1996.

11. Ersoy K, Kavuncubasi S, Ozcan YA, Harris JM. Technical efficiencies of Turkish hospitals: DEA approach. *Journal of Medical Systems* 1997;21(2):67-74.

12. Parkin D, Hollingsworth B. Measuring production efficiency of acute hospitals in Scotland 1991-94: validity issues in data envelopment analysis. *Applied Economics* 1997;29(11):1425-1433.

13. Hollingsworth B, Parkin D. The efficiency of Scottish acute hospitals - an application of data envelopment analysis. *IMA J Math Appl Med Biol.* 1997;12:161-173.

14. Thanassoulis E, Boussfofiane A, Dyson RG. Exploring output quality targets in the provision of perinatal-care in England using data envelopment analysis. *European Journal of Operational Research* 1995;80(3):588-607.

15. Kooreman P. Nursing-home care in the Netherlands - a nonparametric efficiency analysis. *Journal of Health Economics* 1994;13:345-346.

16. Majumdar SK. Assessing firms capabilities - theory and measurement - as study of Indian pharmaceutical industry. *Economic and Political Weekly* 1994;29:M83-M89.

17. Ozcan YA, Bannick RR. Trends in department-of-defence hospital efficiency. *Journal of Medical Systems* 1994;18:69-83.

18. Ozcan YA, Mccue MJ, Okasha AA. Measuring the technical efficiency of psychiatric hospitals. *Journal of Medical Systems* 1996;20:141-150.

19. Huang Y-GL. An application of data envelopment analysis: measuring the relative performance of Florida general hospitals. *Journal of Medical Systems* 1990;14:191.

20. Huang Y-GL. *An evaluation of the efficiency of rural primary care programs: an application of data envelopment analysis in Chapel Hill, North Carolina.* PhD thesis, University of North Carolina, School of Public Health; 1986.

21. Kirigia JM, Sambo LG, Scheel H. Technical efficiency of public clinics in Kwazulu-Natal Province of South Africa. *East African Medical Journal* 2001;78(3 Suppl):S1-S13.

22. Eyob ZA. *Hospital efficiency in sub-Saharan Africa: evidence from South Africa. Working paper No. 187.* World Institute for Development Economics Research, United Nations University; 2000.

23. Kirigia JM, Sambo LG, Lambo E. Are public hospitals in Kwazulu/Natal Province of South Africa technically efficient? *African Journal of Health Science* 2000;7(3-4):24-31.

24. Emrouznejad A. Ali Emrouznejad's Data Envelopment Analysis HomePage 1995-2001, www.DEAzone.com.

25. Boussofiane A, Dyson RG, Thanassoulis E. Applied data envelopment analysis. *European Journal of Operational Research* 1991;52(1):1-15.

26. Carrin G, Desmet M, Basaza R. Social health insurance development in low-income developing countries: new roles for government and non-profit health insurance organizations in Africa and Asia. In: Xenia Scheil-Adlung X, editor. *Building social security: the challenge of privatisation.* New Brunswick, NJ: Transaction Publishers; 2000. p125-153.

27. Mwabu GM, Ainsworth M, Nyamete A. Quality of medical care and choice of medical treatment in Kenya: an empirical analysis. *Journal of Human Resources* 1993;28(4):838-862.

28. Jones AM, Kirigia JM. Health knowledge and smoking behaviour among South African women. *Health Economics* 1999;12(8):165-169.

29. Kirigia JM, Muthuri LHK. Predictors of women's decision to ask new partners to use condoms to avoid HIV/AIDS in South Africa. *East African Medical Journal* 1999;76(9):484-489.

30. Jones AM, Kirigia JM. The determinants of the use of alternative methods of contraception among South African women. *Applied Economics Letters* 2000;7:501-504.

31. Kirigia JM, Kainyu LH. Predictors of toilet ownership in South Africa. *East African Medical Journal* 2000;77(12):40-45.

32. Mansfield E. *Managerial economics: theory, applications, and cases.* New York: W.W. Norton & Company; 1999.

-8-

Technical Efficiency of Peripheral Health Units in Pujehun District of Sierra Leone: *A DEA Application**

Ade Renner, Joses M. Kirigia, Eyob Z. Asbu, Saidou P. Barry, Doris G. Kirigia, Clifford Kamara and Lenity Kainyu Muthuri

ABSTRACT

The data envelopment analysis (DEA) method has been fruitfully used in many countries in Asia, Europe, and North America to shed light on the efficiency of health facilities and programmes. There is, however, a dearth of such studies in countries in sub-Saharan Africa. Since hospitals and health centres are important instruments in the efforts to scale up pro-poor cost-effective interventions aimed at achieving the United Nations Millennium Development Goals, decision-makers need to ensure that these health facilities provide efficient services. The objective of this study was to measure the technical efficiency (TE) and scale efficiency (SE) of a sample of public peripheral health units (PHUs) in Sierra Leone.

This study applied the data envelopment analysis approach to investigate the technical efficiency and scale efficiency among a sample of 37 PHUs in Sierra Leone. Twenty-two (59%) of the 37 health units analysed were found to be technically inefficient with an average score of 63% (standard deviation = 18%). On the other hand, 24 (65%) health units were found to be scale inefficient with an average scale efficiency score of 72% (standard deviation=17%).

It was concluded that with the existing high levels of pure technical and scale inefficiency, scaling up of interventions to achieve both global and regional targets such as the MDG and Abuja health targets becomes far-fetched. In a country with per capita expenditure on

* The original article appeared in *BMC Health Services Research* 2005;5(77):1-11. Reproduced with the permission of BioMed C entral Ltd.

health of about US$7, and with only 30% of its population having access to health services, it was demonstrated that efficiency savings can significantly augment the government's initiatives to cater for the unmet health care needs of the population. Therefore, we strongly recommend that every country in the Region should institutionalise health facility efficiency monitoring at the Ministry of Health headquarters (MoH/HQ) and at each health district headquarters.

BACKGROUND

Public health is the science and art of preventing disease, prolonging life and promoting health and efficiency through organised community effort. [1,p.23]

Located in West Africa, Sierra Leone has a population of 4.6 million and a total fertility rate of 6.5. Its health indicators are poor. For example, life expectancy at birth is 34.2 years and the probability of dying (per 1,000 live births) before the age of 5 years is 313 and between 15 and 59 years is 619 [2]. The number of maternal deaths per 100,000 live births is 2,000 [3]. These dismal health indicators are a reflection of poor governance [4], poor macroeconomic performance [5], and poor national health system performance [6].

The total expenditure on health as a percentage of the gross domestic product (GDP) increased from 2.6% in 1996 to 4.3% in 2000 [2]. General government expenditure on health constituted 60% of the total expenditure on health; the remaining 40% came from private households and out-of-pocket spending. The fact that health indicators had continued to decline [7] inspite of health expenditure increases could be partly due to an inefficient public health system.

Peripheral health units (PHUs) are a vital part of Sierra Leone's public health system. Given their strategic location in the midst of communities, they constitute an invaluable vehicle for "organising community effort for the sanitation of the environment, the control of communicable infections, the education of the individual in personal hygiene and the organisation of medical and nursing services for the early diagnosis and preventive treatment of disease" [1]. PHUs are instrumental in efforts to scale up a pro-poor package of cost-effective interventions aimed at achieving the United Nations Millennium Development Goals [8,9]. We concur with the father of public health, C.E.A. Winslow [1], that part of the mandate of the public health discipline ought to be promotion of efficiency, i.e., to maximise the benefit of health interventions (promotion, prevention, and preventive treatment) to communities at large from available resources. Therefore, decision-makers need to ensure that PHUs (and all other branches of the public health system) provide services efficiently.

In Sierra Leone, no studies of the efficiency of health facilities had been conducted using data envelopment analysis (DEA). This study was therefore significant in assessing efficiency using more robust techniques and generating information that would be useful for policy, planning, and operational management. The objectives of this study were (i) to measure the technical and scale efficiency among a sample of public PHUs in Sierra Leone employing the DEA method; and (ii) to demonstrate how its results could be used in the pursuit of the public health objective of promoting efficiency in health facilities.

METHODS

Overview of Sierra Leone's Healthcare Delivery System

The Ministry of Health and Sanitation (MOHS) provides about 50% of healthcare services. The remainder is provided by the private sector (private-for-profit institutions and traditional healers) and national (e.g., Christian Health Association of Sierra Leone) and international NGOs (e.g., German Leprosy Rehabilitation Association and *Medecins Sans Frontieres*) [10]. The country has 13 health districts each with a District Health Management Team responsible for the implementation, supervision, and monitoring of health programmes in the district. Sierra Leone has a total of 31 government hospitals, 22 mission hospitals/clinics, 78 private hospitals/clinics and a network of 788 PHUs. As indicated in Table 8.1, there are geographical inequities in the distribution of health facilities in the country [10].

Table 8.1   Functioning PHUs and hospitals

Health District	Government PHUs	Government hospitals	Mission hospitals/clinics	Private hospitals/clinics
Bo	87	1	2	3
Kenema	85	2	3	3
Moyamba	95	1	3	5
Port Loko	74	2	2	1
Bombali	66	1	2	9
Kailahun	57	1	2	3
Koinadugu	51	1	0	0
Kono	61	1	2	1
Tonkolili	60	1	2	1
Kambia	35	2	1	1
Pejehun	46	5	0	0
Bonthe	34	1	2	3
Western area	37	12	1	48
Total	788	31	22	78

Source: WHO Regional Office for Africa [10]

Table 8.2 provides estimates of the number and ratio of human resources for health in 2002. Approximately 63% of the health workers were employed by the government and the remaining by NGOs and private-for-profit institutions.

Table 8.2   Estimated number and ratio of health personnel in 2002

Categories of human resources	Number employed by Government	Number employed by NGOs and private sector	Total number of human resources	Population per health worker
Doctors	169	131	300	15,290
Nurses	406	200	606	7,569
Other nursing personnel	1,655	1,500	3,155	1,454
Pharmacists	11	-	11	417,000
Dispensing technicians	124	-	124	36,992
Environmental health officers	168	36	204	22,485
Endemic disease control assistant	332	-	332	13,816
Community health officers	194	90	284	16,151
Laboratory technicians	28	12	40	114,675
Radiographers	4	8	12	38,2250
Sanitary Engineers	2	0	2	2,293,500
Health education officers	4	1	5	917,400
Other health workers	294	-	294	15,602

Source: WHO Regional Office for Africa [10]

Data

Input and output data were analysed for the year 2000. Due to research resource constraints, the planning and information department at the MOHS decided to choose one health district for the study of PHUs. The choice of the study district was done using a simple random sampling technique. This process led to the choice of Pujehun District. Even though there are 46 PHUs in Pujehun today, in the year 2000 there were only 39 PHUs. The data were collected by Pujehun District Health Team using the primary healthcare facility efficiency analysis data collection instrument of the WHO Regional Office for Africa [11].

Overview of a Public Health System

Turnock [12] developed a conceptual framework that ties together the mission and functions of public health to the inputs, processes, outputs, and outcomes of the system (see Figure 8.1). He stated that health systems combine inputs (human, organisational, informational, financial, and other resources) to produce outputs (programmes or services or interventions) intended to ultimately yield health or quality-of-life outcomes. In terms of measurability, the author posits that many inputs such as human, financial, and organisational resources are easily counted or measured. He further explains that outputs (such as number of antenatal care visits, number of immunisations provided, number of people who receive health education, and number of condoms distributed) are also generally easy to recognise and count. Following Turnock [12], a public health practice, such as a health centre, employs multiple inputs to produce multiple outputs.

Data envelopment analysis (a non-parametric method) defines efficiency as the ratio of the weighted sum of outputs of a health centre to its weighted sum of inputs [13]. It is particularly useful in public sector organisations (e.g., health facilities) that lack the profit maximisation motive and employ a multiple input, multiple output production process. The technical efficiency (TE) of PHUs was found by solving the following linear programming problem for each health unit in the sample:

$$\text{Max } h_0 = \sum_{r=1}^{s} u_r y_{rj_0}$$

Subject to

$$\sum_{i=1}^{m} v_i x_{ij_0} = 1$$

$$\sum_{r=1}^{s} u_r y_{rj} - \sum v_i x_{ij} \leq 0, \quad j = 1,...,n$$

$$u_r, v_i \geq 0$$

Where:

y_{rj} = amount of output r from health centre j

x_{ij} = amount of input i to health centre j

u_r = weight given to output r

v_i = weight given to input i

n = number of hospitals
s = number of outputs
m = number of inputs

This mathematical programming technique establishes a production possibilities frontier based on relatively efficient health centres and measures how far the inefficient health centres are from this "best" practice frontier [14]. The efficient health centres lie on the frontier and are assigned a score of 1 or 100%. Inefficient health centres are allocated a score that is less than 1 (or less than 100%). The higher the score, the greater the efficiency and vice versa.

Model Specification

The variable returns to scale (VRS) model was estimated to facilitate the estimation of scale efficiency. It assumed that changes in inputs would lead to disproportionate changes in outputs. In other words, a percentage increase in input can yield less than a percentage change in output signifying diseconomies of scale, or more than a percentage increase of output implying existence of economies of scale. The scale efficiency (SE) is the ratio of constant returns to scale technical efficiency (TE_{CRS}) to variable returns to scale technical efficiency (TE_{VRS}), i.e., $SE = (TE_{CRS})/ (TE_{VRS})$ [15]. All the analysis was undertaken using DEAP, the software developed by Coelli [16].

Output Orientation

The output-oriented DEA model was used for the analysis because the management of PHUs had no control over inputs, especially the deployment of human resources. However, given their public health orientation, PHU staff had a duty to induce demand (through health promotion strategies) for preventive healthcare services such as antenatal care, family planning services, immunisations, etc. Through their outreach public health work among communities, PHU staff were also supposed to mobilise community efforts and other resources to provide clean water and hygienic human waste disposal facilities, e.g., vented improved pit latrines especially in rural areas and slums.

Table 8.3 on health indicators for Sierra Leone shows serious population under-coverage of the various interventions. This is mainly due to critical resource constraints, e.g., per capita total expenditure on health in Sierra Leone is only US$7 compared to US$34 per person recommended by the WHO Commission for Macroeconomics and Health [8]. This implies that although the communities might want more of the services, budgetary pressures make it difficult to increase inputs even assuming that PHUs had control over input (which they do not have). Even where inputs (e.g., labour) might be underutilised it is not within the power of PHUs to dispose of excess inputs. We felt that output maximisation is the most appropriate orientation for health centres which are given a fixed input and requested to produce as much output as possible. Thus, an output-oriented approach focused on the amount by which health unit outputs could be expanded with the same level of inputs.

Furthermore, the output- and input-oriented models will estimate exactly the same frontier, and therefore, by definition identify the same set of PHUs (firms) as being efficient. It is only the efficiency measures associated with the inefficient firms that may differ between the two methods [16]. In fact, under the assumption of constant returns to scale, even the efficiency scores will not change. We, therefore, felt that the choice of model was not going to affect the results significantly.

Table 8.3   Manifestations of inaccessibility to basic health services in Sierra Leone

Health manifestation	Percentage of population without access
Pregnant women without access to prenatal/ antenatal care	32.0
Pregnant women without access to trained attendants during childbirth	58.0
Married women aged 15-49 years not using contraceptives	96.0
Newborns weighing less than 2.5 kg at birth	22.0
Children (0-59 months) whose weight falls below minus two standard deviations of the median of the international (NCHS) reference population	27.2
Children (0-59 months) whose weight falls below minus three standard deviations of the median of the international (NCHS) reference population	8.7
Children (0-59 months) suffering moderate stunting	33.9
Children (0-59 months) suffering severe stunting	15.8
Children (0-59 months) suffering moderate wasting	9.8
Children (0-59 months) suffering severe wasting	1.9
Infants not fully immunised with:	
BCG	61.0
DPT3	76.0
OPV3	74.0
Measles	57.0
TT2	80.0
Population without access to safe water	57.0
Population without access to sanitation facilities	57.0
Population without access to healthcare services	70.0
Per capita total expenditure on health (US$)	7.0

Sources: UNICEF [19] and WHO/AFRO [20]

DEA Inputs and Outputs

The DEA model was estimated with a total of eight variables: six outputs and two inputs. The six outputs for each individual PHU were as follows: (*a*) number of antenatal plus post-natal visits; (*b*) number of child deliveries; (c) nutritional/child growth monitoring visits; (*d*) number of family planning visits; (*e*) number of children under the age of 5 years immunised plus pregnant women immunised with tetanus toxoid (TT); and (*f*) total number of health education sessions conducted through home visits, public meetings, school lectures, and outpatient department. Peripheral health units in Sierra Leone did not provide curative care; they were dedicated fully to the provision of health promotion and disease prevention services. The two inputs were (*a*) technical staff (community health nurse, vaccinator, and maternal and child health aide); and (*b*) subordinate staff (including traditional birth attendants, porters, and watchmen). The choice of inputs and outputs was guided by the public health conceptual framework and past studies.

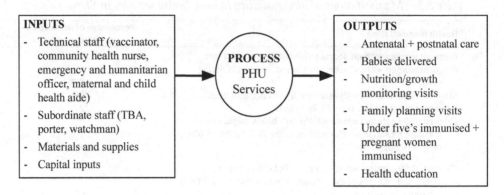

INPUTS		OUTPUTS
- Technical staff (vaccinator, community health nurse, emergency and humanitarian officer, maternal and child health aide)	**PROCESS** PHU Services	- Antenatal + postnatal care - Babies delivered - Nutrition/growth monitoring visits
- Subordinate staff (TBA, porter, watchman)		- Family planning visits - Under five's immunised + pregnant women immunised
- Materials and supplies		- Health education
- Capital inputs		

Figure 8.1   Relationship between inputs and the production process and resulting outputs

RESULTS

Data for two of the sampled PHUs was incomplete, and thus analysis was based on data from 37 health units of Pujehun District. Table 8.4 presents descriptive statistics for the outputs and inputs of the 37 public PHUs. The TE and SE scores for individual PHUs are given in Table 8.5. Out of the 37 PHUs, 15 (41%) were found to be technically efficient with a TE score of 100%. The remaining 22 (59%) were technically inefficient since they had a TE score of less than 100%. Seven (47%) of the inefficient PHUs had a TE score of less than 50%. The overall sample average TE score was 78% (standard deviation (SD) = 23%). This implies that if the inefficient PHUs were to operate as efficiently as their peers on the efficient frontier, outputs could be increased by about 22% without changing the quantity of inputs used. The average TE score among the inefficient PHUs was 63% (SD=18%).

About 65% of the PHUs were found to be scale inefficient, that is, they suffered from inefficiencies emanating from inappropriate size, i.e., being too small or too large. The average SE score for the sampled PHUs was 82%. The scale inefficient PHUs had an average SE score of 72% (SD=17%). This implies that if all inefficient PHUs had an optimal size, output would have increased by about 28% without increasing the input consumption. Thirteen (35%) PHUs manifested constant returns to scale, 21 (57%) showed decreasing returns to scale, and 3 (8%) showed increasing returns to scale.

Table 8.4   Means and standard deviations for public PHUs outputs and inputs

Variables	Total	Mean	Standard deviation	Maximum	Minimum
Outputs					
Antenatal plus postnatal care visits	25,099	678	749	4,080	130
Number of deliveries	4,863	131	99	445	14
Nutrition/growth monitoring visits	29,633	801	1 045	4,555	0
Family planning visits	2,958	80	55	252	10
Number of children under the age of 5 years and pregnant women fully immunised	33,399	903	846	4,422	193
Health education sessions	7,458	202	118	434	55
Inputs					
Technical staff	78	2	1	5	1
Subordinate staff	27	1	1	3	0

Table 8.5   Technical and scale efficiency scores for public PHUs

DMU (Health Unit)	Technical efficiency	Scale efficiency	DMU (Health unit)	Technical efficiency	Scale efficiency
Potoru	100	100	S/Malen	77	54
Gbahama	100	100	Karlu	77	48
Jendema	100	100	Futa Peje	72	62
Saama P	100	100	Kpowubu	72	96
Geoma	100	100	Falaba	71	58
Gissiwulo	100	100	Gbaa	70	84
S/Griema	100	100	Sulima	65	85
Sengema	100	100	Bomu Sa	64	58
Massam	100	100	Vaama	60	100
Static Pu	100	93	Pehala	55	93
Gbondapi	100	88	Gofor	55	64
Zimmi	100	86	T/Barri	49	100
Banjadum	100	84	Saahun	49	100
Bandajum	100	75	Fairo	46	60
Taninahu	100	59	Waiima	45	100
B/Massaq	97	62	Bumpeh	45	57
Dandabu	90	44	Kowama	37	80
S/Kpaka	87	99	S/Bessima	26	85
Njaluahu	82	57			

DISCUSSION

The findings of this study revealed that more than half of the PHUs were operating at less than optimal levels of pure technical and scale efficiency. The performance of some of the PHUs in the sample was actually observed to be very low and raises much concern for planners and policy makers. With the existing levels of inefficiency, the achievement of the health policy objectives and health-related global and regional targets such as the Millennium Development Goals (MDGs) and Abuja targets will be compromised. Hence, greater focus should be placed on efficient use of the existing resources. The results obtained in Sierra Leone were similar to those obtained from the efficiency analysis of Kenyan health centres [17]. A study found 56% health centres in Kenya to be technically inefficient with an average TE score of 65%. The average scale efficiency score among inefficient PHUs was 72% in Sierra Leone and 70% in Kenya. Seventy per cent of primary healthcare clinics in Kwazulu-Natal province in South Africa were found to be technically inefficient and 84% scale inefficient [18].

Table 8.6 shows the total output increases needed to make inefficient public PHUs efficient. In order to become efficient, the 22 inefficient PHUs combined would need to increase their current output levels by 57% more antenatal and postnatal care visits, 50% more deliveries, 85% more nutrition/growth monitoring visits, 45% more family planning visits, 40% more children and pregnant women who are fully immunised, and 36% more health education sessions. This potential of providing more preventive health services to those currently without access, at no extra cost, would be of great public health importance in a poor country like Sierra Leone where large numbers of women do not have access to contraceptives, antenatal care, and trained attendants during childbirth; where a large percentage of children are underweight, stunted and wasted; and where a large proportion of children do not have access to the Expanded Programme on Immunisation (EPI) that targets diphtheria, tetanus, whooping cough, polio, tuberculosis, and measles (see Table 8.3). Also, over 50% of the population in the country does not have access to safe water, sanitation facilities, and healthcare services. Thus, it is irrational, immoral, and unethical to deny needy people access to essential health services through inefficiencies.

Table 8.6   Total output increases needed to make inefficient public PHUs efficient

Outputs	Radial movement (A)	Slack movement (B)	Total value (A+B=C)
Antenatal plus postnatal care visits	5,819	8,509	14,327
Number of deliveries	1,328	1,095	2,423
Nutrition/growth monitoring visits	5,903	19,398	25,301
Family planning visits	835	502	1,338
Number of children under the age of 5 years and pregnant women fully immunised	8,430	4,945	13,375
Health education sessions	1,964	744	2,708

The predominant form of scale inefficiency is decreasing returns to scale, which is also known as diseconomies of scale. A PHU operating at decreasing returns to scale has an inefficiently large size. A percentage increase in all inputs is followed by less than a percentage change in outputs. To improve the efficiency of the inefficiently large PHUs, there is a need to have more health units of a relatively smaller size. Judging from the various statements contained in the national health policy and plan and the health sector reforms that the Ministry of Health has been implementing, there is clearly a willingness to optimise the use of the scarce health resources. While the scope for staff reduction in Pujehun District of Sierra Leone was almost non-existent as revealed by this study, there was certainly scope for providing essential public PHUs to a significantly larger number of people than the health units were actually providing. This could be achieved through a conscious pursuit of health promotion strategies [19] to create or induce demand for essential preventive public health services that were being under-utilised. Examples of such demand-inducing strategies might include:

1. *Health information*: Improve people's ability to access health information to increase their capacity to make informed choices concerning their health-related behaviours (e.g., making available at community level information on the benefits of antenatal care, family planning, use of condoms to prevent HIV infection or transmission, immunisation, safe water, hygienic sanitation facilities, abstinence from use of addictive substances (e.g., tobacco, alcohol and illicit drugs), physical activity, and healthy diet. This strategy was important for primary prevention, which aimed at keeping a disease from ever developing or a trauma from ever occurring [20].

2. *Health education*: Communicating information concerning the underlying social, economic, and environmental conditions impacting on health as well as individual risk factors and risk behaviours and use of the health system. In addition, health education was meant to foster motivation, skills, and confidence among communities to take action to improve their health [19].

3. *Screening and individual risk assessment:* Identifying and assisting individuals at special risk to seek secondary prevention, which involves early detection and early intervention against disease before it developed fully, e.g., cervical cancer screening (pap smears) to identify pre-malignant cell changes [20], screening for intestinal nematode infections, ascariasis, trichuriasis, hookworm disease, or tropical diseases (e.g., trypanosomiasis, schistosomiasis, lymphatic filariasis, and onchocerciasis).

4. *Social marketing:* Attempting to influence communities living in the vicinity of health units on how to think and behave (with respect to utilisation of preventive health services) by using marketing techniques [19]. The object of social marketing would be to cultivate positive attitudes, values, and behaviours towards participation in disease prevention services.

The findings indicate that the amount of outputs could be increased tremendously without increasing the quantity of inputs used. Table 8.6 shows that each of the outputs exhibits a tremendous increase – more than 50% in some cases. This includes both radial and slack movements. Radial movements indicate the proportional increase in outputs, that is, an increase without changing the mix of the outputs. The slack movements, which arise because of the sections of the piece-wise linear frontier that run parallel to the axes are also reported in order to give an accurate indication of the technical efficiency of the health centres. It should, however, be noted that sometimes slacks are treated as issues of allocative efficiency and therefore the focus is on the radial efficiency score. Thus, with the potential increase in outputs from the current sample of health centres, it is possible for the health system to significantly increase coverage by the different health interventions and contribute to the achievement of the various national and global health targets.

The extent to which the PHUs can increase their outputs depends on whether the health workers contract renewal and remunerations (especially annual increments) are linked to their performance. Currently, the health workers are paid salaries that are not linked to performance. Efforts to improve health facility efficiency will need to be undertaken in tandem with reforms in health workers' terms of employment. Such reforms are contemplated within the ongoing public sector reforms, which are being supported by bilateral and multilateral development partners.

Limitations of the Study

Our study had some limitations. Firstly, in this study we used the total number of health education sessions conducted through home visits, public meetings, school lectures, and outpatient department as a proxy for health promotion. By so doing we may have underestimated the health promotion work done by health centre staff within communities, such as public health inspection of commercial food outlets, coaching communities on personal hygiene, and advice to communities on the protection of water sources and construction of vented improved pit latrines (in rural areas and shanties) among others.

Secondly, the inputs and outputs data were collected for only one time period; thus, it was not possible to determine whether the health sector reforms had any impact on the efficiency of PHUs. Thirdly, data on drug expenditure at many PHUs were missing; as a result we were forced to drop the variable from the analysis, which may result in shifting the frontier because of outlier figures. Fourthly, we did not manage to collect information on input prices and thus we could not estimate the allocative efficiency of the PHUs. Fifthly, given that the study was conducted in only one district, it would not be advisable to generalise the findings to the whole country. Thus, it is recommended that the study should be replicated in the remaining twelve districts. Lastly, DEA has been criticised for attributing any deviation from the estimated frontier to inefficiency since it is deterministic or non-stochastic

[21,22]. In other words, it does not capture random noise, such as epidemics, civil war, and natural and technological disaster.

To increase the relevance of the study for management purposes, it would have been useful to undertake a second stage analysis of the factors influencing inefficiency using a tobit-censored dependent variable model regression analysis. However, because of the absence of good quality data on the factors often hypothesised to influence inefficiency it was not possible to undertake the analysis.

Implications for Further Applications of DEA in sub-Saharan Africa

A national health system performs the functions of stewardship (oversight), health financing, creating resources/inputs (including human resources for health) for producing health, and delivering (providing) health services with a view to improving responsiveness to people's non-medical expectations, ensuring fair financial contribution to health systems, and ultimately improving health (the three being goals of a health system) [6].

The *World Health Report 2000* ranked the 191 Member States on the basis of their overall goal performance. Table 8.7 provides the ranking of the 46 countries in the WHO African Region. Three countries were ranked between 83 and 99; nine countries were ranked between 118 and 147; and the remaining countries were ranked between 151 and 191. The Sierra Leone health system performed the worst (in these rankings). After the publication of these macro-performance results, countries in the region have been asking what they can do to improve the performance of their health systems, or even the performance of their individual hospitals and health centres which absorb over 80% of recurrent and capital budgets of the Ministries of Health. The starting point in addressing the poor health system performance is measuring which decision-making units (tertiary hospitals, provincial hospitals, health centres, clinics/health posts, and programmes) of the present system are operating efficiently.

These measurements can help identify the efficient DMUs (which can be emulated by inefficient ones), the inefficient DMUs (whose performance needs to be improved), the inputs that are being wasted and the magnitude of waste, and the output increases needed to make inefficient DMUs efficient. This kind of evidence would empower the health policy makers and managers to develop concrete strategies for boosting efficiency of DMUs. As demonstrated in the current study, DEA is a versatile tool/approach for analysing the efficiency of complex DMUs (e.g., hospitals and health centres) that employ multiple inputs to produce multiple outputs with a view to generating the information mentioned above.

Efficiency improvement is a major strategy for mobilising more domestic resources for the massive expansion in coverage of health interventions envisaged in the Millennium Development Goals. Thus, while striving to mobilise more domestic and external resources, it is important to ensure that the available resources are optimally used, that is, ensure that it is not possible by reallocation of available resources to make someone's health status better off without making someone else worse off (economists refer to this situation as Pareto-optimality). If it is possible through reallocation of resources, to improve at least one person's health status without reducing the health status of another person, then there is waste within the health system, health facility, or programme.

Table 8.7   Ranking of WHO African Region countries on the basis of overall health system goal attainment (out of 191 WHO Member States in 2000)

Member State	Rank	Member State	Rank
Seychelles	83	Swaziland	164
Mauritius	90	Namibia	165
Algeria	99	Madagascar	167
Senegal	118	Botswana	168
Cape Verde	126	Mauritania	169
Comoros	137	Rwanda	171
Sao Tome and Principe	138	Guinea	172
Ghana	139	Lesotho	173
Kenya	142	Zambia	174
Benin	143	Eritrea	176
Gabon	147	Chad	177
Zimbabwe	147	Mali	178
South Africa	151	Democratic Republic of Congo	179
Equatorial Guinea	152	Guinea-Bissau	180
Gambia	153	Angola	181
Congo	155	Malawi	182
Togo	156	Nigeria	184
Cote d'Ivoire	157	Mozambique	185
United Republic of Tanzania	158	Ethiopia	186
Burkina Faso	159	Liberia	187
Burundi	161	Niger	188
Uganda	162	Central African Republic	190
Cameroon	163	Sierra Leone	191

Source: WHO [6].

Therefore, we strongly recommend that every country in the region should institutionalise health facility efficiency monitoring at the Ministry of Health headquarters (MoH/HQ) and at each health district headquarters. In the process of institutionalisation, there will be need to observe the following:

(*a*) familiarise the policy makers (ministers, permanent secretaries, directors of medical services), managers (MoH/HQ departmental heads, provincial medical officers of health, district medical officers of health, hospital superintedents), and economists (and planners) at the Ministry of Health with the concepts of technical efficiency, allocative efficiency, and total factor productivity; (*b*) acquire computers (where they do not exist) and software (parametric and non-parametric) for estimating efficiency; (*c*) organise hands-on training for MoH economists and planners (and where possible provincial and district health managers) in the use of the efficiency measurement software; (*d*) adapt the available efficiency data collection questionnaires/ instruments; (*e*) undertake a pilot study among a few different level health facilities and revise the data collection instruments accordingly; (*f*) make the data collection instruments part of the national health information systems; (*g*) decide on the frequency of reporting of the inputs (quantities and prices) and outputs by those in charge of health facilities; (*h*) undertake analysis at the district level (with MoH/HQ support) with a view to identifying causes of inefficiencies, develop strategies for improving efficiency and implementing them; and (*i*) establish efficiency databases at MoH/HQ and at each health district headquarters.

CONCLUSIONS

Data envelopment analysis has been fruitfully used in many countries in Asia [23,24] and Europe [25-30] and in the United States [31-35] to shed light on the efficiency of health facilities and programmes. The current study adds to this literature. The study has revealed the prevalence of high levels of combined pure technical and scale inefficiencies. In a country with very low levels of per capita expenditure on health (US$7) and very limited access to health services, the current levels of inefficiency would seriously impede the government's initiatives to increase the population's access to quality healthcare services. Furthermore, progress towards the achievement of the cherished health policy objectives and global and regional health targets would be seriously hampered. It is therefore recommended that the causes of the inefficiencies be unpacked and necessary efficiency measures be instituted to augment the government's efforts to address the healthcare access issues in the country. To estimate the level of efficiency savings in the overall health system, it is also advisable to undertake a similar study in all types of health facilities in the country.

In any efficiency analysis studies to be conducted in Sierra Leone in the future, more emphasis should be laid on collecting information on the quantities of all the main outputs and inputs (including drugs) and the average or median prices per unit of each input, from all public and private health facilities (health centres and hospitals), to facilitate measurement of total economic efficiencies (i.e., technical plus allocative efficiencies). Furthermore, in order to aid monitoring and evaluation of the effects of different healthcare reforms [36] on the efficiency of individual healthcare facilities over time through the Malmquist productivity index analysis [16,37], it would be necessary to collect data for a year (or more) before the introduction of specific reforms and for subsequent years. The Malmquist productivity index helps to measure explicitly total factor productivity. It decomposes productivity growth into efficiency change and technical change. The former component is considered to be evidence of catching up to the efficiency frontier, while the latter component is considered to be evidence of innovation [37].

ACKNOWLEDGEMENT

We owe profound gratitude to the Sierra Leone MoHS for authorising and facilitating this study. Pujehun District Health Team collected the data. We received commendable editorial support from A Kochar. This paper benefited greatly from the comments and suggestions of the two peer reviewers, Dr. Robert Rosenman and Dr. Antonio Giuffrida. We are indebted to Jehovah Shamah for all round support and guidance at all stages of the study. The findings, interpretations and conclusions contained in this paper and any remaining errors are entirely those of the authors and should NOT be attributed in any manner to the MoHS, the World Health Organization, the University of New South Wales or any of the acknowledged. All authors read and approved the final manuscript.

REFERENCES

1. Winslow CEA. The untilled field of public health. *Modern Medicine* 1920;2:183-191.

2. World Health Organization. *World health report 2002: reducing risks, promoting healthy life*. Geneva: World Health Organization; 2002.

3. World Health Organization. *World health report 2005: make every mother and child count*. Geneva: World Health Organization; 2005.

4. United Nations Development Programme. Human development report 2003: Millennium Development Goals: a compact to end human poverty. New York: UNDP; 2003.

5. The World Bank. *World development report 2003*. Washington DC: World Bank; 2003.

6. World Health Organization. *World health report 2000 – improving performance of health systems*. Geneva: World Health Organization; 2000.

7. World Health Organization. *World health report 2001 - mental health*. Geneva: World Health Organization; 2000.

8. World Health Organization. *Macroeconomics and health: Investing in health for economic development.* Geneva: World Health Organization; 2001.

9. United Nations Organization. *Millennium Development Goals.* New York: UN; 2000.

10. World Health Organization Regional Office for Africa. *WHO country cooperation strategy: Sierra Leone.* Brazzaville: World Health Organization; 2005.

11. World Health Organization Regional Office for Africa. *Primary health care facility economic efficiency analysis data collection instrument.* Brazzaville: World Health Organization; 2001.

12. Turnock BJ. *Public health: what it is and how it works.* Gaithersburg: Aspen Publishers; 1997.

13. Charnes A., Cooper WW, Rhodes E. Measuring the efficiency of decision-making units. *European Journal of Operational Research* 1978;2(6):429-444.

14. Hollingsworth B, Parkin D. The efficiency of the delivery of neonatal care in UK. *Journal of Public Health Medicine* 2001;23(1):47-50.

15. Linna M, Nordblad A, Koivu M. Technical and cost efficiency of oral health care provision in Finnish health centers. *Social Science and Medicine* 2002;56:343-353.

16. Coelli T. A *guide to DEAP version 2.1: a data envelopment analysis (computer) program,* Centre for Efficiency and Productivity Analysis (CEPA) Working Paper 96/08. Department of Econometrics, University of New England; Armidale, NSW Australia; 1996.

17. Kirigia JM, Emrouznejad A, Sambo LG, Munguti N, Liambila W. Using data envelopment analysis to measure the technical efficiency of public health centers in Kenya. *Journal of Medical Systems* 2004;28(2):155-166.

18. Kirigia JM, Sambo LG, Scheel H. Technical efficiency of public clinics in Kwazulu-Natal Province of South Africa. *East African Medical Journal* 2001;78(3 Suppl):S1-S13.

19. Egger G, Spark R, Lawson J, Donovan R. *Health promotion strategies and methods.* Roseville, Australia: McGraw-Hill; 2002.

20. Jenkins CD. *Building better health: a handbook of behavioural change.* Washington DC: Pan African Health Organization; 2003.

21. Lovell CAK. Production frontiers and productive efficiency. In: Fried HO, Lovell CAK, Schimdt SS, editors. *The measurement of productivity efficiency: techniques and application.* New York: Oxford University Press; 1993. p 3-67

22. Zere EA, Addison T, McIntyre D. Hospital efficiency in sub-Saharan Africa: Evidence from South Africa. *South African Journal of Economics* 2000;69(2):336-358.

23. Chang H: Determinants of hospital efficiency: the case of central government-owned hospitals in Taiwan. *Omega International Journal of Management Science* 1998;26(2):307-317.

24. Wan TTH, Hsu N, Feng R, Ma A, Pan S, Chou M. Technical efficiency of nursing units in a tertiary care hospital in Taiwan. *Journal of Medical Systems* 2002;26(1):21-27.

25. Salinas-Jimenez J, Smith P. Data envelopment analysis applied to quality in primary health care. *Annals of Operational Research* 1996;67:141-161.

26. Giuffrida A, Gravelle H. Measuring performance in primary care: econometric analysis and DEA, *Applied Economics* 2001;33:163-175.

27. Zavras AI, Tsakos G, Economou C, Kyriopoulos J. Using DEA to evaluate efficiency and formulate policy within a Greek national primary healthcare network. *Journal of Medical Systems* 2002;26(4):285-292.

28. Ersoy K, Kavuncubasi S, Ozcan YA, Harris II JM. Technical efficiencies of Turkish hospitals: DEA approach. *Journal of Medical Systems* 1997;21(2): 67-74.

29. Jacobs R. Alternative methods to examine hospital efficiency: data envelopment analysis and stochastic frontier analysis. *Health Care Management Science* 2001;4:103-115.

30. Johnston K, Gerard K. Assessing efficiency in the UK breast screening programme: does size of screening unit make a difference? *Health Policy* 56:21-32.

31. Chattopadhy S, Ray CS. Technical, scale, and size efficiency in nursing home care: a nonparametric analysis of Connecticut homes. *Health Economics* 1996;5:363-373.

32. Shroff HFE, Gulledge TR, Haynes KE, Oneill MK. Siting efficiency of long-term healthcare facilities. *Socio-Economic Planning Science* 1998;32(1):25-43.

33. White KR, Fache RN, Ozcan YA. Church ownership and hospital efficiency. *Hospital and Health Services Administration* 1996;41(3):297-310.

34. Harris J, Ozgen H, Ozcan YA. Do mergers enhance the performance of hospital efficiency? *Journal of the Operational Research Society* 2000;51:801-811.

35. Pai C-W, Ozcan YA, Jiang HJ. Regional variation in physician practice pattern: an examination of technical and cost-efficiency for treating sinusitis. *Journal of Medical Systems* 2000;24(2):103-117.

36. Lambo E, Sambo LG. Health sector reform in sub-Saharan Africa: a synthesis of country experiences. *East African Medical Journal* 2003;80(6 Suppl): S1-S20.

37. Fare R, Grosskopf S, Norris M, Zhang Z. Productivity, technical progress, and efficiency change in industrialised countries. *American Economic Review* 1994;84(1):66-83.

-9-

Are Public Hospitals in Kwazulu-Natal Province of South Africa Technically Efficient?*

Joses M. Kirigia, Eitayo Lambo and Luis G. Sambo

ABSTRACT

Generally, policy makers and researchers in South Africa acknowledge that hospitals absorb a disproportionate share of health sector resources. The latter, to a certain extent, have failed to provide the evidence needed to guide the former's decisions. Albeit in an *ad hoc* manner, the post-apartheid policy makers have been reducing hospital budgets to make available the resources needed to strengthen the hitherto neglected primary healthcare system. Since political will exists to reduce (if not eliminate) wastage of resources within the hospitals, micro-efficiency analyses (like the one reported here) are needed to guide the policy makers. This study employed data envelopment analysis (DEA) methodology to identify and measure individual hospital's inefficiencies. The key results were as follows: 40% of the hospitals had some degree of technical inefficiency; 58% were scale inefficient. In total, the following inputs were wasted and not utilised in the production of hospital outputs in Kwazulu-Natal public hospitals: 117.4 doctors (8.0%); 2,709 nurses (11.9%); 61 paramedics (11.5%); 58 technicians (13.1%); 295 administrative staff (11.1%); 835 general staff (11.3%); 1,193 labour provisioning staff (14.3%); 38 other staff (10.7%); and 1,752 beds (7.1%). These are the specific input reductions required to make inefficient hospitals technically efficient. In conclusion, the DEA results constitute a strong guide to healthcare decision-making especially with regard to practical ways of increasing efficiency and rational use of healthcare resources.

---

* The original article appeared in *African Journal of Health Sciences* 2000; 5(77):1-11. Reproduced with the permission of Kenya Medical Research Institute.

INTRODUCTION

A myriad of healthcare reforms are currently being implemented across sub-Saharan Africa (SSA). Some of the reforms relate to alternative financing mechanisms (e.g., user fees and insurance), public/private mix (mainly relating to sub-contracting the provision of certain services in public health facilities to the private sector), and management (e.g., decentralisation of decision-making to health districts) [1,2]. Efficiency improvement is often cited by proponents of healthcare reforms as one of the key rationales for reforming (of course equity being the other one). Unfortunately, there is no assurance that public hospitals will be efficient as a result of implementing those reforms. Infact, apart from theoretical conjectures, there has been no published evidence that healthcare reforms, as implemented to date in SSA, would indeed improve the efficiency of health systems.

Healthcare reforms implementation in SSA has hardly been preceded by economic analyses and gathering of baseline data against which to monitor and evaluate their effects. The goal of this study is to make available some baseline data against which to judge the effects of healthcare reforms in the public hospital sector in Kwazulu-Natal Province of South Africa. The specific objective is to employ data envelopment analysis (DEA) approach to identify and measure hospital efficiencies. So, the study attempts to find out what portion of general hospitals are operating efficiently and, for those inefficient hospitals, what inputs and outputs contribute most to inefficiency.

MATERIALS AND METHODS

Data and Data Sources

Input and output data were obtained from the Provincial Department of Health, Kwazulu Natal, Health Informatics Bulletin (HIB). The data are for the period March 1995 to April 1996. There were 56 provincial hospitals. Fifty-five of these hospitals had inputs and outputs greater than zero and therefore were included in the study. In this study, hospitals were assumed to produce mainly four types of outputs as follows: (1) inpatient days, (2) outpatient department visits, (3) surgical operations, and (4) live births. Nine inputs were included in the computation of efficiency scores as follows: (1) number of medical doctors, (2) number of nurses, (3) number of paramedics, (4) number of technicians, (5) number of administrative staff, (6) number of general staff, (7) number of labour provisioning staff, (8) other types of staff, and (9) number of beds. The selection of the above-mentioned variables was influenced by availability of data on these hospitals in public reports. Data on health technology resources (such as drugs, medical supplies, biomedical equipment, etc) were not available in the HIB.

Analytical/Conceptual Framework

What is efficiency?

Mooney [3, p.9] defines efficiency as maximising the benefit (however defined) to society at large from the resources available (however constrained). Culyer [4] sees efficiency as providing such a mix of effective services at least resource cost and on such a scale that the benefit from having more resources is no larger than their cost. The overall or total economic efficiency (TEE) of a hospital consists of two components: technical efficiency (TE), which reflects the ability of a hospital to produce maximum output (e.g., inpatient days, outpatient department visits, number of surgical operations, and number of live births) from a given set of inputs (e.g., supplies, labour, and medical technology); and allocative efficiency (AE), which reflects the ability of a hospital to use the inputs in optimal proportions given their respective prices. Total economic efficiency is the product of *TE* and *AE*. Thus, a hospital is defined to be technically inefficient if it could have produced the same amount and quality of patient care with fewer resources than it consumed or if it could have produced greater amounts of its outputs with the same amount of resources it used [5]. This study concentrates only on the measurement of TE due to inaccessibility of input prices.

The DEA model

Data envelopment analysis is a linear programming technique for measuring the relative performance of organisational units (e.g., hospitals) where the presence of multiple incommensurate inputs and outputs makes comparison difficult [6]. DEA simultaneously analyses the efficiency with which each decision-making unit (the hospital in this study) uses inputs to produce its outputs. DEA identifies the optimal input/output combination and represents it with the "best practice frontier" or data envelope. DMUs that compose this frontier are assigned a score of one and are technically efficient relative to their peers. All other DMUs are assigned a score of between zero and one. The higher the TE score, the greater the TE of the DMU.

According to Boussofiane et al [6], if a DMU (i.e., a hospital) has a single input and a single output, *TE* is simply defined as:

$$TE = Output / Input \qquad (1)$$

However, in a more typical scenario of multiple hospitals with multiple inputs and outputs, the equation is modified as follows:

$$Efficiency = Weighted\ sum\ of\ outputs / Weighted\ sum\ of\ inputs \qquad (2)$$

Algebraically, the efficiency (E_k) score of a target hospital k can be obtained by solving the model developed by Charnes *et al* [7]:

$$Maximum \quad E_k = \left(\sum_{r=1}^{t} \mu_r Y_{rjk} \bigg/ \sum_{i=1}^{m} v_i X_{ijk} \right) \tag{3}$$

Subject to:

$$\left(\sum_{r=1}^{t} \mu_r Y_{rjk} \bigg/ \sum_{i=1}^{m} v_i X_{ijk} \right) \leq 1, j = 1, 2, ..., n \quad hospitals$$

$$\mu_r, v_i \geq \varepsilon, \quad \forall r \quad \text{and} \quad i$$

Where:

k = the hospital being evaluated in the set of $j = 1, ..., n$ hospitals

Y_{rj} = observed amount of rth ($r = 1, .., s$) output for the jth hospital

X_{ij} = observed amount of ith ($i = 1, .., r$) input for the jth hospital.

u_r = coefficient/weight for output r to be determined from the data by the above model

v_i = coefficient/weight for input i to be determined from the data by the above model

n = number of hospitals in the sample

t = the number of outputs

m = the number of inputs

ε = a small positive number

This study used the DEAP Version 2.1 computer programme developed by Coelli [8] to estimate equation (3) repetitively with each hospital in the sample to derive individual efficiency ratings. These efficiency ratings are presented in the following section. However, the hospital names are disguised, but real names can be made available to the Kwazulu-Natal Provincial Department of Health leadership for information.

RESULTS

The DEA results are summarised in Table 9.1, which indicates that 60% out of 55 hospitals are technically efficient, while 40% are relatively inefficient compared with the other hospitals in the data set; that is, they have a TE rating of less than 1.0. The technically inefficient hospitals should be able to produce their same level of services (outputs) with fewer inputs, and therefore, at lower cost. Average technical efficiency (TE) is 0.906. That is, on average the hospitals should be able to reduce the consumption of all inputs by 9.4 per cent without reducing output levels.

The meaning of the inefficient rating derived from DEA can be understood by examining the results for hospital 9. Data envelopment analysis indicates that hospital 9 is inefficient with a pure technical inefficiency rating of 0.597. Generally, this means that hospital 9 should be able to produce its actual outputs levels using 40.3% ([1.000 – 0.597] × 100) less of each input. More specifically, DEA indicates that the inefficiency was located and measured by comparing hospital 9 with its efficiency reference set (ERS) hospitals 23, 25, 26, 48, and 55 noted in Table 9.1. The efficiency reference set is the group of hospitals against which DEA located the inefficient hospitals and the magnitude of inefficiency.[1] This information is a direct output of DEA.

By identifying the efficiency reference set, DEA allows one to focus on a subset of these hospitals to understand better the inefficiencies present. This comparison is illustrated in Table 9.2, which indicates that a weighted composite of the ERS hospitals would yield a hypothetical hospital that produces as much or more outputs as the inefficient hospital 9 but also uses less inputs than hospital 9. In this example, the composite is constructed by applying the weights (the dual variables from the DEA-linear programme) of 0.313, 0.020, 0.115, 0.338, and 0.213 respectively to the actual outputs and inputs of hospitals 23, 25, 26, 48, and 55. Columns F, G, and H of Table 9.2 indicate that a combination of the actual operations of these five hospitals would result in a hypothetical hospital that would use 1.6 fewer medical doctors, 53 fewer nurses, 4 fewer paramedics, 0.4 fewer technicians, 14.7 fewer administrative staff, 29.8 fewer general staff, 56.6 fewer labour provisioning staff, 1 fewer other staff, and 73.1 fewer beds to produce the same amount of patient care than were produced by the inefficient hospital 9.

---

[1] These ERS hospitals are the basis vectors of the linear programme solution; that is, a convex combination of the actual outputs and inputs of these ERS hospitals results in a composite hospital that produces as much or more outputs as the inefficient hospital while using fewer inputs than the inefficient hospital (Table 9.2).

Table 9.1   DEA efficiency rating of general hospitals in Kwazulu-Natal Province

Hospital	Technical efficiency Score	Scale efficiency Score	Efficiency reference set/ peers
1,2,4,5,7,8,14,15,18, 20,23, 25,26,28,34,39, 44,46,48,50,53,54,55	1.000	1.000	
3	0.987	0.967	48,46,7,26,54
6	0.757	0.999	54,50,7,4,46,26
9	0.597	0.971	26,55,23,25,48
10	1.000	0.702	10
11	0.994	0.740	50,35,44,54,28
12	0.801	0.962	26,45,14,50,48
13	0.589	0.997	25,48,2,23,4,50,7
16	0.984	0.957	26,48,55,45
17	1.000	0.996	17
19	0.818	0.996	7,26,46,28,54
21	0.852	0.884	53,41,20,28,10,54,50
22	0.528	0.921	55,25,41,28,2,7
24	0.532	0.985	50,26,54,2,28,23
27	0.823	0.998	48,50,28,26,55,7,2
29	0.874	0.977	15,26,50,45,28,48
30	0.916	0.986	23,7,2,50,28
31	1.000	0.933	31
32	1.000	0.877	32
33	1.000	0.906	33
35	1.000	0.789	35
36	0.795	0.954	15,44,14,28
37	0.549	0.998	4,50,25,46,26,54,48
38	1.000	0.804	38
40	0.533	0.992	15,44,26,28,50,48
41	1.000	0.859	41
42	0.699	0.978	45,50,28,7,26
43	0.842	0.883	10,54,50,38,28
45	1.000	0.941	45
47	0.929	0.973	48,26,55,25
49	0.780	0.745	14,44,26,48
51	0.643	0.894	7,50,48,28,45
52	1.000	0.807	52
Mean	0.906	0.953	

Table 9.2   Comparison of Hospital 9 with its efficiency reference set hospitals 23, 25, 26, 48, and 55

Inputs	(A) Hospital 23	(B) Hospital 25	(C) Hospital 26	(D) Hospital 48	(E) Hospital 55	(F) Composite = A+B+C+D+E	(G) Hospital 9	H=(G)-(F) Excess Inputs
Doctors	3^a x 0.313^b	0^a x 0.020^b	7^a x 0.115^b	0^a x 0.338^b	3^a x 0.213^b	2.38	4^a	1.62
Nurses	71^a x 0.313^b	80^a x 0.020^b	175^a x 0.115^b	17^a x 0.338^b	136^a x 0.213^b	78.66	132^a	53.34
Paramedics	1^a x 0.313^b	0^a x 0.020^b	2^a x 0.115^b	0^a x 0.338^b	2^a x 0.213^b	0.97	5^a	4.03
Technicians	0^a x 0.313^b	1^a x 0.020^b	5^a x 0.115^b	0^a x 0.338^b	0^a x 0.213^b	0.60	1^a	0.40
Administrative staff	12^a x 0.313^b	2^a x 0.020^b	22^a x 0.115^b	2^a x 0.338^b	20^a x 0.213^b	11.26	26^a	14.74
General staff	32^a x 0.313^b	22^a x 0.020^b	57^a x 0.115^b	10^a x 0.338^b	65^a x 0.213^b	34.24	64^a	29.76
Labour provisioning staff	43^a x 0.313^b	56^a x 0.020^b	81^a x 0.115^b	16^a x 0.338^b	71^a x 0.213^b	44.43	101^a	56.57
Other staff	0^a x 0.313^b	0^a x 0.020^b	0^a x 0.115^b	0^a x 0.338^b	0^a x 0.213^b	0.000	1^a	1
Beds	134^a x 0.313^b	96^a x 0.020^b	205^a x 0.115^b	44^a x 0.338^b	120^a x 0.213^b	107.87	181^a	73.13

Notes:

Hospital 9's DEA technical efficiency rating = 0.597

[a] Actual inputs and outputs as per Appendix 1

[b] Lambda weights (dual variables) from DEA

Table 9.3 Input reductions needed to make inefficient hospitals efficient in Kwazulu-Natal Province

Hospital Code	Doctors	Nurses	Paramedics	Technicians	Administrative staff	General staff	Labour provisioning staff	Other staff	Beds
					Excessive inputs based on DEA evaluation				
3	1.835	1.509	1.738	0.231	0.176	3.667	11.628	0.013	13.419
6	8.132	92.616	0.917	3.99	9.166	19.224	19.711	4.356	101.239
9	1.614	53.246	4.03	0.403	14.724	29.726	56.529	1.000	73.011
11	0.238	232.402	2.09	14.741	23.439	125.157	146.914	3.145	2.747
12	3.251	28.227	1.53	2.813	5.335	16.31	15.961	1.626	36.974
13	3.568	135.316	0.823	0.823	12.487	23.043	69.72	0.41	152.594
16	0.062	1.63	0.647	0.259	2.967	8.162	8.151	0.000	1.987
19	1.834	35.102	0.364	3.251	7.112	13.114	20.424	0.546	66.709
21	6.955	179.14	0.741	1.037	6.373	17.785	89.26	0.909	185.17
22	2.832	308.605	1.986	1.888	13.169	51.441	70.514	0.944	225
24	4.788	125.401	3.521	1.404	36.842	59.381	88.117	1.449	168.449
27	1.088	34.982	0.353	0.53	4.616	15.194	23.246	0.582	40.635
29	1.14	25.765	0.88	1.336	3.142	9.552	48.512	0.272	31.546
30	0.82	13.172	3.441	0.168	11.082	7.497	36.872	0.084	22.644
36	25.854	498.261	9.438	4.566	25.598	145.666	210.064	7.539	38.955
37	4.061	121.262	2.538	2.708	20.059	39.712	71.021	2.534	151.629
40	26.365	269.596	13.48	7.475	20.086	76.138	74.659	4.653	156.947
42	2.605	99.456	1.583	2.955	9.514	20.456	24.066	1.602	84.841
43	12.857	297.743	9.272	1.424	38.649	54.599	45.044	3.973	96.181
47	2.239	55.93	0.071	0.141	10.953	33.375	30.028	0.000	8.843
49	3.075	27.444	0.468	4.572	7.572	38.507	13.33	0.794	22.395
51	2.22	72.463	1.278	1.071	12.137	27.633	19.634	1.573	69.967

DISCUSSION

Key Findings Related to Technical Efficiency

The overall average level of TE among Kwazulu-Natal hospitals is 90.6%. Forty per cent of the hospitals had some degree of technical inefficiency. Twenty-seven per cent of the technically inefficient facilities had a TE score of between 0.51 and 0.60; nine per cent between 0.61 and 0.70; eighteen per cent between 0.71 and 0.80; twenty-three per cent between 0.81 and 0.90; and twenty-three per cent between 0.91 and 0.99. These results imply that the facilities in the above-mentioned inefficiency groups should be able to reduce the use of all inputs by 44.5%, 34.5%, 24.5%, 14.5%, and 5% respectively without reducing levels of their outputs. The specific amounts of input reductions required to make inefficient hospitals technically efficient are listed in Table 9.3. In connection with these excess resources that are currently wasted and not utilised in the production of hospital outputs, there are a number of policy options available to the provincial health system managers:

1. Do nothing and continue the wasteful status quo situation.

2. Options related to excess beds and space are to either (*a*) sell the excess beds and the space they are occupying or (*b*) rent the excess beds and space to private health practitioners if there is demand.

3. Options related to excess non-technical staff include (*a*) voluntary retrenchment with "golden-hand-shakes"; (*b*) forced retrenchment with severance packages; (*c*) reallocate the excess labour force to underserved areas of the province; and (*d*) reallocate the excess labour force to understaffed primary healthcare facilities. The decision criteria would be to opt for retrenchment, if and only if, the cost (in terms of severance packages) is less than or equal to the benefits (in terms of personnel cost savings). The magnitude of savings will depend on the number of years remaining before retirement (for each of the employees concerned), the magnitudes of remunerations, the nature of contracts, and cooperation of the trade unions among others.

4. Options related to excess technical staff; the four options mentioned under (3) would also be applicable here. It is the opinion of these authors that given the infancy state of primary health care in the Province and in South Africa in general [9], it would NOT be cost-effective to offer technical staff the option of early retirement. Instead, excess technical staff should be transferred to the Primary Healthcare System either within or outside the province which would increase coverage and quality of services provided in the peripheral health facilities.

5. Closure of some hospitals: holding equity and political concerns constant, the policy makers could opt to close down those healthcare

facilities with efficiency scores below a certain threshold (to be decided upon by the policy makers).

6. Conversion of hospitals into PHC facilities; this last option would entail conversion of hospitals into community health centres or clinics. Of course, if this option were to be pursued there would be need to work out the details of the conversion process.

Key Findings Related to Scale Efficiency

Hospitals with a scale efficiency (SE) of one are said to have the most productive size for that particular input-output mix [10,11]. In this study, the average SE was ninety-five per cent (see Table 9.1). Of the 55 hospitals in the data set, 24 exhibited constant returns to scale (CRS); which means they were operating at their most productive scale sizes. Of the rest, 16 exhibited increasing returns to scale (IRS) and the other 16 operated under decreasing returns to scale (DRS). Thus, in total thirty-two of the hospitals in the province had some degree of scale inefficiency. Three per cent of those facilities had a scale efficiency ranging between 0.51 and 0.60; three per cent between 0.61 and 0.70; nine per cent between 0.71 and 0.80; twenty-two per cent between 0.81 and 0.90; and sixty-three per cent between 0.91 and 0.99. When scale efficiency is less than one, the implication is that the hospital is not operating at the most productive scale size for its observed input mix. In order to operate at the most productive scale size (MPSS), a hospital exhibiting DRS should scale down both outputs and inputs. Similarly, if a hospital is showing IRS it should expand both outputs and inputs.

Limitations of the Study

1. We were not able to verify whether the ERS facilities had exactly the same standards in terms of type of services provided, severity of cases treated, qualification and number of staff, working schedules (number of work days, length of working days, and daily work patterns), functional building capacity, healthcare technology, etc.

2. The analysis assumes that the case mix of a specific hospital and its ERS hospitals is similar. We were not able to verify whether that assumption was plausible. However, given that the hospitals in the data set were all non-teaching and non-specialist hospitals, the above assumption would most likely hold.

3. It could rightly be argued that the objective function of the hospital sector is to maximise health gains from the available resources, and that the ideal output indicator would be the one that captures in a sensitive, valid, reliable, and culturally acceptable manner changes in both quantity and health-related quality of lives of those who interact with public hospitals. Given the unavailability of data on either disability-adjusted life years (DALYs) saved or quality-adjusted life years (QALYs) [12]

gained due to care in each of the hospitals in the data set, we opted to use proxies that have been used in similar studies.

4. Hospitals could be argued to produce deaths through negligence, human errors, and nosocomial infections. In this study we did not include the number of hospital deaths.

5. As noted by Professor Mills [13], hospitals have an important supportive role in terms of supervision of lower level facilities and referrals. However, given that this analysis was based on secondary data, it was not possible to quantify the amounts of hospital inputs used when executing their supervisory role. The patients referred from clinics to the hospitals are included in the latter's caseload; and thus, there is no need for special consideration.

6. There may be variation in quality of care from one health facility to another (e.g., those facilities offering higher quality of care may require more personnel time and other inputs than those offering low quality of care). Given that this study was based on secondary data, it was not possible to determine whether there was any variance in quality of care across the facilities.

7. If a hospital is effective in providing preventive care (better health promotion activities; better hygiene, better human environment management, better disposal of human waste, etc) in the catchment area, the demand for curative care would be expected to decrease and such a hospital could be wrongly interpreted as being inefficient. In addition, if a hospital is effectively supporting PHC facilities in its vicinity, this would most likely increase the perceived quality of the latter and in the process reduce demand for services from the former. This implies that there is need to extend TE analysis of hospitals beyond the hospital compounds into the catchment areas and, specifically, into the peripheral healthcare facilities supported by such hospitals. The authors of this study were not able to do the above.

Suggestions for Further Research

There is urgent need for:

1. A facility-based survey to determine whether there is any systematic relationship between efficiency score and the level of quality of care (as perceived by both patients and clinicians).

2. Analysis of both technical and allocative efficiency of PHC facilities in Kwazulu-Natal Province.

3. Analysis of both technical and allocative efficiency of hospitals and PHC facilities in all other provinces of South Africa.

4. Conducting similar studies in other SSA countries with a view to informing policy action.

5.   Application of DEA to test the hypothesis that health facilities run by non-governmental organisations (NGOs) are more efficient than those run by government.

6.   Monitoring and evaluation of different forms of healthcare reforms on efficiency of healthcare facilities.

CONCLUSION

In this study we analysed the input-output data from fifty-five non-teaching/non-specialist public hospitals from Kwazulu-Natal Province of South Africa. We attempted to find out what proportion of those hospitals were operating technically efficiently and for those inefficient hospitals, what inputs and outputs contributed most to inefficiency. Sixty per cent out of the fifty-five hospitals were technically efficient. Forty per cent of the hospitals had some degree of technical inefficiency. Fifty-eight per cent were scale inefficient.

A summary of the total amounts of specific inputs that were wasted and not utilised in the production of hospital outputs in Kwazulu-Natal Province public hospitals were as follows:

- 117.4 doctors (8.0%);

- 2,709 nurses (11.9%);

- 61 paramedics (11.5%);

- 58 technicians (13.1%);

- 295 administrative staff (11.1%);

- 835 general staff (11.3%);

- 1,193 labour provisioning staff (14.3%);

- 38 other staff (10.7%); and

- 1,752 beds (7.1%).

Those are the specific input reductions required to make inefficient hospitals technically efficient. It would be economically rational for policy makers to consider compulsory retirement of the excess administrative, general, labour provisioning, and other general support staff. The doctors, nurses, paramedics, and technicians could (with some orientational training) be reallocated to the primary healthcare system (especially in the underserved rural areas). It would be unwise to offer the technical staff the option of early retirement; simply because their services are needed in other parts of the province and country.

In a nutshell, this study has demonstrated that 40% of public hospitals in Kwazulu-Natal are using more resources than is necessary for an effective impact, which is wasteful and inconsistent with the objective of maximising communities' health gains from the available healthcare resources. Thus in the words of Professor Anthony J. Culyer [4], it is unethical to be inefficient (and ethical to be efficient). For if more than necessary is used, the excess could have been used at no cost to the patients in question in order to further the health of some other patients. Thus, overall community health (whose maximisation is our postulated ethical imperative) is lower than it need be.

As researchers, we are well aware, of course, that efficiency analyses (like the one reported in this paper) are only a guide to decision making and ultimately the property rights over decision making lies with the policy makers at the Provincial and National Departments of Health. However, in deciding whether or not to take necessary measures to reduce the inefficiencies revealed by efficiency analyses, policy makers should take note of Professor Gavin Mooney's caution that "The price of inefficiency, inexplicitness and irrationality in health care is paid in death and sickness" [3, p.55].

ACKNOWLEDGEMENT

We owe profound gratitude to the leadership of the Department of Health, Kwazulu-Natal Province, for having sent Kirigia the data set used in this study while he was still teaching at the University of Cape Town. We dedicate this paper to the South African National and Provincial Departments of Health who are striving to maximise health gains from the available resources for the benefit of all South Africans. Lastly, we would like to thank Jehovah Rapha for ultimately being our healer. The opinions expressed in this paper and any mistakes are the authors' and should not be attributed to either the WHO or to any of the acknowledged persons.

REFERENCES

1. Gilson L, Mills A. Health sector reforms in sub-Saharan Africa: lessons of the last 10 years. *Health Policy* 1995;32:215-243.

2. Gilson L. Managem*ent and healthcare reform in Sub-Saharan Africa.* Social Science and Medicine 1995;40(5):698-710.

3. Mooney GH. *Economics, medicine and health care*. New York: Harvester Wheatsheaf; 1986.

4. Culyer AJ. The morality of efficiency in health care: some uncomfortable implications. *Health Economics* 1992;1(1):7-18.

5. Sherman HD. Hospital efficiency measurement and evaluation. *Medical Care* 1984;22(10):922-938.

6. Bussofiane A, Dyson RG, Thanassoulis E. Applied data envelopment analysis. *European Journal of Operational Research* 1991;52(1):1-15.

7. Charnes A, Cooper WW, Rhodes E. Measuring the efficiency of decision making units. *European Journal of Operational Research* 1978;2(6):429-444.

8. Coelli T. *A guide to DEAP version 2.1: a data envelopment analysis (computer) program*, Centre for Efficiency and Productivity Analysis (CEPA) Working Paper 96/08. Department of Econometrics, University of New England, Armidale, NSW Australia; 1996.

9. Kacheing'a MO. *Healthcare technology assessment in sub-Saharan Africa: a cross-national study of Kenya and South Africa* [PhD Thesis]. Cape Town (South Africa): University of Cape Town, Department of Biomedical Engineering; 1999.

10. Banker RD, Charness A, Cooper WW. Some models for estimating technical and scale efficiencies in data envelopment analysis. *Management Science* 1984;30(1):1078-1092.

11. Banker RD, Conrad RF, Strauss RP. A comparative application of data envelopment analysis and translog methods: an illustrative study of hospital production. *Management Science* 1986;32(1):30-44.

12. Kirigia JM. Health impacts of epidemiological environment change: measurement issues. *Environment and Development Economics* 1996;1(3):359-367.

13. Mills A. The economics of hospitals in developing countries: part II: costs and sources of income. *Health Policy and Planning* 1990;5(3):203-218.

-10-

Technical Efficiency of Public Clinics
in Kwazulu-Natal Province of South Africa*

Joses M. Kirigia, Luis G. Sambo and Helga Scheel

ABSTRACT

Background: In sub-Saharan Africa (SSA) much of the attention of policy makers, healthcare managers, health systems researchers, and donors is focussed almost solely on mobilising additional resources and not on efficiency in their use.

Objective(s): To investigate the technical inefficiencies among 155 primary healthcare clinics in Kwazulu-Natal Province of South Africa and to draw policy implications.

Design: Cross-sectional provincial health clinic survey.

Setting: Kwazulu-Natal Provincial Department of Health Clinics survey, 1996.

Subjects: The analysis is based on 155 public clinics.

Interventions: Non-intervention data envelopment analysis (DEA) study.

Main outcome measures: Technical and scale efficiency scores.

Results: Forty-seven (30%) public clinics were found to be technically efficient. Among the 108 (70%) technically inefficient facilities, 16% had an efficiency score of 50% or less. The presence of inefficiencies indicates that a clinic has excess inputs or insufficient outputs

---

* The original article appeared in *East African Medical Journal* 2001;78(3):S1-S13. Reproduced with the permission of East African Medical Journal (EAMJ).

compared to those clinics on the efficiency frontier. To achieve technical efficiency, Kwazulu-Natal clinics would, in total, have to decrease inputs by 417 nurses and 457 general staff. Alternatively, outputs would have to be increased by 115,534 antenatal visits, 1,010 births (deliveries), 179,075 childcare visits, 5,702 dental visits, 121,658 family planning visits, 36,032 psychiatric visits, 56,068 sexually transmitted disease visits, and 34,270 tuberculosis visits.

Conclusion: There is need for more detailed studies in a number of the relatively efficient clinics to determine why they are efficient with a view to documenting attributes of "best practice" that other clinics can emulate. The potential benefit of replicating this kind of study in other provinces, and indeed, other SSA countries cannot be overemphasised.

Key words: data envelopment analysis, technical efficiency, scale efficiency

INTRODUCTION

In every developing country decisive steps are needed to correct the pervasive inefficiency of clinical health programmes and facilities and especially of government services. World Bank [1]

As we begin the twenty-first century, sub-Saharan Africa (SSA) healthcare systems are still facing numerous threats including increasing demands for quality care; severe budgetary constraints; over-concentration of resources on high-level health facilities that benefit relatively few people [1]; skewed distribution of healthcare resources between geographical regions [2]; health inequalities; limited responsiveness to clients' rational expectations; unfair financing systems [3,4]; and inefficient use of healthcare resources leading to inflation in costs of service delivery, and hence, undermining health sector reform benefits [5].

In spite of the above threats, we do believe that this century offers opportunities for improving health, reducing health inequalities, enhancing the level and distribution of responsiveness to clients' rational expectations, and developing fair systems of financing in SSA. In our opinion, the greatest challenge facing health policy makers is the extent to which health systems are using the available resources without wastage in achieving the above-mentioned health system goals. Our concern with efficient use of resources derives from the immorality of inefficiency. An inefficient health system is unethical because it denies other people an opportunity to improve their health status at no extra cost to the providers.

One of the key challenges facing health systems analysts in this century is to conduct micro-level efficiency analyses that would enable health policy makers and managers to identify the magnitudes by which some inputs in individual health facilities or programmes could be reduced without a reduction in output(s). So far, the attention of policy makers, healthcare managers, health systems analysts, and donors has been focussed on mobilising additional resources and not on efficiency in their use. This explains the dearth of literature on the subject of health sector micro-level efficiency analyses in sub-Saharan Africa.

In 1995/1996 financial year, the overall South African health budget amounted to 16.1 billion rand. Sixty-eight per cent of the budget was allocated to tertiary, regional, community, and specialised (e.g., psychiatric, TB, etc) hospitals; and 19% to primary health care [2]. Thus, in general health facilities absorbed over 80% of the total budget. This is why we have chosen to focus on technical efficiency of health facilities. Our first analysis dealt with technical efficiency of public hospitals in Kwazulu-Natal Province [5]. This study deals with the same problem, but among primary health care clinics.

Efficiency of a health facility consists of two strands: technical efficiency (TE) and allocative efficiency (AE) [6]. Technical efficiency reflects the ability of a facility to obtain maximum output(s) from a given set of inputs. Thus, a facility is said to be technically inefficient if it is possible to either increase output without increasing any input or decreasing any output. Allocative efficiency reflects the ability of a facility to use inputs in optimal proportions given their respective prices [7].

The objectives of this study were to investigate the technical inefficiencies among PHC clinics in Kwazulu-Natal Province of South Africa and to draw policy implications. The paper describes the data and DEA conceptual framework and presents the empirical results. The last section contains some implications for policy, suggestions for further research, and the conclusion.

MATERIALS AND METHODS

Conceptual Framework

The two principal methods for estimating the production frontiers are (*a*) the parametric approach that uses econometric methods [8-10] and (*b*) the non-parametric approach that uses linear programming techniques [6,7] such as data envelopment analysis (DEA). In this study, we used the DEA approach because it focuses on each clinic in contrast to parametric population or sample averages; produces a single efficiency measure for each clinic in terms of input-output relationships; can simultaneously handle multiple inputs and multiple outputs without the requirement for homogeneous measurement units; can adjust for exogenous variables that are beyond the control of the decision-making unit; does not require an assumption of a functional form relating inputs to outputs; produces estimates for desired changes in inputs and outputs for getting the inefficient clinics onto the efficient frontier; and focuses on observed best-practice frontiers rather than on central tendency properties of frontiers [11,12].

The following two linear programming problems were estimated using EMS DEA software [13]. The first problem (1) is a standard constant returns to scale (CRS) model [11]:

$$Max \quad h_0 = \sum_{r=1}^{t} u_r y_{rj^0} \tag{1}$$

Subject to: $\sum_{r=1}^{m} v_i x_{ij^0} = 1$

$$\sum_{r=1}^{t} u_r y_{rj} - \sum_{=r}^{m} v_i x_{ij} \leq 0, \quad j = 1,...,n,$$

$$-u_r \leq -\varepsilon, \quad r = 1,...,t$$

$$-v_r \leq -\varepsilon, \quad r = 1,...,m$$

Where:

y_{rj} = the amount of output r produced by clinic j,

x_{ij} = the amount of input i used by clinic j,

u_r = the weight given to output r,

v_i = the weight given to input i,

n = the number of clinics,

t = the number of outputs,

m = the number of inputs,

ε = a small positive number.

The last constraint means that all clinics (i.e., decision-making units) are either on or below the frontier. The second problem (2) is a variable returns to scale model:

$$Max \quad h_0 = \sum u_r y_{rj^0} + u_0 \tag{2}$$

Subject to: $\sum v_i x_{ij^0} = 1$

$$\sum u_r y_{rj} - \sum v_i x_{ij} + u_0 \leq 0, \quad j = 1,...,N$$

$$u_r v_i \geq 0$$

From (2) it is possible to derive scale efficiency; that is, whether the clinics are operating on an optimal scale of production or not. In this study, following the guidance provided by Coelli [7], the scale efficiency score for each individual clinic was obtained by dividing its constant returns to scale efficiency score by the corresponding variable returns to scale efficiency score.

Data

Input and output data were obtained from the Provincial Department of Health, Kwazulu-Natal, Health Informatics Bulletin [14]. The data cover the period between March 1995 and April 1996. The 155 clinics in the province which had inputs and outputs greater than zero were included in the study. In this study, clinics were assumed to produce mainly eight types of intermediate outputs as follows: antenatal visits, number of births/deliveries, child health visits, dental care visits, family planning visits, psychiatry visits, sexually transmitted disease visits, and tuberculosis treatment visits. The two inputs included in the estimation of efficiency scores were number of nurses and number of general staff (including administrative, subordinate, and labour provisioning staff). The selection of the above-mentioned variables was guided by the availability of data in the Health Informatics Bulletin.

Data Entry and Analysis Procedure

Step A: The inputs and outputs data were entered on Excel spreadsheet as follows: names of clinics in column 1; Input1{I}, i.e., number of nurses in column 2; Input2{I}, i.e., number of general staff (including administrative, subordinate, and labour provisioning staff) in column 3; Output1{O}, i.e., antenatal care visits in column 4; Output2{O}, i.e., number of deliveries/births in column 5; Output3{O}, i.e., number of child healthcare visits in column 6; Output4{O}, i.e., number of dental care visits in column 7; Output5 {O}, i.e., number of family planning visits in column 8; Output6 {O}, i.e., number of psychiatry visits in column 9; Output7 {O}, i.e., number of sexually transmitted diseases-related care visits in column 10; and Output8 {O}, i.e., number of tuberculosis-related visits in column 11.

Step B: Click on **Start, Program,** and **EMS** - this will open a window containing five items (File, Edit, DEA, Window, and Help) at the top right-hand corner.

Step C: Click on **File** and then on **Load Data** - you will be prompted to type "Filename", e.g., C:\HEC\WHO8.XLS and to indicate "File Type", e.g. "Excel 5.0 (*.xls)" or "Text (*.txt)".

Step D: At the EMS menu click on **Open**. If the data retrieval process has been successful, "Input Output Data C:\HEC\WHO8.XLS" will appear at the bottom left-hand corner of the window.

Step E: Click on **DEA** and then on **Run Model**. This will lead you to a window titled "E Run Model Window". At the menu, select **Model**. The programme will take you to a window containing "Structure" with a choice between convex and non-convex models; "Returns to Scale", that is, constant, variable, non-increasing, or non-decreasing; "Distance", that is, radial or additive; and "Orientation" - input or output. Once you have made your choices, click on the **Start** icon for the model to run. The EMS, in a few seconds, will produce a sheet containing results, which include DMU name, efficiency score, DEA weights/multipliers, peers/benchmarks, slacks per input, and slacks per output.

Step F: Note that in an input-oriented DEA model, excess input equals radial reduction plus slacks. Firstly, add individual variable's slacks across all the DMUs or clinics. If you are using Excel software simply go to the bottom of the column containing slacks for a specific input and click on the summation sign (Σ). Of course, if there are some empty cells, having clicked on Σ in the menu, one will need to manually specify the range [e.g., =sum(P2:P156)]. Secondly, since the technical efficiency score indicates how the DMUs or clinics can reduce their inputs, the radial reduction (RR) is defined as specific input's absolute quantity (Q) minus efficiency score (TE) times specific input's absolute quantity (Q), that is, $RR = [Q - (TE \times Q)]$.

Step G: Scale efficiency score = CRS score ÷ VRS score. Thus, to obtain scale efficiency score, you will need to run the EMS model twice (i.e., using CRS and VRS model specifications). After the technical efficiency estimations, the following null hypothesis, "H0: vectors of variable means are equal for the two groups (efficient and inefficient) of clinics", was tested using 2-group Hotelling's T-squared generalised means test. The tests were conducted using STATA [15] software.

RESULTS

The means and standard deviations of input and output variables for both efficient and inefficient clinics are presented in Table 10.1. The 2-group Hotelling's T-squared generalised means test yielded a T-squared of 39.39 which was greater than $F_{(10,144)}$ test statistic of 3.707 at 0.0002% level. This result indicates that the means for efficient and inefficient groups are significantly different at the 0.0002% level.

Table 10.1 Means and standard deviations for various variables

Variable	Efficient clinics (n=47)		Inefficient clinics (n=108)	
	Mean	Standard deviation	Mean	Standard deviation
Number of nursing staff	11.43	19.24	7.57	9.08
Number of general staff (including administrative, general, and labour provisioning staff)	10.92	14.53	8.67	8.90
Number of antenatal visits	4,788.23	6,380.23	2,124.66	1,869.87
Number of births	199.09	489.17	63.19	81.85
Number of child health visits	5,900.79	6,127.09	3,510.95	2,486.2
Number of dental care visits	999.28	3,171.88	57.21	229.56
Number of family planning visits	4,704.38	15,261.75	1,927.71	2,260.74
Number of psychiatry visits	472.09	668.29	330.23	449.09
Number of sexually transmitted disease visits	1,672.64	3,106.04	681.01	750.23
Number of tuberculosis visits	1,536.62	4,594.29	350.17	962.34

Table 10.2 summarises the distribution of clinics by their technical and scale efficiency scores. Forty-seven (30%) of the clinics were technically efficient since their efficiency scores were equal to one. Twenty-five (16%) of these facilities manifested 100% scale efficiency. Among the 108 (70%) technically inefficient facilities, 16% had an efficiency score of 50% or less. To enhance readers' understanding of these results, let us use Clinic 1 as an example. We note that the technical efficiency score for Clinic 1 (in Appendix 10.1) is 60%. This implies that, Clinic 1 should be able to reduce the utilisation of all inputs by 40% without reducing any output. Technical efficiency and scale efficiency scores for individual clinics are presented in Appendix 10.1. Table 10.3 shows total output increases and input reductions needed to make inefficient clinics efficient. Output increases and input reductions needed to make each inefficient clinic efficient are presented in Appendices 10.2 and 10.3.

Appendices 10.4 and 10.5 summarise the linear probability and logistic model results of the regression analyses conducted to determine the causal-effect relationship between technical efficiency score and various explanatory variables. The linear probability model (LPM) results summarised in Appendix 10.4 should be interpreted as describing the probability that an individual clinic will be efficient given information about its output and input characteristics. The coefficients of an LPM represent the effect of a unit change in the concerned explanatory variable on the probability of a clinic being found relatively efficient. For instance, the slope coefficient for general staff was -0.097. It means that on average an increase in the total number of general staff by one would lead to a reduction in a clinic's probability of being efficient by 9.7%.

The slope coefficient for a logit model shows the impact of a unit increase in an explanatory variable (holding other factors constant) on the log of odds in favour of a clinic being relatively efficient. For example, in Appendix 10.5, the coefficient for general staff was -0.143. This means that a unit increase in number of general staff will lead to a decrease of 0.143 in the log of odds of a clinic being relatively efficient.

Table 10.2 Distribution of clinics by their technical and scale efficiency scores

Efficiency brackets (%)	Number of clinics in various technical efficiency brackets (%)	Number of clinics in various scale efficiency brackets (%)
1 – 10	1 (0.6)	0 (0.0)
11 – 20	3 (1.9)	5 (3.2)
21 – 30	4 (2.6)	10 (6.5)
31 – 40	8 (5.2)	15 (9.7)
41 – 50	8 (5.2)	26 (16.8)
51 – 60	19 (12.3)	6 (3.9)
61 – 70	31 (20.0)	16 (10.3)
71 – 80	21 (13.5)	19 (12.3)
81 – 90	9 (5.8)	11 (7.1)
91 – 99	4 (2.6)	22 (14.2)
100	47 (30.3)	25 (16.1)
Total	**155 (100)**	**155 (100)**

Note: The technical efficiency scores reported in Table 10.2 are for variable returns to scale (VRS) specifica-tion. That specification was chosen because it permits the calculation of TE devoid of these SE effects [7].

Table 10.3 Total increases in outputs and input reductions needed to make inefficient clinics efficient

Output (number of visits)	Output increases required
Antenatal care	115,534
Births	1,010
Child care	179,075
Dental care	5,702
Family planning	121,658
Psychiatric care	36,032
Sexually transmitted diseases care	56,068
Tuberculosis care	34,270

Total input reduction needed	
Input (numbers)	Excess number of inputs
Nurses	417
*General staff	457

* Includes administrative, general, and labour provisioning staff

DISCUSSION

This study used data envelopment analysis (DEA) - a mathematical programming method - to estimate technical efficiency of 155 clinics of Kwazulu/Natal Province in South Africa. Forty-seven (30%) of the clinics were found to be technically efficient. However, a significant number of the clinics (70%) were found to have varying degrees of technical inefficiency. The presence of inefficiencies indicates that a clinic has excess inputs or insufficient outputs compared to those clinics operating on the efficiency frontier. To achieve technical efficiency, Kwazulu-Natal clinics would, in total, have to reduce inputs by 417 (30.8%) nurses and 457 (31.5%) general staff (including administrative, casual and labour provisioning staff). Alternatively, outputs would have to be increased by 115,534 (25.4%) antenatal visits, 1,010 (6.2%) births (deliveries), 179,075 (27.3%) childcare visits, 5,702 (10.7%) dental visits, 121,658 (28.3%) family planning visits, 36,032 (62.3%) psychiatric visits, 56,068 (36.8%) sexually transmitted disease visits, and 34,270 (31.1%) tuberculosis visits. The prevalence and magnitudes of technical inefficiencies in the clinics are significantly smaller than those found in the public hospitals of Kwazulu/Natal Province [5].

With regard to excess inputs, the policy makers have a number of options that are not necessarily mutually exclusive:

1. Transfer the excess nurses to more efficient clinics. It would not be sensible to retrench this cadre of staff for three reasons. Firstly, society has invested a substantial amount of resources in their training. Two, given the apartheid legacy of over-investment in high-level hospital care at the expense of primary health care, it would not make sense to deplete the PHC resources further. Thirdly, in general PHC facilities offer more cost-effective services than the hospitals. Thus, as the World Bank [1,p.65] advocates: "reforms [should] entail shifting new government spending for health away from specialised personnel, equipment, and facilities at the apex of health systems and down the pyramid toward the broad base of widely accessible care in community facilities and health centres".

   Thus, it would be counter-intuitive to even contemplate transferring excess technical staff to higher-levels of care. Lastly, past studies have revealed significant technical inefficiencies in the use of the same cadre of staff among the hospitals [5].

2. Excess general staff could be sent on early retirement. The accruing savings could be used to improve terms and working conditions for the remaining staff.

3. In this century, it would make lots of economic sense to replace jobs-till-old-age-retirement with fixed shorter duration (e.g., 5 years) renewable contracts so as to give the Department of Health a greater degree of flexibility regarding employment of personnel. The renewal of contracts would then be based on objective and transparent performance appraisal and continuing need for the services of specific cadres of staff. For instance, if this kind of human resource contracting system were in place, at the end of the contractual period the excess staff (whose services are not needed in the system) would be paid their pension entitlements without the early retirement premiums.

Alternatively, the Department of Health could embark on a campaign to boost demand for antenatal visits, number of births/deliveries, child health visits, dental care visits, family planning visits, psychiatry visits, sexually transmitted disease visits, and tuberculosis treatment visits. However, such a course of action ought to be (*a*) for those services with an unmet need and (*b*) preceded by demand analyses that would enable the Department of Health to identify variables that could be changed using policy instruments to induce demand for selected services.

Limitations of the Study

1. The study did not include healthcare inputs such as pharmaceuticals, non-pharmaceutical supplies and buildings among others in the analysis.

2. The study focussed only on technical efficiency and not allocative efficiency. Thus, the scores do not capture total efficiencies or inefficiencies.

3. Since the data used are for only one year, the study does not calculate total factor productivity change and technological change.

4. The study used proxy outcome measures. One of the intrinsic goals of health systems is to improve beneficiaries' health status, and thus, the ultimate outcome of a healthcare system ought to be its effect on life expectancy and health-related quality of life of all those who come into contact with it. Therefore, ideally, we should have used indices that combine the two dimensions of health into a unitary measure. The reader can refer to Kirigia [16] for details relating to the application of quality-adjusted-life year (QALY) index in Africa and to Murray [17] for the disability-adjusted life year (DALY) index. We opted for proxy health outcome measures because of the dearth of facility-level information needed to calculate QALYs or DALYs for individual clinics.

Suggestions for Further Research

There is need for health systems researchers to conduct:

1. Detailed investigative studies in a sample of the relatively efficient health facilities to document key attributes of the "best practice". Such best practices could then be emulated by the inefficient clinics.

2. Efficiency studies in all other South African provinces and other SSA countries. Such studies should, whenever feasible, include a more exhaustive list of inputs (e.g., capital, pharmaceutical, and non-pharmaceutical supplies) than those considered in the present study.

3. Cost and allocative efficiency studies whenever data on prices of inputs are available.

4. Studies to calculate indices of total factor productivity change, technological change, technical efficiency change, and scale efficiency change [7] in countries where panel data (on more than one year) are available using the *Malmquist* DEA approach.

CONCLUSION

Data envelopment analysis not only helps healthcare policy makers and managers to answer the question, "How well are the clinics doing?" but also, "How much and in what areas could they improve?" It suggests performance targets. In addition, it identifies the clinics which are performing best and their operating practices can then be examined to establish a guide to best practice for others to emulate. The potential benefit of replicating this kind of study in other provinces, and indeed other countries in SSA, cannot be overemphasised.

REFERENCES

1. World Bank. *World development report 1993: investing in health.* Oxford: Oxford University Press; 1993.

2. Makan B, Valentine N, Kirigia JM. Looking back and looking ahead: South Africa's 1995/96 health budget. *Budget Watch* 1996;2(1):4.

3. Murray CJL, Frenk J. A WHO framework for health systems performance assessment. GPE Discussion Paper No. 6. Geneva: World Health Organization; 1996.

4. World Health Organization. *World health report 2000: health systems - improving performance.* Geneva: World Health Organization; 2000.

5. Kirigia JM, Sambo LG, Lambo E. Are public hospitals in Kwazulu/Natal Province of South Africa technically efficient? *African Journal of Health Sciences* 2000;7(3-4):25-32.

6. Farrell MJ. The measurement of productive efficiency. *Journal of the Royal Statistical Society* 1967;120:253-281.

7. Coelli T. A *guide to DEAP version 2.1: a data envelopment analysis [computer] program*, Centre for Efficiency and Productivity Analysis (CEPA) Working Paper 96/08. Department of Econometrics, University of New England; Armidale, NSW Australia.

8. Anderson DL. A statistical cost function study of public general hospitals in Kenya. *Journal of Developing Countries* 1980;14:223-235.

9. Bitran-Dicowsky R, Dunlop DW. The determinants of hospital costs: an analysis of Ethiopia. In: Mills A , Lee K, editors. Health Economics Research in Developing Countries. Oxford: Oxford University Press; 1993.

10. Wouters A. The cost and efficiency of public and private health facilities in Ogun State, Nigeria. *Health Economics* 1993;2:31-42.

11. Charness A, Cooper WW, Rhodes E. Measuring the efficiency of decision making units. *European Journal of Operational Research* 1978;2(6):429-444.

12. Nunamker TR. Using data envelopment analysis to measure the efficiency of non-profit organizations: a critical evaluation. *Managerial and Decision Economics* 1985;6(1):50-58.

13. Scheel H. *EMS data envelopment software.* Operations Research & Wirtschaftsinformatik. Dortmund: University of Dortmund; 1998.

14. South Africa Department of Health. *Health Informatics Bulletin: March 1995 to April 1996.* Pietermaritzburg: Department of Health Kwazulu-Natal; 1996.

15. STATA. *Reference Manual (STATA Release 4.0).* Texas: Stata Corporation; 1997.

16. Kirigia JM. Cost-utility of schistosomiasis intervention strategies in Kenya. *Environment and Development Economics* 1998;3:319-346.

17. Murray CJL. Quantifying the burden of disease: the technical basis for disability-adjusted life years. *Bulletin of the World Health Organization* 1994;72(3):429-445.

Appendix 10.1   *Efficiency score, scale efficiency score and excess numbers of staff*

Name of Clinic	Technical Efficiency Score	Scale Efficiency Score	Name of Clinic	Technical Efficiency Score	Scale Efficiency Score
Hlokozi	0.60	0.43	Oliviershoek	0.96	0.98
Mabaleni	1.00	0.60	Wembesi	0.36	0.98
Madlala	1.00	0.37	Dengeni	0.53	0.17
Morrison's Post	1.00	0.94	Ekubungazeleni	0.62	0.72
Ndelu	1.00	0.41	Hlengimpilo	0.62	0.13
Ntimbankulu	0.58	0.35	Mahashini	0.62	0.48
Nyangwini	1.00	0.86	Maphophoma	0.66	0.65
Pungashe	0.72	1.00	Ngqeku	0.52	0.21
St. Faiths	0.65	0.92	Njoko	0.72	0.62
Umzinto CHC	1.00	0.77	Usuthu	0.74	0.49
Bomela	0.50	0.70	Mobile 1	1.00	1.00
Gamalakhe	0.31	0.99	Dlebe	0.74	0.47
Gcilima	1.00	0.99	Ezimfabeni	0.75	0.42
Izingolweni	0.95	0.77	Altona	0.62	0.53
Ludimala	0.70	0.41	Friesgewaagt	0.63	0.80
Ntabeni	1.00	1.00	Hartland	0.84	0.62
Pisgah	0.58	0.49	Kwashoba	0.54	0.65
Caluza	0.40	0.99	Ncotshana	0.68	0.85
Gcumisa	1.00	1.00	Tobolsk	0.73	0.30
Mpophomeni	0.50	0.91	Kwamame	0.66	0.64
Mpumalanga	1.00	1.00	Lomo	0.79	0.46
Mpumuza	1.00	1.00	Mabedlana	0.78	0.43
Msunduzi	1.00	0.90	Makhosini	0.61	0.28
Ndaleni	0.82	0.70	Mpungamhlophe	0.88	0.70
Taylors Halt	0.71	0.83	Ncemane	0.68	0.39
Mobile	1.00	1.00	Nhlungwane	0.55	0.21
Imbalenhle	1.00	0.44	St. Francis	0.17	0.63
Richmond	0.66	0.98	Ulundi A	0.36	0.80
Underberg	0.28	0.74	Zilulwane	0.65	0.47
Ehlanzeni	0.35	0.39	Jozini	1.00	1.00
Cwaka	1.00	0.68	Madonela	1.00	0.47
Ethembeni	0.52	0.50	Makhathini	0.63	0.47
Gunjana	1.00	0.40	Mhlekazi	0.58	0.49
Mazebeko	0.72	0.27	Ophansi	0.81	0.62
Ngubevu	0.70	0.17	Kwamsane	1.00	1.00
Nocomboshe	0.69	0.21	Mpukunyoni	1.00	0.95
Brunville	0.41	0.90	Phelindaba	0.71	0.56
Driefontein	0.57	0.73	Zamazama	0.91	0.71
Ekuvukeni	1.00	1.00	Emanyiseni	0.89	0.44
Ezakheni No. 2	1.00	0.65	Gwaliweni	0.70	0.47
Limehill	0.77	0.55	Ndumu	0.64	0.90
Rockcliff	0.79	0.72	Shemula	0.68	0.40
Mobile 1	0.61	0.91	Mbazwana	0.70	0.54
Amazizini	0.52	0.89	Ntshongwe	0.85	0.44
Dukuza	0.55	0.77	Comm. City FP	1.00	1.00
Injisuthi	0.39	0.78	Inanda FP	0.09	0.38
Ncibindane	0.52	0.72	Goodwins	1.00	1.00
Ntabamhlophe	0.57	0.98	Kwamashu	1.00	0.91

... /cont.

Appendix 10.1 (cont.)

Name of Clinic	Technical Efficiency Score	Scale Efficiency Score	Name of Clinic	Technical Efficiency Score	Scale Efficiency Score
Lindelani	0.28	0.75	Ntinini	1.00	1.00
Molweni	0.52	0.39	Naasfarm	0.86	0.78
Ndwedwe	0.30	1.00	Osizweni 1	1.00	0.80
Ntuzuma	1.00	0.87	Thembalihle	0.45	0.98
Qadi	0.75	0.93	Madadeni 1	0.40	1.00
Rydalvale	1.00	1.00	Madadeni 5	0.47	1.00
Phoenix CHC	1.00	0.75	Dkodweni	0.52	0.28
Baniyena	1.00	0.38	Ndulinde	1.00	0.71
D State	0.62	0.98	Mobile	1.00	0.35
Dudulu	1.00	1.00	Manyane	1.00	0.26
Ekuphileni	1.00	1.00	Mfongosi	1.00	0.27
Imfume	0.68	0.62	Mntungweni	1.00	0.44
Jolivet	0.62	0.40	Mobile	0.29	0.95
Kwamakhutha	0.87	0.92	Gezinsila	0.70	0.12
Kwadengezi	0.33	0.76	Ngudwini	0.70	0.25
Magabheni	0.50	0.46	Ntumeni	0.70	0.19
Mntungwane	0.44	0.32	Osungulweni	0.73	0.31
Nkwali	0.62	0.41	Melmoth	0.99	1.00
Odidini	0.75	0.97	Dondotha	0.18	0.66
Osizweni	0.41	0.83	Ndlangubo	0.72	0.68
Umbumbulu	1.00	1.00	Ndundulu	1.00	1.00
Umlazi "V"	0.74	0.99	Ngwelezane	0.80	0.77
Umzomuhle	0.63	0.35	Nomponjwana	1.00	1.00
Zwlibomvu	0.55	0.31	Nseleni	0.11	0.84
Isandlwana	1.00	0.52	Ntambanana	0.80	0.86
Mangeni	1.00	0.43	Ntuze	0.52	1.00
Masotsheni	0.61	0.99	Halambu	1.00	1.00
Mondlo 1	0.90	0.99	Vumanhlamvu	0.60	0.69
Mondlo 2	0.79	0.47	Mthandeni	1.00	0.46
Ntababomvu	1.00	0.43			

Appendix 10.2   Input reductions needed to make inefficient clinics efficient

Name of clinic	Excess no. of nurses	Excess no. of general Staff	Name of clinic	Excess no. of nurses	Excess no. of general staff
Hlokozi	1.62	2.83	Maphophoma	1.38	2.06
Mabaleni	0.00	0.13	Ngqeku	2.38	2.86
Madlala	0.00	0.53	Njoko	1.14	1.71
Morrison's Post	0.00	0.00	Usuthu	0.77	1.54
Ndelu	0.00	0.00	Mobile 1	0.00	0.00
Ntimbankulu	1.67	2.93	Dlebe	0.77	1.53
Nyangwini	0.00	0.00	Ezimfabeni	0.76	1.53
Pungashe	1.69	2.39	Altona	1.50	2.25
St. Faiths	1.41	2.47	Friesgewaagt	1.48	2.22
Umzinto CHC	0.00	0.00	Hartland	0.47	0.94
Bomela	2.52	4.03	Kwashoba	2.28	2.74
Gamalakhe	7.55	21.43	Ncotshana	1.62	1.95
Gcilima	0.00	0.00	Tobolsk	0.80	1.60
Izingolweni	0.66	1.28	Kwamame	1.70	2.04
Ludimala	0.89	2.08	Lomo	0.64	1.29
Ntabeni	0.00	0.00	Mabedlana	0.67	1.33
Pisgah	1.67	2.93	Makhosini	1.97	2.36
Caluza	8.44	5.43	Mpungamhlophe	0.47	0.71
Gcumisa	0.00	0.00	Ncemane	1.29	1.94
Mpophomeni	4.00	2.50	Nhlungwane	2.23	2.67
Mpumalanga	0.00	0.00	St. Francis	66.58	66.58
Mpumuza	0.00	0.00	Ulundi A	6.99	5.09
Msunduzi	0.00	0.00	Zilulwane	1.39	2.09
Ndaleni	0.71	0.36	Jozini	0.00	0.00
Taylors Halt	1.43	1.15	Madonela	0.00	0.00
Mobile	0.00	0.00	Makhathini	1.48	2.58
Imbalenhle	0.00	0.00	Mhlekazi	2.12	2.96
Richmond	5.17	7.38	Ophansi	0.56	1.32
Underberg	8.58	6.44	Kwamsane	0.00	0.00
Ehlanzeni	3.89	9.72	Mpukunyoni	0.00	0.00
Cwaka	0.00	0.00	Phelindaba	1.16	2.03
Ethembeni	2.38	3.34	Zamazama	0.36	0.64
Gunjana	0.00	0.01	Emanyiseni	0.32	0.53
Mazebeko	0.85	1.99	Gwaliweni	1.19	1.79
Ngubevu	0.92	2.14	Ndumu	2.49	2.49
Nocomboshe	0.93	2.17	Shemula	1.29	1.93
Brunville	6.50	8.87	Mbazwana	1.21	1.81
Driefontein	2.55	2.13	Ntshongwe	0.45	1.04
Ekuvukeni	0.00	0.00	Com. City FP	0.00	0.00
Ezakheni No. 2	0.00	0.00	Inanda FP	40.01	20.01
Limehill	0.91	0.91	Goodwins	0.00	0.00
Rockcliff	0.83	1.04	Kwamashu	0.00	0.00
Mobile 1	3.16	0.79	Lindelani	8.63	6.48
Amazizini	3.38	2.41	Molweni	2.38	2.85
Mahashini	1.53	2.29	Ndwedwe	9.81	7.01

…/ cont.

Appendix 10.2 (cont.)

Name of clinic	Excess no. of nurses	Excess no. of general staff	Name of clinic	Excess no. of nurses	Excess no. of general staff
Ntuzuma	0.00	0.00	Naasfarm	1.81	1.39
Qadi	6.44	2.52	Osizweni 1	0.00	0.00
Rydalvale	0.00	0.00	Thembalihle	7.72	4.96
Phoenix CHC	0.00	0.00	Madadeni 1	8.34	5.96
Baniyena	0.00	0.00	Madadeni 5	7.48	5.35
D State	3.77	3.39	Dkodweni	2.38	3.33
Dudulu	0.00	0.00	Ndulinde	0.00	0.00
Ekuphileni	0.00	0.00	Mobile	0.00	0.01
Imfume	1.29	1.61	Manyane	0.00	0.35
Jolivet	1.53	2.30	Mfongosi	0.00	0.40
Kwamakhutha	1.69	1.04	Mntungweni	0.00	0.02
Kwadengezi	8.05	5.37	Mobile	9.99	5.71
Magabheni	2.53	4.04	Gezinsila	0.91	2.11
Mntungwane	4.47	1.68	Ngudwini	0.89	2.08
Nkwali	1.88	1.13	Ntumeni	0.89	2.08
Odidini	2.70	1.47	Osungulweni	0.81	1.88
Osizweni	5.89	4.72	Melmoth	0.02	0.05
Umbumbulu	0.00	0.00	Dondotha	14.02	23.10
Umlazi "V"	3.32	2.04	Ndlangubo	0.83	1.94
Umzomuhle	1.47	2.20	Ndundulu	0.00	0.00
Zwlibomvu	2.27	2.73	Ngwelezane	0.59	1.38
Isandlwana	0.00	0.00	Nomponjwana	0.00	0.00
Mangeni	0.00	0.00	Nseleni	28.43	44.43
Masotsheni	3.10	3.48	Ntambanana	0.61	1.43
Mondlo 1	0.50	0.80	Ntuze	4.29	3.81
Mondlo 2	0.64	1.27	Halambu	0.00	0.00
Ntababomvu	0.00	0.00	Vumanhlamvu	2.83	1.61
Ntinini	0.00	0.00	Mthandeni	0.00	0.46

Appendix 10.3   Increases in outputs needed to make inefficient clinics efficient

Name of clinic	Ante natal	Births	Child	Dental	FP	Mental	STD	TB
Hlokozi	1,423	-	401	-	-	130	434	11
Mabaleni	419	4	494	2	0	207	309	64
Madlala	1,242	34	313	5	401	166	211	63
Morrison's Post	-	-	-	-	-	-	-	-
Ndelu	-	-	-	-	-	-	-	-
Ntimbankulu	724	-	1,431	1	240	95	463	-
Nyangwini	-	-	-	-	-	-	-	-
Pungashe	3,710	86	-	-	1,345	-	312	1,183
St Faiths	76	34	-	-	453	-	446	1,515
Umzinto CHC	-	-	-	-	-	-	-	-
Bomela	441	3	-	-	980	14	-	-
Gamalakhe	2,212	-	-	19	-	-	-	-
Gcilima	-	-	-	-	-	-	-	-
Izingolweni	3,202	58	-	-	3,974	-	1,142	7,912
Ludimala	288	3	1,588	1	420	-	-	-
Ntabeni	-	-	-	-	-	-	-	-
Pisgah	855	6	-	-	963	4	304	-
Caluza	-	107	-	150	5,415	-	-	291
Gcumisa	-	-	-	-	-	-	-	-
Mpophomeni	-	22	-	7	2,268	99	-	-
Mpumalanga	-	-	-	-	-	-	-	-
Mpumuza	-	-	-	-	-	-	-	-
Msunduzi	-	-	-	-	-	-	-	-
Ndaleni	967	9	-	2	1,528	114	578	39
Taylors Halt	343	9	424	12	721	-	823	1,639
Mobile	-	-	-	-	-	-	-	-
Imbalenhle	-	-	-	-	-	-	-	-
Richmond	1,210	96	-	-	3,423	1,564	2,383	2,089
Underberg	-	18	-	4	2,040	538	1,018	82
Ehlanzeni	1,323	-	826	0	706	345	77	25
Cwaka	-	-	-	-	-	-	-	-
Ethembeni	326	-	213	-	1,357	425	414	-
Gunjana	641	8	1,267	0	916	247	161	22
Mazebeko	584	-	1,772	-	1,258	305	274	-
Ngubevu	863	-	1,867	0	772	144	209	-
Nocomboshe	421	-	1,391	0	649	191	165	-
Brunville	962	-	7,477	24	-	738	2,498	239
Driefontein	1,125	-	2,107	15	463	85	619	-
Ekuvukeni	-	-	-	-	-	-	-	-
Ezakheni No 2	-	-	-	-	-	-	-	-
Limehill	681	-	1,783	6	281	276	885	-
Rockcliff	1,417	-	2,483	7	563	164	666	-
Mobile 1	297	0	-	0	1,212	75	-	-
Amazizini	697	-	508	12	-	-	363	74
Dukuza	1,114	-	168	-	406	103	184	67
Injisuthi	443	-	1,841	11	79	170	139	127
Ncibindane	317	-	-	-	-	241	425	34
Ntabamhlophe	2,700	-	3,905	32	-	559	300	307
Oliviershoek	5,072	-	4,527	-	-	292	807	608
Wembesi	653	55	-	8	-	358	-	60

.../cont.

Appendix 10.3 (cont.)

Name of Clinic	Ante natal	Births	Child	Dental	FP	Mental	STD	TB
Dengeni	1,352	-	1,905	2	1,577	409	895	36
Ekubungazeleni	-	-	3,178	7	194	500	271	145
Hlengimpilo	1,170	-	2,033	1	1,304	327	650	34
Mahashini	279	-	-	-	1,161	112	367	10
Maphophoma	-	-	-	2	884	176	465	72
Ngqeku	1,249	3	1,548	2	1,360	315	851	38
Njoko	475	-	1,507	10	-	477	581	95
Usuthu	7	2	-	1	853	46	215	32
Mobile 1	-	-	-	-	-	-	-	-
Dlebe	666	-	215	-	257	36	276	14
Ezimfabeni	750	-	-	1	744	164	239	12
Altona	-	1	-	-	-	249	133	18
Friesgewaagt	278	21	420	-	685	-	97	-
Hartland	-	49	2,024	-	262	264	-	61
Kwashoba	-	33	127	-	1,494	496	-	56
Ncotshana	-	46	2,197	9	1,209	91	-	-
Tobolsk	590	2	874	-	642	216	27	19
Kwamame	-	14	-	-	301	416	460	265
Lomo	647	-	-	-	1,341	347	568	48
Mabedlana	1,088	-	582	-	1,047	258	389	42
Makhosini	1,426	-	2,140	-	1,654	466	838	118
Mpungamhlophe	1,287	-	-	-	1,008	350	403	386
Ncemane	1,342	-	1,039	-	1,527	472	834	73
Nhlungwane	1,628	-	2,330	-	1,196	471	901	66
St Francis	8,380	-	6,304	1,910	3,866	-	1,695	4,393
Ulundi A	708	-	1,357	-	1,990	395	-	102
Zilulwane	1,242	-	99	3	1,416	422	747	64
Jozini	-	-	-	-	-	-	-	-
Madonela	-	-	-	-	-	-	-	-
Makhathini	804	-	1,412	-	829	582	192	-
Mhlekazi	1,906	-	2,823	1	851	614	550	49
Ophansi	677	-	235	-	955	612	-	49
Kwamsane	-	-	-	-	-	-	-	-
Mpukunyoni	-	-	-	-	-	-	-	-
Phelindaba	828	-	2,558	-	893	664	144	82
Zamazama	2,191	-	2,780	-	959	748	421	209
Emanyiseni	415	-	1,634	-	994	403	400	61
Gwaliweni	2,623	-	3,464	1	1,292	523	903	34
Ndumu	3,441	-	6,493	-	1,179	858	417	303
Shemula	1,353	-	1,783	7	1,436	549	722	45
Mbazwana	953	-	1,947	-	896	558	165	109
Ntshongwe	336	-	1,594	-	1,004	524	136	189
Commercial City FP	-	-	-	-	-	-	-	-
Inanda FP	1,941	11	3,094	3	-	520	2,683	54
Goodwins	-	-	-	-	-	-	-	-

.../cont.

Appendix 10.3 (cont.)

Name of Clinic	Ante natal	Births	Child	Dental	FP	Mental	STD	TB
Kwamashu	-	-	-	-	-	-	-	-
Lindelani	-	7	-	2	-	526	320	66
Molweni	1,101	3	520	-	145	410	655	22
Ndwedwe	2,871	-	4,659	74	-	532	477	197
Ntuzuma	-	-	-	-	-	-	-	-
Qadi	3,191	-	5,720	30	-	713	917	218
Rydalvale	-	-	-	-	-	-	-	-
Phoenix CHC	-	-	-	-	-	-	-	-
Baniyena	-	-	-	-	-	-	-	-
D State	-	87	3,678	67	29	-	420	-
Dudulu	-	-	-	-	-	-	-	-
Ekuphileni	-	-	-	-	-	-	-	-
Imfume	192	8	-	2	-	62	649	-
Jolivet	381	-	1,084	-	765	77	559	-
Kwamakhutha	-	-	2,879	372	-	-	1,965	1,329
Kwadengezi	359	-	-	3	-	123	2,163	66
Magabheni	602	-	2,115	1	256	237	530	-
Mntungwane	752	-	2,320	4	917	263	464	-
Nkwali	662	10	1,741	2	638	243	1,159	-
Odidini	1,314	-	1,188	77	4,254	1,070	-	-
Osizweni	-	13	1,122	-	-	-	1,069	861
Umbumbulu	-	-	-	-	-	-	-	-
Umlazi "V"	-	-	7,500	222	179	-	727	2,468
Umzomuhle	663	1	1,727	-	488	370	425	-
Zwlibomvu	869	-	1,347	0	1,471	452	958	50
Isandlwana	96	6	1,588	1	948	277	92	44
Mangeni	-	-	-	-	-	-	-	-
Masotsheni	1,548	-	3,583	33	-	192	228	-
Mondlo 1	472	-	2,733	3	-	148	97	-
Mondlo 2	380	-	813	-	532	355	38	52
Ntababomvu	546	37	1,167	2	119	100	15	79
Ntinini	-	-	-	-	-	-	-	-
Naasfarm	2,772	-	4,985	2,065	3,977	-	-	1,990
Osizweni 1	-	-	-	-	-	-	-	-
Thembalihle	106	-	-	-	3,167	58	-	522
Madadeni 1	1,520	-	3,964	268	6,238	301	-	519
Madadeni 5	371	-	937	127	10,930	-	-	1,187
Dkodweni	1,326	-	1,860	2	1,593	566	850	-
Ndulinde	-	-	-	-	-	-	-	-
Mobile	149	2	1,043	3	343	38	155	25
Manyane	361	19	1,623	0	365	112	219	87
Mfongosi	566	9	1,235	7	760	190	252	59
Mntungweni	432	10	153	1	518	149	114	25
Mobile	710	-	3,167	2	1,048	436	-	51
Gezinsila	1,119	-	1,850	-	848	225	192	7

.../cont.

Appendix 10.3 (cont.)

Name of Clinic	Ante natal	Births	Child	Dental	FP	Mental	STD	TB
Ngudwini	589	-	1,369	-	641	270	44	5
Ntumeni	681	-	1,631	-	804	271	148	11
Osungulweni	1,646	-	2,336	1	1,425	529	465	39
Melmoth	16	-	-	-	-	401	-	-
Dondotha	2,788	-	4,271	13	1,310	772	847	-
Ndlangubo	162	27	-	-	555	254	91	-
Ndundulu	-	-	-	-	-	-	-	-
Ngwelezane	213	-	-	-	1,135	671	469	-
Nomponjwana	-	-	-	-	-	-	-	-
Nseleni	2,944	-	1,646	-	228	868	690	9
Ntambanana	-	-	179	-	401	419	399	-
Ntuze	1,609	-	-	13	-	600	225	-
Halambu	-	-	-	-	-	-	-	-
Vumanhlamvu	-	14	930	17	2,517	398	1,553	350
Mthandeni	677	20	1,928	8	23	74	185	100

Appendix 10.4   Linear probability regression model results

Explanatory Variables	Coefficients	Z	P>|z|
Number of nursing staff	-0.121	-3.099*	0.002
Number of general staff (including administrative, general, and labour provisioning staff)	-0.097	-1.467	0.142
Antenatal care visits	0.00009	1.146	0.252
Number of births	0.00400	2.370*	0.018
Child healthcare visits	0.00009	1.540	0.123
Dental care visits	0.00090	2.057*	0.040
Family planning visits	0.00001	0.469	0.639
Psychiatry care visits	-0.00020	-0.462	0.644
Sexually transmitted diseases care visits	0.00020	1.691	0.091
Tuberculosis care visits	0.00010	1.685	0.092
Constant	-0.288000	-0.727	0.467
Number of observations	155.0000		
$Chi^2(10)$	44.4800		
$Prob > Chi^2$	0.0000		
Pseudo R^2	0.2339		

* Statistically significant at 95% level.

Appendix 10.5   Logistic regression model results

Explanatory Variables	Coefficients	Odds Ratio	Z	P>|z|
Number of nursing staff	-0.249	0.779	-2.802*	0.005
Number of general staff (including administrative, general, and labour provisioning staff)	-0.143	0.867	-1.210	0.226
Antenatal care visits	0.0002	1.000	1.268	0.205
Number of births	0.0050	1.005	1.697	0.090
Child health visits	0.0002	1.000	1.776	0.076
Dental care visits	0.0020	1.002	2.368*	0.018
Family Planning visits	0.00002	1.000	0.405	0.686
Psychiatry care visits	-0.0002	1.000	-0.266	0.790
Sexually transmitted diseases care visits	0.0003	1.000	1.923	0.054
Tuberculosis care visits	0.0002	1.000	1.606	0.108
Constant	-0.5050	-	-0.749	0.454
Number of observations	155.000			
Chi^2(10)	45.2000			
Prob > Chi^2	0.000			
Pseudo R^2	0.2376			
Log Likelihood Ratio	-72.504			

* Statistically significant at 95% level.

-11-

Technical Efficiency of Primary Health Units in Kailahun and Kenema Districts of Sierra Leone*

Joses Muthuri Kirigia, Luis Gomes Sambo,
Ade Renner, Wondi Alemu, Santigie Seasa, Yankuba Bah

ABSTRACT

The objectives of the study reported in this paper were to (*a*) estimate the technical efficiency of samples of community health centres (CHCs), community health posts (CHPs), and maternal and child health posts (MCHPs) in Kailahun and Kenema districts of Sierra Leone; (*b*) estimate the output increases needed to make inefficient MCHPs, CHCs and CHPs efficient; and (*c*) explore strategies for increasing technical efficiency of these institutions.

This study applied the data envelopment analysis (DEA) approach to analyse technical efficiency of random samples of 36 MCHPs, 22 CHCs, and 21 CHPs using input and output data for 2008. The findings indicated that 77.8% of the MCHPs, 59.1% of the CHCs, and 66.7% of the CHPs were variable returns to scale technically inefficient. The average variable returns to scale technical efficiency was 68.2% (SD = 0.272) among the MCHPs, 69.2% (SD = 0.332) among the CHCs, and 59% (SD = 0.347) among the CHPs.

This study revealed significant technical inefficiencies in the use of health system resources among peripheral health units in Kailahun and Kenema districts of Sierra Leone. There is need to strengthen national and district health information systems to routinely track the quantities and prices of resources injected into the healthcare

---

* The original article appeared in *International Archives of Medicine* 2011;4(15):1-14. Reproduced with the permission of BioMed Central Ltd.

systems and health service outcomes (indicators of coverage, quality, and health status) to facilitate regular efficiency analyses.

BACKGROUND

The vision of Sierra Leone is to have a functional national health system delivering efficient and high quality health services that are accessible, equitable, and affordable for everyone [1]. The general objective of the National Health Sector Strategic Plan (NHSSP) is to strengthen the functions of the national health system so as to improve access to health services (i.e., their availability, utilization, and timeliness); quality of health services (i.e., their safety, efficacy, and integration); equity in health services (particularly their access by disadvantaged groups); efficiency of service delivery (i.e., value for resources); and inclusiveness (partnerships) [2] in their delivery.

The first principle stated in the NHSSP [2, p.11] calls for "Accountable central governance and provision of effective and efficient local health services composed of a comprehensive range of primary and secondary health services across the nation". One of the strategic objectives of the country's healthcare delivery is to increase attendance at healthcare facilities by mothers and children, the poor, and other vulnerable groups from the current low level of 0.5 health facility contacts per person per year to 3 contacts per person per year by 2015. The government of Sierra Leone is implementing several health sector reforms to improve efficiency of health services. These reforms deal with decentralisation and devolution of authority to 19 local councils that are now responsible for managing the delivery of both the primary and secondary health care levels, transfer to the local councils of tied grants amounting to a quarter of the national health budget [2], introduction of user fees in public health facilities [3], and experimentation with autonomy for hospitals [4].

One of the three objectives of the Sierra Leone health financing strategy is to ensure equitable and efficient allocation and use of health sector resources by (*a*) developing and implementing equitable, needs-based criteria for allocating financial resources, (*b*) harnessing NGO and private sector resources through contractual arrangements in pursuit of national health development goals, (*c*) developing provider (health facilities and health workforce) payment mechanisms that create incentives for greater effectiveness and efficiency, and (*d*) institutionalising health sector efficiency monitoring [2].

The broad aim of this study was to contribute towards objective (*d*) of the health financing strategy. The 2005 Sierra Leone efficiency study applied the data envelopment analysis (DEA) approach to assess the technical efficiency (TE) of peripheral health units (PHUs) in Pujehun district [5]. The study reported in this paper is the second attempt to apply the DEA approach in measuring the TE of health units in the country. The specific objectives of the study reported in this paper were:

1. To estimate the TE of samples of community health centres (CHCs), community health posts (CHPs), and maternal and child health posts (MCHPs) in two districts of Sierra Leone;

2. To estimate the output increases needed to make inefficient CHCs, CHPs, and MCHPs efficient;

3. To explore the strategies that increase TE of primary health care units.

Review of Literature on Efficiency of Primary Health Care Units

The studies reviewed below demonstrate that the DEA approach has been fruitfully used in Africa, Europe, and North America to monitor and evaluate the efficiency of various primary health care decision-making units (DMUs). Sebastian and Lemma [6] estimated the TE of 60 health posts in rural Tigray, Ethiopia. The inputs were number of health extension workers (HEWs) and of voluntary health workers (traditional birth attendants and community health workers). The outputs for each health post were health education sessions given by HEWs, pregnant women who completed three antenatal care visits, child deliveries, number of persons who repeatedly visited the family planning service, diarrhoeal cases treated in children under-five, visits carried out by community health workers, total number of new patients attended, and malaria cases treated. The mean scores for technical and scale efficiency were 0.57 (SD = 0.32) and 0.95 (SD = 0.11) respectively. Fifteen (25%) health posts were found to be technically efficient and thirty-eight (63.3%) were operating at their most productive scale size.

Halsteinli, Kittelsen, and Magnussen [7] used DEA-Malmquist indices to assess productivity growth in an unbalanced panel of 48–60 Norwegian outpatient child and adolescent mental health service units (CAMHS) over the period 1998–2006. Input variables were full-time equivalent (FTE) university-educated personnel (psychiatrists and psychologists) and FTE college-educated personnel (mainly from the fields of social work, education, and psychiatric nurses). The outputs were treated patients and direct and indirect consultations. This study estimated three models, namely, Model P, an unadjusted model where output was measured as total number of patients; Model PGR, incorporating case-mix adjustment where patients were split into eight groups believed to be clinically meaningful; and Model PDG_C, in which the aggregate numbers of direct and indirect consultations were added as outputs. The range of mean TE scores across the three models was 47–67% in 1998, 50–71% in 1999, 52–72% in 2000, 53–72% in 2001, 52–73% in 2002, 52–75% in 2003, 54–75% in 2004, 58–78% in 2005, and 58–78% in 2006. The mean Malmquist total factor productivity indices for the panel of the 37 CAMHS for Model PGR were 1.069 in 1998–2001 and 1.060 in 2001–2004. For Model PGR_C these scores were 1.105 in 1998–2001 and 1.151 in 2001–2004.

Amada and Santos [8] assessed the performance of 337 health centres in Portugal in 2005. The inputs were doctors, nurses, and administrative and other staff. The outputs were family planning consultations; maternity consultations; consultations by patients grouped in ages of 0–18, 19–64, and 65 and above; home doctor consultations; home nurse consultations; curatives and other nurse treatments; injections given by a nurse; and vaccinations given by a nurse. The mean TE score was 84.4% (SD = 14.7%).

Marschall and Flessa [9] evaluated the relative efficiency of 20 local health centres in rural Burkina Faso. The inputs chosen were personnel costs in 2004, health centre building area (square metres), depreciation of health centre equipment in 2004, and vaccination costs in 2004. The health centres' intermediate outputs were number of general consultations and nursing care cases at the dispensary, deliveries in the maternal ward, immunisation, and special services such as family planning and prenatal and postnatal consultations. Fourteen health centres were technically efficient and scale efficient. The average TE score was 91% (SD = 17). The mean scale efficiency score was 97% (SD = 12%).

Akazili et al. [10] calculated the TE of 89 health centres in Ghana. The inputs used were non-clinical staff including labourers, clinical staff, beds and cots, and expenditure on drugs and supplies. The outputs were general outpatient and antenatal care visits, deliveries, children immunised, and family planning visits. Thirty-one (35%) health centres were technically efficient. The inefficient health centres had an average TE score of 57% (SD = 19%). Nineteen (21%) health centres were scale efficient and the inefficient health centres had an average scale score of 86% (SD = 14%).

Milliken et al. [11] undertook an efficiency comparison of four distinct models of primary health service delivery in Ontario. Their study covered 32 fee-for-service practices (FFS) including family health groups (FHGs), 31 health service organisations (HSOs), 27 family health networks (FHNs), and 19 community health centres (CHCs). The input variables were practice site costs per provider and per patient and provider-patient ratio. The output measures were the average number of visits per patient at the practice site and performance indicators measuring technical quality of care and health service delivery. The study estimated three different scenarios based on the input measure used as follows: scenario 1 used cost per provider, scenario 2 used cost per patient, and scenario 3 used provider-patient ratio. For scenario 1, the efficiency scores were 60.4% (SD = 16.9) for the entire sample (N = 109), 50.4% (SD = 12.2) for CHCs, 69.1% (SD = 17.2) for FFS, 62.8% (SD = 17.2) for FHNs, and 55.9% (SD = 14.4) for HSOs. For scenario 2, the efficiency scores were 43.8% (SD = 22.6) for the entire sample, 25.5% (SD = 16.5) for CHCs, 52% (SD = 22.7) for FFS, 43.9% (SD = 23.3%) for FHNs, and 46.7% (SD = 19.8) for HSOs. The mean technical efficiency score for scenario 3 was

41% (SD = 21.1) for the entire sample, 31% (SD =19.2) for CHCs, 43.9% (SD = 22.4) for FFS, 38.7% (SD = 18.6) for FHNs, and 46% (SD = 21.5) for HSOs.

Kirigia et al. [12] employed the DEA-based Malmquist productivity index to assess the technical and scale efficiency and productivity change over a four-year period (2001–2004) among 17 public health centres in Seychelles. The inputs used were total number of hours for doctors and for nurses. The outputs were patients dressed, domiciliary cases treated, and sum of number of visits for PFMAPIS (pap smear, family planning clinic, maternal and child health, antenatal care and postnatal care, and children immunised and those participating in a school health programme). For the 17 health centres, those that had a variable returns to scale (VRS) TE score of 100% were 10 (59%) in 2001, 9 (47%) in 2002, 9 (53%) in 2003, and 10 (59%) in 2004. The average VRS technical efficiency scores were 93%, 92%, 92%, and 96% respectively during the years under consideration. Out of the 17 health centres 5 (29.4%), 6 (35.3%), 7 (41.2%), and 7 (41.2%) were scale efficient in 2001, 2002, 2003, and 2004 respectively. The average scale efficiency score in the sample was 90% in 2001, 93% in 2002, 92% in 2003, and 95% in 2004. The Malmquist index of total factor productivity change (MTFP) was 1.024, technical change was 1.215, efficiency change was 0.843, pure efficiency change was 1.000, and scale efficiency change was 0.843. This meant that health centre productivity increased by 2.4% over the four years largely due to innovation. Whereas efficiency regressed by 15.7%, technical change (innovation) improved by 21.5% per annum.

Kontodimopoulous, Nanos, and Niakas [13] investigated TE of 17 Greek hospital health centres (HHCs). The inputs used were doctors, nurses, and beds and the outputs were admissions, outpatient visits, and preventive medical services. Seven HHCs were technically efficient. The average TE score was 73.23% (SD = 10.09) and the median score was 77.57%.

Masiye et al. [14] estimated the degree of technical, allocative, and cost efficiency among 40 health centres in Lusaka, Central and Copper-Belt provinces of Zambia 58% of which were government owned and 42% private-for-profit enterprises. The study used the numbers of clinical officers, nurses, and other staff as inputs and the number of outpatient visits as output. The average TE, allocative efficiency (AE), and cost efficiency (CE) scores for the private health centres were 70%, 84%, and 59% respectively. These scores were 56%, 57%, and 33%, respectively for government health centres. For the whole sample the averages were 61.9% for TE, 68.5% for AE, and 44.5% for CE. Of the 17 private health centres, 5 had a TE score of 100 and 4 had AE and CE scores of 100%. Contrastingly, only 1 of the 23 government health centres had TE, AE, or CE scores of 100%.

Renner et al. [5] investigated TE and SE levels among a sample of 37 public PHUs in Sierra Leone. The six outputs for each PHU were (*a*) antenatal plus postnatal visits, (*b*) child deliveries, (*c*) nutritional/child growth monitoring visits, (*d*) family planning visits, (*e*) immunised children under five years and pregnant women immunised with tetanus toxoid (TT), and (*f*) total health education sessions conducted through home visits, public meetings, school lectures, and outpatient departments. In Sierra Leone, PHUs did not provide curative care services but were dedicated to health promotion and disease prevention services. The two inputs were (*a*) technical staff (community health nurse, vaccinators, and maternal and child health aides) and (*b*) subordinate staff including traditional birth attendants, porters, and watchmen. Twenty-two (59%) of the 37 health units analysed were found to be technically inefficient with an average score of 63% (SD = 18%). On the other hand, 24 (65%) health units were found to be scale inefficient with an average scale efficiency score of 72% (SD = 17%).

Osei et al. [15] estimated the TE of 17 district hospitals and 17 health centres in Ghana in 2000. The DEA model was estimated with these four outputs: child deliveries; fully immunised children under the age of five years; maternal visits for antenatal care, postnatal care and family planning, and childcare visits for nutritional and child growth monitoring; and outpatient curative visits. The two inputs were technical staff including medical assistants, nurses, and paramedical staff and support or subordinate staff including cleaners, drivers, gardeners, watchmen, and others. Eight (47%) hospitals were technically inefficient with an average TE score of 61% and an SD of 12%. Ten (59%) hospitals were scale inefficient manifesting an average SE of 81% (SD = 25%). Out of the 17 health centres, 3 (18%) were technically inefficient with a mean TE score of 49% (SD = 27%) and 8 (47%) were scale inefficient with an average SE score of 84% (SD = 16%).

Kirigia, Emrouznejad, Sambo et al. [16] measured the TE of 32 public health centres in Kenya. The six inputs used were clinical officers and nurses; physiotherapists, occupational therapists, public health officers, dental technologists, laboratory technicians and laboratory technologists; administrative staff; non-wage expenditures; and beds. The four outputs were visits for diarrhoea, malaria, sexually transmitted infections, urinary tract infections, intestinal worms, and respiratory disease; visits for antenatal care and family planning; immunisations; and other general outpatient visits. Fourteen (44%) health centres were technically efficient and the average TE score was 65% (SD = 22%). Nineteen (59%) health centres were scale efficient and the average SE score was 70% (SD = 19%).

Linna, Nordblad and Koivu [17] measured the productive efficiency of 228 public dental health centres across Finland. Their study estimated two primal models. Model 1 (*PMODEL1*) was the visit output model whose outputs were total visits to dentists and total visits to hygienists and dental assistants among each of three age groups categorised as 0–18 years, 19–39 years, and >39 years. Input variables included number of FTE dentists, number of other employees (hygienists, dental assistants, and administrative staff), and total cost of materials and equipment. Model 2 (*PMODEL2*) was the patients' model whose outputs were number of patients treated categorised under the three ages groups: 0–18 years, 19–39 years, and >39 years. The inputs for Model 2 were as for primal Model 1. This study, in addition, estimated two cost efficiency models. The cost efficiency Model 1 (*CMODEL1*) used all the outputs used in primal Model 1 plus total operating costs in each health centre as the input variables, while the second model (*CMODEL2*) used all the outputs in primal Model 2 plus total operating costs in each health centre as the input variables. Some 47, 19, 18 and 4 health centres were found to be efficient in *PMODEL1*, *PMODEL2*, *CMODEL1*, and *CMODEL2* respectively. The average efficiency scores were between 72% and 81% in the primal models and between 62% and 79% in the cost models.

Kirigia, Sambo and Scheel [18] investigated the TE of 155 primary health care clinics in Kwazulu-Natal Province of South Africa. The clinics were assumed to produce eight types of intermediate outputs, which were visits for antenatal care, child delivery, child health, dental care, family planning, psychiatry services, sexually transmitted disease, and tuberculosis treatment. Two inputs were included in the model as number of nurses and number of general support staff. Forty seven (30%) of the clinics were technically efficient, 25 (16%) of which manifested 100% scale efficiency.

Johnston and Gerard [19] investigated the relative efficiency of 64 (33 large and 31 small) breast cancer screening units in the UK. The outputs were invitations, screenings, and cancers detected. The inputs were number of FTE radiologists, radiographers, administration staff, medical and nursing staff engaged in assessment work, and number of dedicated mammography machines and assessments performed. The overall sample average TE score was 82.1% (SD = 20) and the median score was 91.2%. Twenty-five units were technically efficient. The average TE score for the large units was 92.1 (SD = 14) and the median was 100%. Thirteen of the large units were efficient. The small units had an average TE score of 84.5% (SD = 84.5) and a median score of 95.6%. Seven of these units were technically efficient.

Salinas-Jimenez and Smith [20] explored the role of quality indicators in primary care and examined the extent to which DEA provides useful insight in the quality of performance of 85 UK family health service authorities (FHSA). The seven indicators of quality used were the number of general medical practitioners per 10,000 patients on a list, the percentage of practices employing a practice nurse, the percentage of general medical practitioners with a patient list of less than 2500, the percentage of general medical practitioners not practising single handedly, the percentage of general medical practitioners who had achieved the higher rate of payments for childhood immunisation, the percentage of females aged 35 to 64 registered with the FHSA and who also had an adequate cervical smear in the previous five-and-half years, and the percentage of practice premises that satisfied the minimum standards set out in paragraph 50.10 of the State of Fees and Allowances, excluding practices exempt under paragraph 51.11. The measure of resource inputs for the FHSAs was gross expenditure on general medical services (in British pounds) per head of resident population. Forty-three (51%) of the FHSAs were deemed efficient. Amongst the inefficient units, the average performance level was 92.6%.

METHODS

Study Area

Sierra Leone is situated on the west coast of Africa, with the North Atlantic Ocean to its west and lies between Guinea and Liberia. It is divided into four major administrative areas (northern, southern, eastern, and western regions) and twelve districts (Bo, Mombali, Bonthe, Kailahun, Kambia, Kenema, Koinadugu, Kono, Moyamba, Port Loko, Pujehun, and Tonkolili). Freetown, the capital city, is in the western region. The current study took place in Kailahun and Kenema districts.

The public health system comprises four levels [2]:

Peripheral level - Peripheral health units, which are the frontline health services, are classified into three levels:

1. At the village level are the MCHPs, which serve less than 5,000 people. They are staffed by MCH aides (supported by community health workers (e.g., traditional birth attendants and volunteers) who are trained to provide antenatal care, supervised delivery, postnatal care, family planning, child growth monitoring, immunisation, health education, management of minor ailments, and referral of cases to the next level.

2. Community health posts, which operate in small towns, serve 5,000 to 10,000 people, and are staffed by state enrolled community health nurses (SECHNs) and MCH aides. They provide similar services as MCHPs in addition to prevention and control of communicable diseases and rehabilitation.

3. Community health centres, situated at the chiefdom level, cover 10,000 to 20,000 people and are staffed by a community health officer (CHO), SECHNs, MCH aides, an epidemiological disease control assistant, and an environmental health officer (EHO). They provide

production process, and resulting outputs is described in Figure 11.1. Since health centres and health posts employ multiple inputs to produce multiple outputs, we chose to employ the DEA approach, which is versatile in this kind of production scenario.

DEA is a functionalist, linear programming methodology for evaluating the relative efficiency of each production unit among a set of fairly homogeneous decision-making units (DMUs) such as MCHPs, CHPs, and CHCs. Technical efficiency is a measure of the ability of a DMU to provide maximum quantities of health services (outputs) from a given set of health system resources (inputs). Technical efficiency is affected by the size of operations (scale efficiency) and by managerial practices (non-scale technical efficiency or pure technical efficiency) [25].

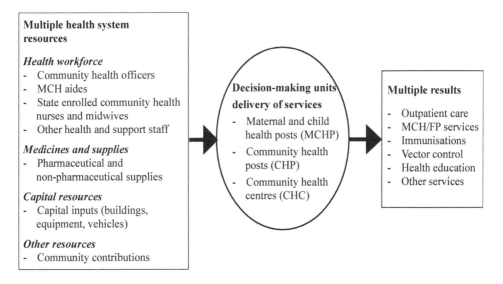

Figure 11.1   Relationship between inputs and the production process and resulting outputs outputs

DEA plots an efficient frontier using combinations of inputs and outputs from the best performing health facilities. Health facilities that compose the "best practice frontier" are assigned an efficiency score of one (or 100%) and are deemed technically efficient compared with their peers. The efficiency of the health facilities below the efficiency frontier is measured in terms of their distance from the frontier. The inefficient health facilities are assigned a score between zero and one. The higher the score the more efficient a health facility is. Since MCHPs, CHPs, and CHCs employ multiple inputs to produce multiple outputs, their individual TE can be defined as [26]:

$$\text{Technical efficiency score} = \frac{\text{Weighted sum of outputs}}{\text{Weighted sum of inputs}}.$$

The TE score of each MCHP, CHC, or CHP in the sample was obtained by solving models 1 and 2 (Figure 11.2) [16]. We need to explain what we mean by constant returns to scale and variable returns to scale. Returns to scale refers to the changes in output as all inputs change by the same proportion. For example, if an MCHP, CHC, or CHP increased all its health system inputs by the same proportion, the health service outputs might have one of the following outcomes: increase by the same proportion as the inputs (i.e., constant returns to scale, CRS); increase less than proportionally with the increase in inputs (i.e., decreasing returns to scale, DRS); or increase more than proportionally with the increase in inputs (i.e., increasing returns to scale, IRS). Health centres or posts manifesting CRS can be said to be operating at their most productive scale sizes. In order to operate at the most productive scale size, a health facility displaying DRS should scale down both outputs and inputs. If a health facility is exhibiting IRS, it should expand both outputs and inputs in order to become scale efficient [15].

Model 1	Model 2
DEA weights model for input-oriented, constant returns to scale	**DEA weights model for input-oriented, variable returns to scale**
$\text{Efficiency} = \underset{u_r, v_i}{\text{Max}} \sum_r u_r y_{rj0}$	$\text{Efficiency} = \underset{u_r, v_i}{\text{Max}} \sum_r u_r y_{rj0} + u_0$
Subject to	Subject to
$\sum_r u_r y_{rj} - \sum_i v_i x_{ij} \leq 0 \quad ; \forall j$	$\sum_r u_r y_{rj} - \sum_i v_i x_{ij} + u_0 \leq 0 \quad ; \forall j$
$\sum_i v_i x_{ij0} = 1$	$\sum_i v_i x_{ij0} = 1$
$u_r, v_i \geq 0 \quad ; \forall r, \forall i$	$u_r, v_i \geq 0 \quad ; \forall r, \forall i$

Figure 11.2 DEA models

Where:

$\sum$ = summation

y_{rj} = the amount of output r produced by health centre j,

x_{ij} = the amount of input i used by health centre j,

u_r = the weight given to output r (r = 1,..., t and t is the number of outputs),

v_i = the weight given to input i (i = 1, ..., m and m is the number of inputs),

n = the number of health centres, and

j_0 = the health centre under assessment.

Output Orientation

Managers of MCHs, CHPs, and CHCs have no control over inputs, especially staffing. However, given the orientation of these units to primary health care with a strong bias towards health promotion and disease prevention and control, they can influence a great number of people; for example, people seeking antenatal and postnatal care, family planning services, birthing services, child growth monitoring, immunisation, health education, treatment of common diseases and injuries, and vector control (water, sanitation, insecticide-treated bed nets) through their public health outreach work among communities. It is for this reason that we estimated an output-oriented DEA model.

Variables

The DEA model for MCHPs, CHCs, and CHPs was estimated with a total of five variables; three of which were outputs and two were inputs. The three outputs for each individual health centre were the number of outpatient, maternal, child health, and family planning visits plus immunisation visits (OMFE); the number of vector control activities; and the number of health education sessions. The two inputs were the number of community health officers, MCH aides, and state enrolled community health nurses (CHO + MA + SECHN); and the number of support staff (including cleaners, drivers, gardeners, watchmen and others). The choice of inputs and outputs for the DEA analysis was guided in part by the availability of data and previous DEA healthcare studies in the African Region.

Data

The data used in this study are for 2008. Data were collected from random samples of functional MCHPs (36), CHCs (22), and CHPs (21) using an efficiency questionnaire developed by the WHO African Regional Office for primary health level facilities [27]. The data were analysed using DEAP software developed by Professor Tim Coelli [28].

Limitations of the Study

Interpretation of the results of this study ought to take cognisance of the limitations of the study. Firstly, the DEA analytical methodology attributes any deviation from the best practice frontier to inefficiency even though some level of deviation could be due to statistical noise such as epidemics, natural disasters, internal displacement of people by civil wars, or measurement errors. Secondly, given that DEA is underpinned by a functionalist paradigm using a deterministic/non-parametric technique, it is difficult to use in statistical tests of hypotheses dealing with inefficiency and structure of the production function. Thirdly, it could be argued that the output of MCHPs, CHCs, and CHPs is the change in beneficiaries' health status as a result of receiving health services from these institutions. Fourthly, the only health system input used in the current study was health workforce owing to unavailability of data on non-personnel expenditures. The inputs that were not included in the model include medicines, non-pharmaceutical supplies, buildings, equipment, etc. Fifthly, the study did not give due consideration to social, cultural, and behavioural inputs, which can strongly influence the outcome or outputs of health systems in a functional or deterministic manner. Lastly, the productivity of the health workforce is likely to be influenced by their emotions, perceptions, cultural background, and various human motivation factors that were not captured in this study.

RESULTS

Appendix 11.1 presents the descriptive statistics for the CHCs and CHPs and MCHPs. The average number of outpatient curative and preventive care visits was higher among CHCs than CHPs and MCHPs. This might partially be attributed to the fact that CHCs have higher health workforce endowment than CHPs and MCHPs.

Technical Efficiency of MCHPS

Appendix 11.2 presents the technical and scale efficiency scores for MCHP clinics. The average score for CRS technical efficiency (CRSTE) was 42.7% (SD = 43.6); for VRS technical efficiency (VRSTE) the average score was 68.2% (SD = 27.2), and for scale efficiency (SE) the average score was 52.8% (SD = 50.6). The average of 68.2% for VRSTE implies that the inefficient MCHPs would need to increase their outputs by 31.8% to become efficient. For CRS, of the 36 MCHPs 17 had a TE of 0%, 1 a TE of 31–40%, 1 a TE of 41–50%, 1 a TE of 51–60%, 3 a TE of 61–70%, 2 a TE of 71–80%, 2 a TE of 81–90%, 3 a TE of 91–99%, and 6 a TE of 100%. Thus, as far as CRS was concerned, 30 MCHPs were relatively technically inefficient and the remaining 6 were technically efficient. For VRS, out of the 36 MCHPs 5 had a TE of 31–40%, 3 a TE of 41–50%, 5 a TE of 51–60%, 3 a TE of 61–70%, 4 a TE of 71–80%, 2 a TE of 81–90%, 4 a TE of 91–99%, and 8 a TE of 100%.

Therefore, for VRS, 28 MCHPs were relatively technically inefficient and 8 were technically efficient. Seventeen MCHPs were scale inefficient and nineteen were scale efficient. Nineteen MCHPs manifested constant returns to scale and seventeen experienced decreasing returns to scale.

Technical Efficiency of CHCs

Appendix 11.3 presents the technical and scale efficiency scores for CHCs. The average score for CRSTE was 62.4% (SD = 32.7), for VRSTE it was 69.2% (SD = 32.7), and for scale efficiency it was 88.8% (SD = 13.5). The mean of 69.2% for VRSTE implies that the inefficient CHCs ought to increase their output by 30.8%. The CRSTE scores for the 22 CHCs were distributed as follows: 3 had a CRSTE of 11–20%, 3 a CRSTE of 21–30%, 1 a CRSTE of 31–40%, 1 a CRSTE of 41–50%, 3 a CRSTE of 51–60%, 2 a CRSTE of 71–80%, 3 a CRSTE of 81–90%, and 6 a CRSTE of 100%. Thus, in the CRS DEA model 72.3% of the CHCs were found to be technically inefficient. The distribution of VRSTE scores was as follows: 1 had a VRSTE score of 11–20%, 4 a score of 21–30%, 1 a score of 31–40%, 1 a score of 41–50%, 3 a score of 51–60%, 1 a score of 61–70%, 2 a score of 91–99%, and 9 a score 100%. Therefore, in the VRS DEA model 59.1% of the CHCs were technically inefficient. In terms of SE, the 22 CHCs were distributed as follows: 2 had an SE of 51–60%, 1 an SE of 61–70%, 2 an SE of 71–80%, 3 an SE of 81–90%, 7 an SE of 91–99% and 7 SE of 100%. Thus, 68.2% of CHCs were scale inefficient.

Technical Efficiency of CHPs

Appendix 11.4 portrays the technical and scale efficiency scores for CHPs. The average scores among the CHPs were 57.2% (SD = 35.8) for CRSTE, 59% (SD = 34.7) for VRSTE, and 95.5% (SD = 9.4) for scale efficiency. The VRSTE score of 59% indicates that the inefficient CHPs will need to increase their health service output by 41% in order to become technically efficient. The 21 CHPs had CRSTE scores distributed as follows: 1 had a CRSTE score of 1–10%, 2 a score of 11–20%, 3 a score of 21–30%, 3 a score of 31–40%, 3 a score of 41–50%, 1 a score of 51–60%, 1 a score of 91–99%, and 7 had a score of 100%. Thus, in the CRS DEA model 67% of the CHPs were technically inefficient relative to their peers.

The VRSTE scores among the 21 CHPs were distributed as follows: 1 had a VRSTE score of 1–10%, 2 a score of 11–20%, 2 a score of 21–30%, 2 a score of 31–40%, 4 a score of 41–50%, 2 a score of 51–60%, 1 a score of 91–99% and 7 a score of 100%. Thus, in the VRS DEA model 67% of the community health posts were technically inefficient relative to their peers. Of the 21 CHPs, 14 had an SE score of 100%. The remaining seven were scale inefficient: 1 had an SE of 61–70%, 1 an SE of 71–80%, 2 an SE of 81–90%, and 3 an SE of 91–99%. Seven CHPs manifested DRS, implying that they were too big for their size. The other 14 manifested CRS indicating that their size was optimal.

DISCUSSION

Key Findings

The findings show that 28 (77.8%) MCHPs, 14 (59.1%) CHCs, and 14 (66.7%) CHPs had VRSTE scores of less than 100%, an indication that they were technically inefficient. The average TE scores were 68.2% (SD = 0.272) among MCHPs, 69.2% (SD = 0.332) among CHCs, and 59% (SD = 0.347) among CHPs. Thus, the TE of CHCs was higher than that of either MCHPs or CHPs. The average SE scores were 52.8% (SD = 50.6) among MCHPs, 88.8% (SD = 13.5) among CHCs, and 95.5% (SD = 9.4) among CHPs. It is worth noting that average SE scores for CHPs were higher than those for both CHCs and MCHPs.

The TE of PHUs in Sierra Leone of between 59% and 69.2% was within the ranges for Canada (60.4%) [11], Ethiopia (57%) [6], Ghana (57%, 49%) [10,15], Kenya (65%) [16], Norway (58–78%) [7], Sierra Leone (63%), and Zambia (61.9%) [14]. However, the TE of Sierra Leone's PHUs was lower than those of Burkina Faso (91%) [9], Finland (72–81%) [17], Greece (73.23%) [13], Portugal (84.4%) [8], Seychelles (92–96%) [12] and UK (82.1%, 92.6%) [19,20]. The SE of primary care units in Sierra Leone of between 52.8% and 95.5% was in the same range as those of Ethiopia (95%) [6], Finland (62–79%) [17], Ghana (86%, 84%) [10,15], Kenya (70%) [16] and Sierra Leone (72%) [5]. However, the SE score was lower than that of Burkina Faso of 97% [9].

Scope of Output Increases and Implications for Policy

Were the inefficient MCHPs, CHCs, and CHPs to operate as efficiently as their peers on the production possibilities frontier (efficiency frontier), there would be scope to increase health service outputs. Appendix 11.5 presents output increases needed to make inefficient MCHPs efficient. The inefficient MCHPs combined would need to increase the number of OMFE visits by 36,848, vector control activities by 7,150, and health education sessions by 3,660 in order to become efficient. Appendix 11.6 depicts the output increases needed to make inefficient CHCs efficient. To achieve this, the inefficient CHCs combined would need to increase the number of OMFE visits by 70,334 (74%), vector control activities by 4,042 (30%), and health education sessions by 7,330 (145%).

Appendix 11.7 portrays the output increases needed to make inefficient CHPs efficient. The inefficient CHPs combined would need to increase the number of OMFE visits by 57,493 (105%), vector control activities by 9,688 (122%), and health education sessions by 2,966 (74%) in order to become efficient. In relation to the health units (MCHPs, CHCs and CHPs) with outputs falling short of the variable returns to scale DEA targets, the Ministry of Health and Sanitation could improve their efficiency by boosting demand for underutilised services, i.e., outpatient care, maternal and child health services, family planning services, routine immunisation, vector control activities, and health education sessions. This might be achieved by leveraging several strategies.

First, the financial barriers to effective access to health services such as the need to make out-of-pocket payments can be addressed through a number of ways: (*a*) planned abolishment of official and unofficial user fees in public health facilities [29]; (*b*) provision of free ambulance services; (*c*) improvement of transport in rural areas where most of the primary healthcare units are situated; (*d*) improvement in health workforce motivation and supervision to make them more responsive to non-medical expectations of patients and by so doing reduce patient waiting, diagnosis, and treatment time and so improve perceived quality of care; (*e*) implementation of universal coverage policy, which seeks access to key promotive, preventive, curative, and rehabilitative health interventions for all residents at an affordable cost through either tax-funded health services or national social health insurance [30–33]; (*f*) increase of people's access to microfinance and lending programmes to help households to self-insure for consumption of basic services [34]; and (*g*) increase demand for underutilised preventive health services by making direct cash transfers to poor households contingent on them utilising those services [35–37].

Second, the demand for MCHP, CHC, and CHP services can be created through leveraging behaviour change community health programmes to move groups and individuals one step at a time (by providing knowledge, motivation, and skills) through the stages (pre-contemplation, contemplation, preparation, action, maintenance) of behaviour change [38]. Third, judicious use should be made of health promotion to stimulate demand for underutilised PHU services. It is important to remember that health promotion is any combination of health education with appropriate legal, fiscal, economic, environmental, and organisational interventions in programmes to attain health and prevent disease [39]. Health promotion action can contribute towards optimal utilisation of PHU services by:

1. Increasing individual knowledge and skills using health information, education, and communication (IEC) [40];

2. Strengthening community action through social mobilisation and social marketing [39];

3. Using mediation and negotiation to create environments that are protective and supportive of health [39];

4. Developing public health policies, legislation, and economic and fiscal controls that enhance health and development through lobbying and advocacy [39];

5. Reorienting health services by emphasising prevention and promotion of healthy behaviour and lifestyle patterns.

In short, health promotion methods using IEC, social mobilisation, social marketing, mediation, lobbying, and advocacy are especially relevant in mobilising non-health sectors such as agriculture, commerce, culture, education, industry, information technology, sanitation, transport and water to contribute to health development through action on the broad determinants of health [39].

CONCLUSION

This study estimated TE of samples of peripheral health units in Kailahun and Kenema districts of Sierra Leone and the output increases needed to make inefficient units efficient. The findings indicate that 28 (77.8%) MCHPs, 14 (59.1%) CHCs, and 14 (66.7%) CHPs were variable returns to scale technically inefficient.

In line with the Ouagadougou Declaration on Primary Health Care and Health Systems in Africa: Achieving Better Health for Africa in the New Millennium [41], there is need to strengthen national and district health management information systems to routinely capture data on input quantities, prices of health systems, and outputs of health services to facilitate regular efficiency analyses. Institutionalisation of health facility efficiency monitoring will arm health decision-makers with the vital information needed to take appropriate actions to reduce waste of scarce health systems resources. Institutionalisation of monitoring of health facility efficiency will strengthen health sector advocacy for increasing domestic and external resources for health.

Acknowledgements

We are grateful to the Ministry of Health and Sanitation of Sierra Leone for having authorised this study to be carried out. The data were collected by Dr Santigie Seasay from Kailahun District and Dr Yankuba Bah from Kenema District. The two are district medical officers in charge of the two districts. We owe profound gratitude to Jehovah Jireh for sustenance during the entire study.

This article contains the perceptions and views of the authors only and does not represent the decisions or the stated policies of either the World Health Organization or the Ministry of Health and Sanitation of Sierra Leone.

REFERENCES

1. Government of Sierra Leone, Ministry of Health and Sanitation. *National health policy.* Freetown: Government Printer; 2009.

2. Government of Sierra Leone, Ministry of Health and Sanitation. *National health sector strategic plan: 2010–2011.* Freetown: Government Printer; 2009.

3. Government of Sierra Leone, Ministry of Health and Sanitation. *Cost-sharing policy.* Freetown: Government Printer; 2006.

4. Government of Sierra Leone. *Hospital Boards Act.* Freetown: Government Printer; 2003.

5. Renner Ade, Kirigia JM, Zere AE, Barry SP, Kirigia DG, Kamara C, Muthuri HK. Technical efficiency of peripheral health units in Pujehun district of Sierra Leone: a DEA application. *BMC Health Services Research* 2005; 5:77. Available at: http://www.biomedcentral.com/1472–6963/5/77

6. Sebastian MS, Lemma H. Efficiency of the health extension programme in Tigray, Ethiopia: a data envelopment analysis. *BMC International Health and Human Rights* 2010; 10:16. Available at: http://www.biomedcentral.com/1472-698X/10/16

7. Halsteinli V, Kittelsen SA, Magnussen J. Productivity growth in outpatient child and adolescent mental health services: the impact of case-mix adjustment. *Social Science & Medicine* 2010;70: 439–446.

8. Amado CAEF, Santos SP. Challenges for performance assessment and improvement in primary health care: the case of the Portuguese health centres. *Health Policy* 2009; 91:43–56.

9. Marschall P, Flessa S. Assessing the efficiency of rural health centres in Burkina Faso: an application of data envelopment analysis. *Journal of Public Health* 2009; 17(2):87–95.

10. Akazili J, Adjuik M, Jehu-Appiah C, Zere E. Using data envelopment analysis to measure the extent of technical efficiency of public health centres in Ghana. *BMC International Health and Human Rights* 2008;8:11. Available at: http://www.biomedcentral.com/1472-698X/8/11

11. Milliken O, Devlin RA, Barham, Hogg W, Dahrouge S, Russell G. *Comparative efficiency assessment of primary care models using data envelopment analysis.* Department of Economics Working Paper #0802E. Ottawa (Ontario): University of Ottawa; 2008.

12. Kirigia JM, Emrouznejad A, Vaz RG, Bastiene J, Padayachy J. A comparative assessment of performance and productivity of health centres in Seychelles.

International Journal of Productivity and Performance Management 2008; 57(1):72–92.

13. Kontodimopoulous N, Nanos P, Niakas D. Balancing efficiency of health services and equity of access in remote areas in Greece. *Health Policy* 2006;76:49–57.

14. Masiye F, Kirigia JM, Emrouznejad A, Sambo LG, Mounkaila A, Chimfwembe D, Okello D: Efficient management of health centres human resources in Zambia. *Journal of Medical Systems* 2006;30:473–481.

15. Osei D, George M, d'Almeida S, Kirigia JM, Mensah AO, Kainyu LH. Technical efficiency of public district hospitals and health centres in Ghana: a pilot study. *Cost Effectiveness and Resource Allocation* 2005;3:9. Available at: http://www.resource-allocation.com/content/3/1/9.

16. Kirigia JM, Emrouznejad A, Sambo LG, Munguti N, Liambila W. Using data envelopment analysis to measure the technical efficiency of public health centres in Kenya. *Journal of Medical Systems* 2004;28(2):155–166.

17. Linna M, Nordblad A, Koivu M. Technical and cost efficiency of oral healthcare provision in Finnish health centres. *Social Science & Medicine* 2003;56: 343–353.

18. Kirigia JM, Sambo LG, Scheel H. Technical efficiency of public clinics in Kwazulu-Natal Province of South Africa. *East African Medical Journal* 2001;78 (3 Suppl): S1–S13.

19. Johnston K, Gerard K. Assessing efficiency in the UK breast screening programme: does size of screening unit make a difference? *Health Policy* 2001;56: 21–32.

20. Salinas-Jimenez J, Smith P. Data envelopment analysis applied to quality in primary health care. *Annals of Operations Research* 1996;67:141–161.

21. World Health Organization: *National health accounts: country information.* Geneva:World Health Organization; 2009. Available (http://www.who.int/ nha/country)

22. African Union. *African Union Summit on HIV/AIDS, Tuberculosis and other related diseases.* Decision OAU/SPS/Abuja/3. Addis Ababa: African Union; 2001.

23. World Health Organization: *Macroeconomics and health: investing in health for economic development.* Geneva: World Health Organization; 2001.

24. World Health Organization: *World health statistics report.* Geneva: World Health Organization; 2010.

25. Commonwealth of Australia. Steering Committee for the Review of Commonwealth/State Service Provision: Data envelopment analysis: a technique for measuring the efficiency of government service delivery. Canberra: AGPS; 1997.

26. Charnes A, Coopers W, Rhodes E. Measuring the efficiency of decision making units. *European Journal Operational Research* 1978;2(6):429–444.

27. World Health Organization, Regional Office for Africa. *Primary health care facility economics efficiency analysis data collection instrument.* Brazzaville: World Health Organization; 2000.

28. Coelli TJ: *A guide to DEAP version 2.1: a data envelopment analysis (computer) program,* Centre for Efficiency and Productivity Analysis (CEPA) Working Paper 96/08. Department of Econometrics, University of New England, Armidale, NSW Australia; 1996.

29. Yates R. Universal health care and the removal of user fees. *The Lancet* 2009;373:2078–81.

30. Carrin G, Doetinchem O, Kirigia J, Mathauer I, Musango L. Social health insurance: how feasible is its expansion in the African Region? *DevIssues* 2008;10(2):7–9.

31. Carrin G, Mathaur I,Xu K, Evans D. Universal coverage of health services: tailoring its implementation. *Bulletin of the World Health Organization* 2008;86(11):857–863.

32. McIntyre D, Garshong B, Mtei G, Meheus F, Thiede M, Akazili J, Ally M, Aikins M, Mulligan J-A, Goudge J. Beyond fragmentation and towards universal coverage: insights from Ghana, South Africa and the United Republic of Tanzania. *Bulletin of the World Health Organization* 2008;86(11):871–876.

33. World Health Organization. World health report: health systems financing – the path to universal coverage. Geneva: World Health Organization; 2010.

34. Leive A, Xu K. Coping with out-of-pocket health payments: empirical evidence from 15 African countries. *Bulletin of the World Health Organization* 2008;86(11):849–856.

35. Morris SS, Flore R, Olinto P, Medina JM. Monetary incentives in primary health care and effects on use and coverage of preventive healthcare interventions in rural Honduras: cluster randomized trial. *The Lancet* 2004;364:2030–37.

36. Lim SS, Dandona L, Hoisington JA, James SL, Hogan MC, Gakindu E. India's Janani Suraksha Yojana, a conditional cash transfer programme to increase births in health facilities: an impact evaluation. *The Lancet* 2010;375:2009–23.

37. Save the Children UK. *Lasting benefits: the role of cash transfers in tackling child mortality.* London: Save the Children; 2009.

38. Jenkins CD. *Building better health: a handbook of behavioural change.* Washington, D.C.: Pan American Health Organization; 2003.

39. World Health Organization Regional Office for Africa. *Health promotion: a strategy for the African Region.* AFR/RC51/12. Brazzaville: World Health Organization; 2003.

40. Mushi D, Mpembeni R, Jahn A. Effectiveness of community based safe motherhood promoters in improving the utilisation of obstetric care. The case of Mtwara Rural District in Tanzania. *BMC Pregnancy and Childbirth* 2010;10:14. Available at: http://www.biomedcentral.com/1471–2393/10/14

41. World Health Organization, Regional Office for Africa. *Ouagadougou declaration on primary health care and health systems in Africa: achieving better health for Africa in the new millennium.* Brazzaville: World Health Organization; 2008.

Appendix 11.1   Descriptive statistics for community health posts, maternal, child health and family planning centres, and community health centres.

	OMFE	Vector control activities	Health education sessions	Number of CHOs + MCH aides + SECHNs	Number of other health staff
Community health posts					
Mean	2,604.3	377.6	190.1	1.8	4.2
SD	2,444.9	402.2	301.4	0.4	4.6
Median	1,885.0	294.0	130.0	2.0	2.0
Maternal and child health and family planning centres (MCHP)					
Mean	1,715.1	318.8	152.6	1.2	1.9
SD	947.1	194.9	101.0	0.8	2.9
Median	1,710.5	346.0	120.0	1.0	1.0
Community health centres (CHC)					
Mean	4,330.5	615.2	230.5	2.5	5.6
SD	2,750.4	546.8	325.7	0.9	4.6
Median	3,892.5	475.0	128.5	2.0	5.5

Note: OMFE is the number of outpatient care visits plus maternal, child health and family planning visits plus immunisation visits

Appendix 11.2   Technical and scale efficiency scores for maternal, child health, and family planning clinics

MCHP units	CRSTE	VRSTE	Scale	Returns to scale
Kpayama	1	1	1	–
Gbo Kakajama	0.782	0.782	1	–
Gbo Lambayama	0.921	0.921	1	–
Woyama	0	0.373	0	DRS
Nyagbebu	0	0.334	0	DRS
Gendema	1	1	1	–
Kondebalihun	0	0.578	0	DRS
Nyandehun Koya	0	0.936	0	DRS
Gbado	0	0.323	0	DRS
Gbagaima	0	1	0	DRS
Sembehun	0	0.784	0	DRS
Gandorhun	0	0.407	0	DRS
Jui	0	0.344	0	DRS
Gelehun	0	0.555	0	DRS
Samai Town	0.619	0.619	1	–
Masahun	0.323	0.323	1	–
Ngelehun	0	0.54	0	DRS
Sandaru Gaura	0.924	0.924	1	–
Konabu	0	0.73	0	DRS
Njagbahun	1	1	1	–
Diamei Dama	0.604	0.604	1	–
Perrie Gaura	0.887	0.887	1	–
Jao Tunkia	0	1	0	DRS
Guala	0.681	0.681	1	–
Semewahun	0.616	0.616	1	–

.../cont.

Appendix 11.2 (cont.)

MCHP units	CRSTE	VRSTE	Scale	Returns to scale
Sembeima	0.759	0.759	1	–
Ngiehun	1	1	1	–
Bomie	0.838	0.838	1	–
Massayeima	0	0.43	0	DRS
Fola	1	1	1	–
Gbeika	0	0.188	0	DRS
Pendembu Njiegbla	0.44	0.44	1	–
Niahun Gboyama	0	0.557	0	DRS
Ngiehun	1	1	1	–
Jikibu	0.973	0.973	1	–
Mende Buima	0	0.122	0	DRS
Mean	**0.427**	**0.682**	**0.528**	
SD	**0.436**	**0.272**	**0.506**	
Median	**0.382**	**0.706**	**1.000**	

Note: CRSTE = technical efficiency from CRS DEA; VRSTE = technical efficiency
from VRS DEA; scale = scale efficiency = CRSTE/VRSTE

*Appendix 11.3   Technical and scale efficiency score for community
health centres (CHCs)*

Firm	CRSTE	VRSTE	Scale	Returns to scale
Dodo	1	1	1	–
Blama	0.14	0.243	0.578	DRS
Baoma Koya	0.214	0.223	0.962	DRS
Levuma	0.767	1	0.767	DRS
Sendumei	1	1	1	–
Boajibu	0.531	0.57	0.932	DRS
Largo	0.296	0.493	0.601	DRS
Bendu	1	1	1	–
Tungai	1	1	1	–
Hangha	1	1	1	–
Ngegbwema	0.879	0.947	0.928	DRS
Tongo	0.876	1	0.876	DRS
Bandajuma	0.576	0.659	0.874	DRS
Pejewa	0.186	0.188	0.992	DRS
Lalehun Kovoma	0.212	0.212	1	–
Dia	0.462	0.509	0.909	DRS
Daru	0.728	1	0.728	DRS
Gbahama	0.306	0.326	0.94	DRS
Kailahun Town	0.82	0.984	0.833	DRS
Pendembu	1	1	1	–
Mobai	0.189	0.283	0.667	DRS
Baiwalla	0.554	0.59	0.939	DRS
Mean	**0.624**	**0.692**	**0.888**	
SD	**0.327**	**0.332**	**0.135**	
Median	**0.652**	**0.803**	**0.936**	

Note: CRSTE = technical efficiency from CRS DEA
VRSTE = technical efficiency from VRS DEA
Scale = scale efficiency = CRSTE/VRSTE

Appendix 11.4 *Technical and scale efficiency score for community health posts (CHP)*

Firm	CRSTE	VRSTE	Scale	Returns to scale
Serabu	0.228	0.247	0.923	DRS
Yabaima	0.236	0.37	0.638	DRS
Ngiehun Kojo	1	1	1	–
Konta	1	1	1	–
Jormu	0.405	0.486	0.832	DRS
Benduma	1	1	1	–
Veinema	0.969	0.969	1	–
Kpetema	0.477	0.546	0.874	DRS
Mano Njiegbla	1	1	1	–
Mbowohun	1	1	1	–
Bendu	0.535	0.541	0.989	DRS
Bunumbu	1	1	1	–
Mamboma	0.087	0.087	0.995	–
Mano menima	0.294	0.294	1	–
Bandajuma Kpolihun	0.138	0.138	1	–
Kwellu Ngieya	0.433	0.433	1	–
Ngiehun	0.314	0.314	1	–
Nyandehun	0.404	0.406	0.994	DRS
Mafindor	1	1	1	–
Konjo	0.332	0.414	0.801	DRS
Mano Sewallu	0.15	0.15	1	–
Mean	**0.572**	**0.590**	**0.955**	
SD	**0.358**	**0.347**	**0.094**	
Median	**0.433**	**0.486**	**1.000**	

Appendix 11.5 *Output increases needed to make inefficient maternal and child health posts efficient*

MCHP units	OMFE	Vector control activities	Health education sessions
Kpayama	0	0	0
Gbo Kakajama	637	77	51
Gbo Lambayama	221	40	13
Woyama	2,555	399	181
Nyagbebu	2,255	407	199
Gendema	0	0	0
Kondebalihun	1,275	257	215
Nyandehun Koya	2,313	30	23
Gbado	1,081	419	241
Gbagaima	0	0	0
Sembehun	664	126	210
Gandorhun	1,290	583	111
Jui	2,157	381	204
Gelehun	2,116	379	92
Samai Town	929	238	85

../cont.

Appendix 11.5 (cont.)

MCHP unit	OMFE	Vector control activities	Health education sessions
Masahun	1,663	460	84
Ngelehun	1,478	241	227
Sandaru Gaura	209	35	13
Konabu	962	231	280
Njagbahun	0	0	0
Diamei Dama	1,008	240	93
Perrie Gaura	338	44	48
Jao Tunkia	0	0	0
Guala	819	168	68
Semewahun	927	231	86
Sembeima	665	118	62
Ngiehun	0	0	0
Bomie	477	55	82
Massayeima	2,223	306	187
Fola	0	0	0
Gbeika	2,195	770	138
Pendembu Njiegbla	1,632	318	137
Niahun Gboyama	1,260	228	182
Ngiehun	0	0	0
Jikibu	74	0	4
Mende Buima	3425	369	344
Total	**36,848**	**7,150**	**3,660**
Mean	**1,024**	**199**	**102**
SD	**919**	**194**	**95**
Median	**928**	**198**	**85**

Appendix 11.6   Output increases needed to make inefficient community health centres efficient

Community health centre (CHC)	OMFE	Vector control activities	Health education sessions
Dodo	0	0	0
Blama	9,588	344	473
Baoma Koya	7,886	370	470
Levuma	0	0	0
Sendumei	0	0	0
Boajibu	3,812	321	605
Largo	5,946	564	356
Bendu	0	0	0
Tungai	0	0	0
Hangha	0	0	0
Ngegbwema	1,694	51	30
Tongo	0	0	0
Bandajuma	2,448	260	217
Pejewa	8,838	298	630
Lalehun Kovoma	8,614	466	759

…/cont.

Appendix 11.6 (cont.)

Community health centre (CHC)	OMFE	Vector control activities	Health education sessions
Dia	3,991	432	760
Daru	0	0	0
Gbahama	5,631	621	1,297
Kailahun Town	97	21	615
Pendembu	0	0	0
Mobai	8,080	0	434
Baiwalla	3,709	294	684
Total	**70,334**	**4,042**	**7,330**
Mean	**3,197**	**184**	**333**
SD	**3,566**	**215**	**366**
Median	**2,071**	**36**	**287**

Appendix 11.7   *Output increases needed to make inefficient community health posts efficient*

Community health posts (CHP)	OMFE	Vector control activities	Health education sessions
Serabu	4,790	1,048	311
Yabaima	2,077	428	162
Ngiehun Kojo	0	0	0
Konta	0	0	0
Jormu	2,146	790	173
Benduma	0	0	0
Veinema	50	12	32
Kpetema	2,395	686	90
Mano Njiegbla	0	0	0
Mbowohun	0	0	0
Bendu	3,097	1,570	75
Bunumbu	0	0	0
Mamboma	6,532	1,671	157
Mano Menima	5,813	705	192
Bandajuma Kpolihun	7,482	938	142
Kwellu Ngieya	5,736	153	124
Ngiehun	4,390	680	442
Nyandehun	4,008	877	263
Mafindor	0	0	0
Konjo	2,177	0	204
Mano Sewallu	6,800	130	599
Sum	**57,493**	**9,688**	**2,966**
Mean	**2,738**	**461**	**141**
SD	**2,659**	**539**	**160**
Median	**2,177**	**153**	**124**

-12-

Efficient Management of Health Centres
Human Resources in Zambia*

*Felix Masiye, Joses M. Kirigia, Ali Emrouznejad, Luis G. Sambo,
Abdou B. Mounkaila, Davis Chimfwembe and David Okello*

ABSTRACT

This study uses data envelopment analysis (DEA) to estimate the degree of technical, allocative, and cost efficiency in individual public and private health centres and to identify the relative inefficiencies in the use of various inputs among individual health centres. About 83% of the 40 health centres were technically inefficient and 88% of them were both allocatively and cost inefficient. The privately owned health centres were found to be more efficient than public facilities. There is need to undertake these kind of studies among all health facilities (irrespective of proprietorship) in the WHO African Region countries to guide health sector reforms.

Key Words: Health centres management; data envelopment analysis; technical efficiency; Zambia Health

INTRODUCTION

The *World Health Report* (WHR) 2000 [1] and the *Bulletin of the World Health Organization* [2] were devoted to the development and application of a framework for assessing the performance of health systems. The framework includes measurement of three goals of health systems (health, responsiveness, and fairness in financial contribution) and an exposition of four functions of health systems (including financing, service provision, stewardship, and resource generation) [3]. Although the framework and the assessments were heavily criticised on methodological and data grounds [4-7], the WHR created

* The original article appeared in *Journal of Medical Systems 2006;30:473-481*. Reproduced with the permission of Plenum Publishing Corporation.

a heated debate that propelled health systems higher on the priority list of various health development partners. Today, there is a near universal acceptance that in the absence of a functional health system, all piecemeal attempts at addressing priority diseases (e.g., HIV/AIDS, malaria, TB, and childhood diseases) are likely to have dismal, and at most, temporary success.

In that assessment, Zambia ranked number 182 out of 191 Member States of the WHO [1]. Poor countries like Zambia have been asking: What is the point of comparing themselves with rich countries like France, USA, UK, Japan, and others? What is the point of comparing themselves against middle-income countries like South Africa, Botswana, Mexico, and others? Even if Zambia is performing relatively worse off compared to other low-income countries, so what? How can Zambia improve the performance of its health system? How can Zambia measure and improve the performance of its individual health facilities (including hospitals and health centres) that absorb majority of recurrent and capital budgets of the Ministry of Health? The specific objectives of this study were (a) to estimate the degree of technical, allocative and cost efficiency in individual public and private health centres; and (b) to identify the relative inefficiencies in the use of various inputs among individual health centres.

Overview of Zambian Macroeconomic and Health-Related Situation

Socio-economic situation

Zambia is a land-locked, low-income, and highly indebted country located in Southern Africa with a population of 10.4 million people (and growing at annual rate of 2.9%). The economy is largely based on copper mining and agriculture. The collapse of world copper prices in 1970s had devastating effects on the economy. About 86% of the Zambian population lives below the national poverty line and 63.6% live below the income poverty line of US$1 (in 1993 purchasing power parity) per day. The adult illiteracy rate is 21.9%. Thirty-six per cent and 22% of the population do not have access to safe drinking water and adequate sanitation facilities respectively [8].

Health delivery system

Zambia has about 655 doctors, 1,365 clinical officers, and 10,378 nurses working in 84 hospitals and 1,084 health centres [9]. The vision of government has been to provide all Zambians with equitable access to cost-effective quality health care. To realise this vision, government embarked on health sector reform in 1992 whose main thrust was to decentralise the planning, management, and decision-making of health services to the health boards and restructuring of health delivery systems. The process of restructuring culminated in the formation of one Central Board of Health

(CBoH), 72 District Health Boards (DHBs), and 20 Hospital Management Boards (HMBs). The Central Ministry of Health is responsible for policy and strategic direction, while the CBoH is in charge of interpretation and implementation of health policies and overall technical management of health services. The district health system and hospitals are run by the DHBs and HMBs. Inspite of the various forms of health sector reforms that have been introduced, approximately 36% of the population does not have access to essential medicines; 64% of infants do not use oral rehydration; 75% of the eligible population do not use contraceptives; 54% of births are not attended by skilled health attendants; and there are only 7 physicians per 100,000 people [8].

Health profile

Zambian health indicators are generally very poor. Average life expectancy at birth is 41.4 years and the disability-adjusted life expectancy (DALE) is 30.3 years [10]. Maternal mortality ratio (MMR) was recorded at 650 per 100,000 live births [11]. Under-5 mortality rate was 202 per 1,000 [11]. Twenty-five per cent of the children under 5 years of age are underweight [9]. Infant mortality rate was 112 per 1,000 live births [10]. The probability at birth of surviving to age 40 was 53.6% in 2001 [8]. These dismal health indicators have largely been attributed to widespread poverty, which has been widened and deepened by the growing incidence of HIV. Faced with such widespread poverty, the only sustainable option the country has is to improve quality and coverage of health services through enhanced efficiency in the use of health sector resources at all levels of the national health system.

Rationale for focusing on health centres

This study focuses on health centres for a number of reasons: *(a)* they are a critical part of primary healthcare system; *(b)* they are a vital part of the so-called close-to-client (CTC) health service delivery system (or district health system), and thus, important to efforts of scaling-up of pro-poor package of cost-effective interventions to meet the Millennium Development Goals [12], Health-for-All policy in the twenty-first century targets [13], the Commission on Macroeconomics and Health recommendations [14], and the New Partnership for Africa's Development (NEPAD) health targets [15]; *(c)* they serve majority of the rural people (especially the poor) who constitute about 80% of the total population in Zambia (and indeed in majority of other countries in the Region); *(d)* inefficiency among health centres (and all other facilities for that matter) is unethical and immoral [16,17] because it implies lost opportunities of improving an extra person's health status at no additional cost; *(e)* CBoH and DHMTs can evaluate the effect of health sector reforms by scrutinising periodic changes in efficiency scores of both public and private health centres; *(f)* the Zambian hospital efficiency study [9] identified the need for replicating the study among health centres; *(g)* the growing problem of brain-drain in the country (and indeed in the African Region) calls for urgent measures of ensuring that the remaining human resources are utilised optimally; and *(h)* monitoring of efficiency of health centres is part and parcel of the broader stewardship role of the State (through Ministry of Health) [18], especially ensuring that the benefits from health sector investments (by Governments and partners) are optimised.

Previous research/studies

This section does not aim at providing a comprehensive review of the health-related DEA literature. Instead, it attempts to review just a few recent health-related DEA applications to underscore the growing and fruitful use of DEA approaches in shedding light on the efficiency of various aspects of health systems.

USA - Chattopadhy and Ray [19] applied DEA to examine the levels of technical, scale, and size efficiency of 140 nursing homes providing health care to the elderly in Connecticut, USA. Shroff [20] utilised DEA to estimate the relative efficiency of 26 potential sites for a long-term healthcare facility in the Northern Virginia region of USA.

UK - Hollingsworth and Parkin [21] used DEA to analyse data of neonatal services for a sample of 49 units in the United Kingdom to determine technical efficiency, economies of scale, and potential cost savings if the units were to operate efficiently. Jacobs [22] used 232 UK Department NHS hospitals (Trusts) dataset to compare the efficiency rankings of three cost indices (the CCI, 2CCI, and 3CCI) with those obtained using DEA and Stochastic Frontier Analysis (SFA).

Turkey - Ersoy [23] used DEA to find out the portion of a sample of 573 acute general hospitals that were operating efficiently and the inputs (outputs) that contribute most to inefficiency.

Finland - Linna, Nordblad and Koivu [24] used a two-stage procedure to estimate and explain technical efficiency (TE) and cost efficiency (CE) of oral care provision in 228 Finnish health centres.

Taiwan - Chang [25] used DEA to evaluate relative technical efficiency of six central government-owned hospitals in Taiwan utilising panel data for five years. Wan et al [26] explored the technical efficiency of nursing productivity and patient care costs among 57 nursing units in a tertiary care medical centre in Taiwan (Republic of China) using a variable returns to scale DEA model.

South Africa - Kirigia, Sambo, and Lambo [27] employed DEA methodology to identify and measure technical and scale efficiencies among 55 public hospitals in South Africa. Kirigia, Sambo, and Scheel [28] utilised DEA to investigate the technical inefficiencies among 155 primary healthcare clinics in Kwazulu-Natal Province of South Africa. Zere, McIntyre and Addison [29] used DEA to examine technical and scale efficiency of a sample of 86 non-academic acute hospitals in the Eastern, Northern, and Western Cape Provinces of South Africa.

Kenya - Kirigia, Emrouznejad, and Sambo [30] measured relative efficiency of 54 public hospitals in Kenya using input-oriented DEA technique. Twenty-six per cent of the hospitals analysed had some technical inefficiency. The inefficient hospitals could reduce their utilisation of all inputs by about 16% without reducing outputs. About 30% of the hospitals were scale inefficient. The average scale efficiency score in the whole sample was 90% implying that total output could be increased by 10% at the current input levels. The study also estimated the input reductions and/or output increases needed to make the individual inefficient public hospitals efficient.

Zambia - Masiye *et al* [9] used DEA to measure the degree of technical and allocative efficiency of 20 hospitals (including 10 mission, 9 government, and 1 private hospitals) in Zambia. Two models were estimated. The first model used one input (namely total expenditure) and five outputs comprising of outpatient department (OPD) visits for children aged under five years, OPD visits for children aged over five years, number of bed days for under-fives, bed days for over-fives, and number of deliveries. In model 2, the authors used three inputs consisting of non-labour expenditure, number of doctors (including clinical officers), and number of other personnel and three outputs, namely, total OPD visits (under-fives plus over-fives), total number of bed days and number of deliveries. In model 2, they included price variables to enable them to compute allocative efficiency scores.

In model 1, 75% of the hospitals were technically inefficient with an average score of 0.441. In model 2, 50% of the hospitals were found to be technically inefficient with an average score of 0.543. Eighty-five per cent of the hospitals were both allocatively and economically (in overall terms) inefficient with average scores of 0.798 and 0.575 respectively. The latter finding implies that the 17 economically inefficient hospitals could produce their current levels of output with 42.5% less cost. To reduce the inefficiencies in hospitals, it would be necessary to reallocate the excess inputs to the primary healthcare (PHC) facilities, but before such an action is taken there is need to establish the efficiency of individual PHC facilities. This study did not estimate the input reductions and/or output increases needed to make the individual inefficient hospitals efficient. Such information would have been very useful to the policy makers in designing interventions geared toward reducing the inefficient use of individual inputs.

DEA Conceptual Framework

In the production process, health centres turn inputs (factors of production) into outputs (e.g., curative visits, outreach health education visits, MCH visits). Inputs can be divided into the broad categories of labour, materials, and capital each of which might include more narrow subdivisions. Labour inputs include skilled workers (doctors, clinical officers, nurses, pharmacists, laboratory technologists/technicians, etc) and unskilled workers (cleaners, lawn mowers, mesengers, etc) as well as the entrepreneurial efforts of the health centre managers and district health management teams. Materials include pharmaceuticals, non-pharmaceutical supplies, electricity, water, and any other goods that the health centres acquire and transform into final services. Capital includes buildings, vehicles, medical equipment, beds, etc.

The relationship between the quantities of inputs and the resulting quantities of outputs is described by a production function (PF). Production function describes the maximum output feasible for a given set of inputs and a given level of technology (i.e., a given state of knowledge about the various methods that might be used to transform inputs into outputs). Suppose, for example, that the inputs are full-time nursing time and full-time clinical officer time per year and that they are used to produce outpatient care proxied by outpatient visits. That production function can be depicted graphically (Figure 12.1) using an isoquant (IS), (i.e., a curve that shows all the possible combinations of inputs that yield the same output). AB is the isocost, i.e. the minimum cost line.

Technical efficiency (TE) is about ensuring no resources are wasted (i.e., the maximum amount of output is obtained from the available inputs) [31]. Health centres I, Q, and S are technically efficient because they are operating on the production function or isoquant or efficiency frontier. Their efficiency score is one (or 100%). Health centres P and T are inefficient because they are using more nurses' and clinical officers' time to produce the same level of output as health centres I, Q, and S. The extent of technical inefficiency of health centre 'P' can be expressed as [1-(OQ/OP)] [32], which is the amount by which all inputs could be proportionately reduced without a reduction in output.

Allocative efficiency (AE) is about using resources to produce outputs with the highest possible value. Allocative efficiency implies the isoquant (IS) and isocost (AB) lines are tangential. Even though health centres I and Q are technically efficient, they are allocatively inefficient. Health centre S is both technically and allocatively efficient. Allocative efficiency of facility P = OR / OQ.

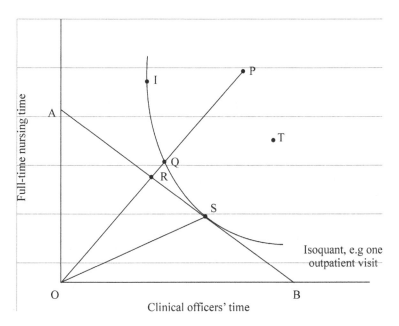

Figure 12.1   Health centre technical and allocative efficiencies

Economic efficiency (or cost efficiency) combines both productive efficiency (producing without waste on the production possibilities frontier) with allocative efficiency (allocating resources to their most highly valued uses) [31]. Cost efficiency of facility P = OR/OP = (OQ/OP) × (OR/OQ) = TE × AE.

The input-oriented frontier production function technical efficiency measurement approach used in this study is that proposed in Farrell [33] and generalised through the use of mathematical programming by Charnes, Cooper and Rhodes [34]. For parametric DEA models see Emrouznejad [35] and Emrouznejad and Thanassoulis [36]. See also Emrouznejad [37] for method of calculation.

Technical efficiency

DEA measures the technical efficiency of health centre *k* compared with *n* peer group of health centres as follows [38]:

Objective function:

$$Max\ E_k = \frac{\sum\limits_{r=1}^{s} u_r y_{rk}}{\sum\limits_{i=1}^{m} v_i x_{ik}}$$

Subject to:

Less-than-unity constraint:

$$\frac{\sum\limits_{r=1}^{s} u_r y_{rj}}{\sum\limits_{i=1}^{m} v_i x_{ik}} \leq 1; j = 1,...,n$$

$$u_r \geq 0; r = 1,...,s,$$

$$v_i \geq 0; i = 1,...,m,$$

where E_k = efficiency score of kth health centre, y_{rj} = observed amount of rth output produced by the jth health centre, x_{ij} = quantity of ith input used by the jth health centre, u_r = the weight given to output r by the DEA programme, v_i = the weight given to ith input by the DEA programme, n = the number of health centres, m = the number of inputs used by health centre k, s = the number of outputs produced by health centre k, and k is the health centre being assessed in the set of $j=1,...,n$ health centres.

The above constraint implies that TE of health centre k is maximised subject to efficiency of all health centres being less than or equal to one. In other words, the relative efficiency of all health centres is constrained between 1 (relatively efficient) and less than 1 (relatively inefficient). The 'Us' and 'Vs' are variables of the problem and are constrained to be greater than or equal to some small positive quantity ϵ in order to avoid any input or output being totally ignored in determining the efficiency [39].

Allocative efficiency

The formula for determining the degree of allocative efficiency for the j_0^{th} health centre is given by estimating the linear program formulation below [40]:

$$\sum_{j=1}^{N} \lambda_j Y_{rj} \geq Y_{rj0}........(r = 1,2,...,R) \tag{1}$$

$$\sum_{j=1}^{N} \lambda_j X_{ij} - Z_i = 0 \ldots (i = 1, 2, \ldots, M') \tag{2}$$

$$\sum_{j=1}^{N} \lambda_j X_{ij} \leq X_{ij0} \ldots (i = M'+1, \ldots, M) \tag{3}$$

$$\sum_{j=1}^{N} \lambda_j \geq 1 \tag{4}$$

$$Min \sum_{i=1}^{M'} P_{ij0} Z_i \tag{5}$$

$$\sum_{i=1}^{M'} P_{ij0} Z_i^* = \sum_{i=1}^{M'} P_{ij0} X_{ij0} \tag{6}$$

$$\sum_{i=1}^{M'} P_{ij0}(X_{ij0} - Z_i^*) \tag{7}$$

$$\frac{\sum_{i=1}^{M'} P_{ij0}(Z_i^*)}{\sum_{i=1}^{M'} P_{ij0} X_{ij0}} \tag{8}$$

Constraint (1) ensures the composite frontier health centre equals or exceeds the level of each output actually obtained by the j_0^{th} health centre; (3) ensures that the frontier health centre enjoys no more of a favourable situation than does the $j0^{th}$ health centre; (4) assumes constant or increasing returns to scale prevail; (5) the objective function; and (2) determines the most cost-effective use of each of the controllable resources so as to meet the specified output vector (Y_1, j_0, $Y_2, j_0, \ldots,$

Y_R, J_0) at minimum total cost, $\sum_{i=1}^{M'} P_{ij0} Z_i^*$.

The goal of the current study was to demonstrate to policy makers, using a sample of Zambian health centres, how data that are routinely collected by a national Health Information System (HIS) can fruitfully be analysed using DEA method to shed light on the performance (efficiency) of individual health centres (HCs). This approach views HCs as productive units that use multiple inputs to produce one or more outputs. The approach yields measures of HCs relative efficiency by deriving an efficiency frontier (a production function) and measuring the distance of HCs to the frontier to get their efficiency scores. Health centres on the frontier get an efficiency score of one (100%) and those below the frontier score less than one (below 100%) depending on how far they are from the frontier.

DATA

Due to budgetary constraints, the current study was based on a sample of 40 health centres (i.e., 3.7% of the total). Fifty-eight per cent of the health facilities in the sample were government owned, while the remaining 42% were private-for-profit. Health centres provide four key services: outpatient visits, basic medical examinations, maternal health services, and outreach preventive care. Cases that require inpatient care are referred to the hospitals. Health centres have a laboratory, pharmacy, consultation room, and a Maternal and Child Health department.

Technical efficiency requires data on quantities of inputs and outputs of health centres. Ultimate health service outcome measures (e.g., number of lives saved or extended, quality-adjusted life years gained, health-adjusted life years gained and disability-adjusted life years saved) are not routinely compiled by either the health centres or the National Health Information System. In fact, even multiple process count information (e.g., number of curative, preventive, and promotive care visits and number of health outreach visits) was not readily available in the records. Therefore, in the current study, the health centres were assumed to produce one output (i.e., number of outpatient healthcare visits) using three inputs, namely, numbers of clinical officers, nurses, and support staff.

The data were collected from 40 health centres in three provinces, namely, Lusaka, Central, and Copperbelt provinces. The data available centrally at the Central Board of Health (CBoH) were found to be outdated. Thus, data had to be collected from health centres using questionnaires prepared for the purpose. The questionnaires were administered by two of the authors (FM and DC). The analysis was accomplished using DEA software developed by Coelli [32]. The main limitations of the current study have to do with lack of quality-adjusted output measures; lack of outpatient visits data broken down by disease to give an indication of case mix differences (if any); and lack of data on non-labour inputs.

RESULTS

Table 12.1 presents the means and standard deviations for input and output variables of 17 private health centres and 23 public health centres. It is important to note that the remunerations in the private sector are more than twice those of the public sector.

Health centres' technical efficiency (TE), allocative efficiency (AE), and cost efficiency (CE) scores are summarised in Table 12.2. Efficiency scores for individual health facilities can be found in Appendix 12.1. The average TE for the whole sample was 0.619, AE was 0.685, and CE was 0.445.

Table 12.1 Descriptive statistics (mean and standard deviation) for the inputs and output

Variable	Privately owned health centres		Government owned health centres	
	Mean	Standard Deviation	Mean	Standard Deviation
Inputs				
Number of clinical officers	3	2	1	1
Number of nurses	3	3	12	7
Number of other staff	2	2	4	2
Clinical officers' average monthly wage plus allowances (in Kwacha)	597,672	136,963	231,903	43,678
Nurses' average monthly wage plus allowances (in Kwacha)	440,265	121,289	205,447	34,184
Other staff average monthly wage plus allowances (in Kwacha)	210,668	95,917	82,014	12,799
Output				
Number of visits	6,322	5,869	11,009	7,899

The TE, AE, and CE scores are constrained between 1 (totally efficient) and 0 (totally inefficient). All those health centres with an efficiency rating of less than one are inefficient. What do the average efficiency scores in Table 12.2 mean? For example, the TE of privately owned health centres is 0.70; this means that those health centres (compared with their peers) on average should be able to produce their actual output level using 30% [(1.00-0.70) × 100] less of each input. As evidenced in Table 12.2 the privately owned health centres are more technically, allocatively, and cost efficient than those owned by the government.

Table 12.2 Descriptive statistics (mean and standard deviation) of efficiency scores

Type of efficiency	Private health centres		Government health centres	
	Mean	Standard deviation	Mean	Standard deviation
Technical	0.70	0.25	0.56	0.21
Allocative	0.84	0.15	0.57	0.25
Cost	0.59	0.27	0.33	0.25

Table 12.3 presents the distribution of health centres across the various efficiency brackets. Twelve (71%) of the 17 privately owned health centres were technically inefficient; 17% of them had a TE score of less than 0.50. There was wide variation in TE of the inefficient health centres ranging from 0.11 to 0.75. Comparatively, 22 (96%) of the 23 government-owned health centres were found to be technically inefficient; 36% of them had a TE score of less than 0.50. There was wide variation in the TE scores among the

inefficient health centres ranging from 0.26 to 0.93. Thirteen (77%) of the 17 privately owned health centres were allocatively inefficient; none of them had an AE score of less than 0.50. The allocative inefficiency ranged from 0.56 to 0.97. Contrastingly, 22 (96%) of the 23 government owned health centres were found to be allocatively inefficient; 59% of them had an AE score of less than 0.50. The allocative inefficiency varied from 0.27 to 0.98.

Thirteen (77%) of the 17 privately owned health centres were cost inefficient; 62% of them had a CE score of less than 0.50. The cost inefficiency ranged from 0.11 to 0.75. On the contrary, 22 (96%) of the 23 government-owned health centres were cost inefficient; 91% of them had a CE score of less than 0.50. The cost inefficiency varied from 0.12 to 0.89. The inefficient health centres should be able to produce their current level of services (outputs) with fewer inputs and, therefore, at lower cost.

Table 12.3 Frequency distribution of health centres efficiency by ownership

Range	Private health centres frequency (%)			Government health centres frequency (%)		
	TE	AE	CE	TE	AE	CE
1	5 (29)	4 (24)	4 (24)	2 (9)	1 (4)	1 (4)
0.90 - 0.99	0 (0)	3 (18)	0 (0)	1 (4)	4 (17)	0 (0)
0.80 - 0.89	1 (6)	2 (12)	0 (0)	1 (4)	1 (4)	2 (9)
0.70 - 0.79	3 (18)	5 (29)	1 (6)	1 (4)	1 (4)	0 (0)
0.60 - 0.69	2 (12)	1 (6)	1 (6)	3 (13)	2 (9)	0 (0)
0.50 - 0.59	4 (24)	2 (12)	3 (18)	7 (30)	1 (4)	0 (0)
0.40 - 0.49	1 (6)	0 (0)	5 (29)	3 (13)	4 (17)	2 (9)
0.30 - 0.39	0 (0)	0 (0)	2 (12	4 (17)	7 (30)	3 (13)
0.20 - 0.29	0 (0)	0 (0)	0 (0)	1 (4)	2 (9)	7 (30)
0.10 – 0.19	1 (6)	0 (0)	1 (6)	0 (0)	0 (0)	8 (35)
Total	17 (100)	17 (100)	17 (100)	23 (100)	23 (100)	23 (100)

DISCUSSION

Table 12.4 portrays the input reductions (or increases) needed to make individual inefficient health centres efficient. The current human resource endowment among the private health centres sub-sample is 43 clinical officers, 43 nurses, and 37 other staff (mainly casual). They can produce their current level of output (a total of 107,477 outpatient visits) with 17 clinical officers, 22 nurses, and 23 other staff. This implies that the private health centres could easily reduce the number of clinical officers by 60%, nurses by 49%, and other staff by 38% while maintaining the current level of health service production. The private proprietors stand to save a total of 27.7 million Kwacha per month by laying off excess clinical officers, nurses, and other staff. Of course, the net saving would be equal to the above estimate minus the affected staff's compensation for premature termination of their employment contract plus any legal fees. The private owners of health centres with excess staff have three options: (*a*) to do nothing (which would amount to continuing the current inefficiencies); (*b*) to terminate contracts of the excess staff; and (*c*) to negotiate with owners of health centres with human resource deficit to take over the excess staff's contract.

It is important to note in Table 12.4 that not all inefficient private health centres have got excess inputs. For example, the "Primary Care Services" health centre has a deficit of 6.8 nurses and "Lime Company Clinic" a deficit of 0.4 nurses. Bank of Zambia Clinic, Mufulira Clinic 6, ZESCO Clinic, and Ajali Clinic together have a deficit of 4 other staff.

The proprietors of those two health centres have three options:

1. To do nothing (which would amount to continuing the current inefficiencies).
2. To negotiate with owners of health centres with excess nurses to have a transfer of staff (and their contracts), that is, if the concerned staff are willing. This option would save all parties concerned some money. The transferring employer may avoid paying the compensation package for terminating contracts of concerned staff; the receiving company would save on recruitment and training costs; and the affected members of staff would retain their contracts, and thus, be saved from income loss and the attendant psychological costs.
3. To recruit from the open market, which may not be feasible in the short-term since there are no unemployed nurses in the country. In the long-term, one possibility is to train more nurses in Zambia.

On the other hand, the current human resource endowment among the public health centres sub-sample is 29 clinical officers, 282 nurses, and 92 other staff. They can produce their current level of output (a total of 253,204 outpatient visits) with 23 clinical officers, 80 nurses, and 54 other staff. This means that the public health centres could easily reduce the number of clinical officers by 21%, nurses by 80%, and other staff by 54% while maintaining the current level of health service provision. The Ministry of Health (MoH) could save a total of 51.6 million Kwacha per month by laying off excess clinical officers, nurses, and other staff.

Table 12.4 Input reductions (or increases) needed to make individual inefficient health centres efficient

	Inputs		
	Clinical Officers	Nurses	Other staff
Private health centres			
Bank of Zambia Clinic	1.0	1.8	-0.5
Mufulira Clinic 6	0.0	3.3	-0.7
Mufulira Clinic 2	0.0	5.8	1.5
Chilanga Cement Clinic	2.0	0.0	1.0
ZESCO Clinic	0.0	6.6	-0.8
ZESCO Clinic 2	1.0	2.0	3.0
TDRC	8.0	7.0	4.0
ZNPF Clinic	1.0	0.2	1.4
Zam. Sugar Co. Clinic	1.0	0.0	2.9
Primary Care Services	6.0	-6.8	2.9
Lever Brothers	1.0	0.3	0.0
Lime Company Clinic	4.0	-0.4	1.3
Ajali Clinic	1.0	1.0	-2.0
Sub-total excess inputs	*26.0*	*21.0*	*13.9*
Public health centres			
Chibuluma Government	0	8.0	0.0
Ngungu	0	14.9	0.1
Kalulushi Main	0	10.0	8.0
Mandevu Clinic	1	2.0	2.0
Kalulushi Government	3	18.4	1.5
Ndola Clinic Limited	0	1.0	-1.0
Kansuswa	0	9.4	-0.8
Ndeke	0	23.5	5.7
Buchi Main	2	11.9	1.6
Kamuchanga	0	10.0	2.0
Bwacha	0	14.1	3.7
Chowa	0	8.7	-0.3
Mukobeko	-1	1.7	0.5
Nakoli	-1	8.5	1.1
Butondo	0	10.4	2.9
Private health centres			
Chibolya	0	6.0	3.0
Chimwemwe	2	11.0	4.9
Bulangililo	0	8.5	1.4
Kawama	0	17.0	1.5
Kwacha	0	2.2	8.5
Luangwa	0	17.2	0.5
Mindolo	0	10.0	2.9
Sub-total excess inputs	*6*	*224.4*	*49.7*
Total excess inputs	**32.0**	**245.4**	**63.6**

Note: A negative sign signifies a deficit.

Regarding public health centres with excess human resources, the MoH has the following policy options:

1. To do nothing (which would amount to continuing the current inefficiencies).

2. To transfer the excess clinical officers to public health centres (e.g., Mukobeko and Nakoli) and hospitals and charitable mission hospitals and health centres which have a deficit. The MoH should opt for early retirement of technical staff only when staffing deficits among the public and charitable health facilities have been bridged.

3. Ndola clinic, Kansuswa, and Chowa combined have a deficit of 2.1 "other staff", which can easily be met from the facilities that have excess casual staff. The remaining "other staff"should be sent on early retirement after the deficits in hospitals and health centres have been met.

Any efficiency savings should be used to improve the remunerations of the remaining staff to reduce the rate of internal brain-drain to the private-for-profit sub-sector and external brain drain to the relatively affluent African countries and developed countries.

CONCLUSION

While DEA has been extensively used in the United States [19,20,41-49), Western Europe [21-24), and Asia [25,26] to study efficiency of health facilities, very few frontier analyses have been conducted in sub-Saharan Africa, yet we believe this is where they are needed most due to severe budgetary constraints. Kirigia, Sambo, and Lambo [27] employed DEA methodology to identify and measure technical and scale efficiencies among 55 public hospitals in South Africa. Forty per cent of the hospitals were found to be technically inefficient. Kirigia, Sambo and Scheel [28] utilised DEA to investigate the technical inefficiencies among 155 primary health care clinics in Kwazulu-Natal Province of South Africa. Seventy per cent of the clinics were technically inefficient. Zere *et al.* [29] used DEA to examine technical and scale efficiency of a sample of 86 non-academic acute hospitals in the Eastern, Northern, and Western Cape Provinces of South Africa. The average technical efficiency was 70%. It was estimated that if the relatively inefficient hospitals operate as efficiently as their peers, efficiency gains in terms of reduction in recurrent expenditure would be about US$47 million.

Kirigia, Emrouznejad and Sambo [30] measured relative efficiency of 54 public hospitals in Kenya using input oriented DEA technique. Twenty six per cent of the hospitals analysed had some technical inefficiencies. About 30% of the hospitals were scale inefficient. Masiye *et al* [9] used DEA to measure the degree of technical and allocative efficiency of 20 hospitals in Zambia. Eighty-five per cent of the hospitals were both allocatively and economically (in overall terms) inefficient. Masiye *et al.* recommended that in order to reduce the inefficiencies in hospitals, it will be necessary to reallocate the excess inputs to the primary health care (PHC) facilities, but before such an action is taken there is need to establish the efficiency of individual PHC facilities.

The current study was partially motivated by the above-mentioned recommendation. Seventy-one per cent of the 17 privately owned health centres were technically inefficient. Ninety-six per cent of the 23 government owned health centres were found to be technically inefficient. Seventy-seven per cent of the 17 privately owned health centres were allocatively inefficient. Ninety-six of the 23 government-owned health centres were found to be allocatively inefficient. Seventy-seven per cent of the 17 privately owned health centres were cost inefficient. Ninety-six per cent of the 23 government owned health centres were cost inefficient. This study identified input reductions needed to make the individual inefficient health centres efficient. The study also identified the policy options available to the policy makers as they ponder how to design interventions geared towards reducing the inefficient use of individual inputs.

We recommended that the current monitoring and evaluation activities going on in the Zambian Ministry of Health and the Central Board of Health should incorporate efficiency measurement and analysis. In addition, it is our hope that the DEA torch shall be taken to all the SSA countries with a view to ensuring that the available resources (and those that will be available in the future) are used to improve access to health services for the greatest number of people possible.

ACKNOWLEDGEMENT

The authors would like to thank the anonymous peer reviewers for their carefully prepared report. All their points have been considered and the paper has been edited accordingly. We owe profound gratitude to Jehovah Jireh for giving us the strength to take this paper to a successful conclusion.

Appendix 12.1   Health centre efficiency scores

Health facility	Technical efficiency	Allocative efficiency	Cost efficiency
Bank of Zambia Clinic	0.536	0.899	0.482
Mufulira Clinic 6	0.7	0.944	0.661
Mufulira Clinic 2	0.525	0.563	0.296
Chilanga Cement Clinic	0.75	0.587	0.44
North Breweries Clinic	1	1	1
Home Clinic	1	1	1
ZESCO Clinic	0.618	0.658	0.406
ZESCO Clinic 2	0.437	0.774	0.339
TDRC	0.111	0.971	0.107
ZNPF Clinic	0.6	0.877	0.526
Zam. Sugar Co. Clinic	0.5	0.894	0.447
Primary Care Services	1	0.748	0.748
Lever Brothers	0.757	0.784	0.594
Lime Company Clinic	0.572	0.797	0.456
Ajali Clinic	0.75	0.715	0.537
ZAMSEED Staff Clinic	1	1	1
Med. Health Centre Clinic	1	1	1
Chibuluma Government	0.5	0.37	0.185
Ngungu	0.5	0.33	0.165
Kalulushi Main	0.375	0.367	0.138
Mandevu Clinic	0.477	0.904	0.431
Kalulushi Government	0.26	0.753	0.196
Ndola Clinic Limited	0.928	0.91	0.844
Kansuswa	0.632	0.467	0.295
Ndeke	0.333	0.679	0.226
Buchi Main	0.338	0.955	0.323
Kamuchanga	0.6	0.27	0.162
Bwacha	0.429	0.283	0.121
Chowa	0.844	0.556	0.469
Mukobeko	1	0.893	0.893
Nakoli	0.75	0.373	0.28
Butondo	0.429	0.373	0.16
Chibolya	0.5	0.447	0.224
Chimwemwe	0.378	0.978	0.37
Bulangililo	0.5	0.379	0.19
Kawama	0.503	0.496	0.25
Kwacha	0.545	0.663	0.362
Luangwa	0.6	0.411	0.247
Mindolo	0.5	0.319	0.16
Ipusukilo	1	1	1
Mean	0.619	0.685	0.443

Note: Allocative efficiency = cost efficiency / technical efficiency.
       Scale assumption: variable returns to scale.

Appendix 12.2   Summary of cost minimising input quantities

Health facility	Clinical officers	Nurses	Other staff
Bank of Zambia Clinic	1	0.167	2.5
Mufulira Clinic 6	1	2.734	2.658
Mufulira Clinic 2	1	0.164	2.508
Chilanga Cement Clinic	1	1	0
North Breweries Clinic	1	0	3
Home Clinic	1	1	0
ZESCO Clinic	1	1.366	2.829
ZESCO Clinic 2	1	1	0
TDRC	1	1	0
ZNPF Clinic	1	0.792	0.625
Zambia Sugar Company Clinic	1	0.965	0.104
Primary Care Services	1	6.8	2.15
Lever Brothers	1	0.671	0.987
Lime Company Clinic	1	2.375	2.703
Ajali Clinic	1	0	3
ZAMSEED Staff Clinic	1	1	0
Medical Health Centre Clinic	1	1	0
Chibuluma Government	1	0	3
Ngungu	1	1.108	2.862
Kalulushi Main	1	0	3
Mandevu Clinic	1	1	0
Kalulushi Government	1	3.625	2.547
Ndola Clinic Limited	1	0.008	2.999
Kansuswa	1	1.608	2.799
Ndeke	1	5.511	2.311
Buchi Main	1	5.054	2.368
Kamuchanga	1	1	0
Bwacha	1	0.908	0.277
Chowa	1	5.283	2.34
Mukobeko	1	4.315	2.461
Nakoli	1	0.494	2.938
Butondo	1	0.64	1.079
Chibolya	1	1	0
Chimwemwe	1	6.959	2.13
Bulangililo	1	0.483	1.552
Kawama	1	3.957	2.505
Kwacha	1	2.844	0.527
Luangwa	1	3.788	2.526
Mindolo	1	0.97	0.09
Ipusukilo	1	8	2

Appendix 12.3 Input reductions or increases needed to make inefficient facilities efficient

Health facility	Clinic officers	Nurses	Other staff
Bank of Zambia Clinic	1	1.833	-0.5
Mufulira Clinic 6	0	3.266	-0.658
Mufulira Clinic 2	0	5.836	1.492
Chilanga Cement Clinic	2	0	1
ZESCO Clinic	0	6.634	-0.829
ZESCO Clinic 2	1	2	3
TDRC	8	7	4
ZNPF Clinic	1	0.208	1.375
Zam. Sugar Co. Clinic	1	0.035	2.896
Primary Care Services	6	-6.8	2.85
Lever Brothers	1	0.329	0.013
Lime Company Clinic	4	-0.375	1.297
Ajali Clinic	1	1	-2
Chibuluma Government	0	8	0
Ngungu	0	14.892	0.138
Kalulushi Main	0	10	8
Mandevu Clinic	1	2	2
Kalulushi Government	3	18.375	1.453
Ndola Clinic Limited	0	0.992	-0.999
Kansuswa	0	9.392	-0.799
Ndeke	0	23.489	5.689
Buchi Main	2	11.946	1.632
Kamuchanga	0	10	2
Bwacha	0	14.092	3.723
Chowa	0	8.717	-0.34
Mukobeko	-1	1.685	0.539
Nakoli	-1	8.506	1.062
Butondo	0	10.36	2.921
Chibolya	0	6	3
Chimwemwe	2	11.041	4.87
Bulangililo	0	8.517	1.448
Kawama	0	17.043	1.495
Kwacha	0	2.156	8.473
Luangwa	0	17.212	0.474
Mindolo	0	10.03	2.91
Total	**32**	**245.411**	**63.625**

Note: The figures in this table represent the difference between the actual inputs quantities and the cost minimising input quantities in Appendix 12.2.

REFERENCES

1. World Health Organization. *The world health report 2000: improving health systems performance*. Geneva: World Health Organization; 2000.

2. World Health Organization. *Bulletin of the World Health Organization*. Special theme issue: Health Systems 2000;78(6). Geneva: World Health Organization; 2000.

3. Murray CJL, Frenk J. A framework for assessing the performance of health systems. *Bulletin of the World Health Organization* 2000;78(6):717-731.

4. Williams A. Science or marketing at WHO? A commentary on 'World Health Report 2000'. *Health Economics* 2000;10(93):93-100.

5. Wagstaff A. *Measuring equity in healthcare financing: reflections on and alternatives to the World Health Organization's fairness of financing index*. Development Research Group and Human Development Network. Washington, D.C: World Bank; 2001.

6. Shaw RP. The world health report 2000 – a financial fairness indicator. useful compass or crystal ball? *International Journal of Health Services* 2002;32(1):195-203.

7. Pedersen KM. The world health report 2000: dialogue of the deaf. *Health Economics* 2002; 11:93-101.

8. United Nations Development Programme. *The human development report 2002*. Oxford: Oxford University Press; 2002.

9. Masiye F, Ndulo M, Roos P, Odegaard K. A comparative analysis of hospitals in Zambia: a pilot study on efficiency measurement and monitoring. In: Seshamani V, Mwikisa CN, Odegaard K, editors. *Zambia's health reforms: selected papers 1995-2000*. Lund: Swedish Institute of Health Economics and University of Zambia, Department of Economics; 2002.p 95-107.

10. World Health Organization. *The world health report 2001 - mental health: new understanding, new hope*. Geneva: World Health Organization; 2001.

11. United Nations Development Programme. *The human development report 2001 - making new technologies work for human development*. Oxford: Oxford University Press; 2001.

12. United Nations. *The millenium international development goals*. New York: UN; 2000.

13. World Health Organization. *Health-for-all policy for the 21st century in the African Region: agenda 2020*. Harare: World Health Organization; 2000.

14. World Health Organization. *Macroeconomics and health: investing in health for economic development*. Geneva: World Health Organization; 2001.

15. New Partnership for Africa's Development. *Human Development Programme: Health*. Pretoria:NEPAD;2000.

16. Mooney GH. *Economics, medicine and health care*. New York; Harvester Wheatsheaf; 1986.

17. Culyer AJ. The morality of efficiency in health care: some uncomfortable implications. *Health Economics* 1992;1(1):7-18.

18. Saltman RB, Ferrousier-Davis O. The concept of stewardship in health policy. *Bulletin of the World Health Organization* 2001;78(6):732-739.

19. Chattopadhy S, Ray CS. Technical, scale, and size efficiency in nursing home care: a nonparametric analysis of Connecticut homes. *Health Economics* 1996;5:363-373.

20. Shroff HFE, Gulledge TR, Haynes KE, Oneill MK. Siting efficiency of long-term healthcare facilities. *Socio-Economic Planning Science* 1998;32(1):25-43.

21. Hollingsworth B, Parkin D. The efficiency of the delivery of neonatal care in the UK. *Journal of Public Health Medicine* 2001;23(1):47-50.

22. Jacobs R. Alternative methods to examine hospital efficiency: data envelopment analysis and stochastic frontier analysis. *Health Care Management Science* 2001;4:103-115.

23. Ersoy K, Kavuncubasi S, Ozcan YA, Harris JM. Technical efficiencies of Turkish hospitals: DEA Approach. *Journal of Medical Systems* 1997;21(2):67-74.

24. Linna M, Nordblad A, Koivu M. Technical and cost efficiency of oral health care provision in Finnish health centres. *Social Science and Medicine* 2003;56(2):343-353.

25. Chang H. Determinants of hospital efficiency: the case of central government-owned hospitals in Taiwan. *Omega International Journal of Management Science* 1998;26(2):307-317.

26. Wan TTH, Hsu N, Feng R, Ma A, Pan S, Chou M. Technical efficiency of nursing units in a tertiary care hospital in Taiwan. *Journal of Medical Systems* 2002;26(1):21-27.

27. Kirigia JM, Lambo E, Sambo LG. Are public hospitals in Kwazulu-Natal Province of South Africa technically efficient? *African Journal of Health Sciences* 2000;7 (3-4):25-32.

28. Kirigia JM, Sambo LG, Scheel H. Technical efficiency of public clinics in Kwazulu-Natal Province of South Africa. *East African Medical Journal* 2001;78(3 Suppl): S1-S13.

29. Zere EA, McIntyre D, Addison T. Technical efficiency and productivity of public sector hospitals in three South African provinces. *South African Journal of Economics* 2001; 69(2):336-358.

30. Kirigia JM, Emrouznejad A, Sambo LG. Measurement of technical efficiency of public hospitals in Kenya: using data envelopment analysis. *Journal of Medical Systems* 2002; 26(1):39-45.

31. Skaggs NT, Carlson JM, Deillingham AE. *Microeconomics: individual choice and its consequences*. London: Blackwell Publishers; 1996.

32. Coelli TJ. *A guide to DEAP version 2.1: a data envelopment analysis [computer] program*, Centre for Efficiency and Productivity Analysis (CEPA) Working Paper 96/08. Department of Econometrics, University of New England, Armidale, NSW Australia; 1996.

33. Farrell MJ. The measurement of productive efficiency. *Journal of the Royal Statistical Society* 1957;120(3):253-281.

34. Charnes A, Cooper WW, Rhodes E. Measuring efficiency of decision making units. *European Journal of Operational Research* 1978;2(6):429-444.

35. Emrouznejad A. An alternative DEA measure: a case of OECD countries. *Applied Economics Letters* 2003;10:779-782.

36. Emrouznejad A, Thanassoulis E. A mathematical model for dynamic efficiency using data envelopment analysis. *J. Appl. Math. Comput.* 2005;160(2):363-378.

37. Emrouznejad A. Measurement of efficiency and productivity in SAS/OR. *Journal of Computor Operatons Research* 2005;32(7):1665-1683.

38. Emrouznejad A, Podinovski V. *Data envelopment analysis and performance management*. Coventry: Warwick Print; 2004.

39. Emrouznejad A: Ali Emrouznejad's Data Envelopment Analysis HomePage 1995-2003, www.DEAzone.com.

40. Morey RC, Fine DJ, Loree SW. Comparing the allocative efficiencies of hospitals. *OMEGA International Journal of Management Science* 1990;18(1):71-83.

41. Ozcan A, Luke RD. A national study of the efficiency of hospitals in urban markets. *Health Services Research* 1993;27(6):719-739.

42. Lynch JR, Ozcan Y. Hospital closure: an efficiency analysis. *Hospital and Health Services Administration* 1994;39(2):205-220.

43. Ozcan Y, Cotter JJ. An assessment of efficiency of area agencies on aging in Virginia through data envelopment analysis. *The Gerontologist* 1994;34(3):363-370.

44. Laura HT, Ozcan YA, Wogan SE. Mental health case management and technical efficiency. *Journal of Medical Systems* 1995;19(5):413-423.

45. Ozcan Y. Efficiency of hospital service production in local markets: the balance sheet of U.S. medical armament. *Socio-Economic Planning Science* 1995;29(2):139-150.

46. White KR, Fache RN, Ozcan Y. Church ownership and hospital efficiency. *Hospital and health services administration* 1996;41(3):297-310.

47. Pai C, Ozcan YA, Jiang HJ. Regional variation in physician practice pattern: an examination of technical and cost efficiency for treating sinusitis. *Journal of Medical Systems* 2000; 24(2):103-117.

48. Harris J, Ozgen H, Ozcan Y. Do mergers enhance the performance of hospital efficiency? *Journal of the Operational Research Society* 2000;5:801-811.

49. Rollins J, Lee K, Xu Y, Ozcan Y. Longitudinal study of health maintenance organisation efficiency. *Health Services Management Research* 2001;14: 49-262.

-13-

A Performance Assessment Method for Hospitals: *The Case of Municipal Hospitals in Angola**

Joses M. Kirigia, Ali Emrouznejad,
Basilio Cassoma, Eyob Z. Asbu and Saidou Barry

ABSTRACT

Over 60% of the recurrent budget of the Ministry of Health in Angola is spent on the operations of the fixed healthcare facilities (health centres and hospitals). However, to date, no study has been attempted to investigate how efficiently those resources are used to produce health services. Therefore, the objectives of this study were to assess the technical efficiency of public municipal hospitals in Angola; assess changes in productivity over time with a view to analysing changes in efficiency and technology; and demonstrate how the results can be used in the pursuit of the public health objective of promoting efficiency in the use of health resources. The analysis was based on a three-year panel data from all the 28 public municipal hospitals in Angola. Data envelopment analysis, a non-parametric linear programming approach, was employed to assess the technical and scale efficiency and productivity change over time using Malmquist index. The results show that, on average, productivity of municipal hospitals in Angola increased by 4.5% over the period 2000-2002 and that growth was due to improvement in efficiency rather than innovation.

Keywords: Hospital performance comparison; efficiency and productivity; data envelopment analysis; Malmquist indices; Angola/Africa.

---

* The original article appeared in *Journal of Medical Systems 2008;32:509-519.* Reproduced with the permission of Plenum Publishing Corporation.

INTRODUCTION

Angola is a country in south-western Africa that emerged from a protracted civil war that lasted for more than two decades. Administratively, Angola is divided into 18 provinces, 164 municipalities, and 557 communes [1]. The country has a population of 15.5 million people, a life expectancy of 40 years, under-5 mortality rate of 260 per 1,000 live births, adult mortality rate of 548 per 1,000, and maternal mortality ratio of 1,700 per 100,000 live births [2]. The country's health and development indicators are dismal [2-4]. The high levels of morbidity and mortality reflect limited access to health services, poverty, nutritional deficiencies, inadequate access to safe sources of water, and poor environmental sanitation [5]. For example, 25% of the urban population and 60% of the rural population do not have access to improved water sources and 84% of the urban population and 44% of the rural population have no access to improved sanitation [6].

The National Health Service is organised into three levels of care: national or specialised hospitals, provincial hospitals, and primary care facilities (municipal hospitals, health centres, and health posts). The country has 8 national referral hospitals, 32 provincial general hospitals, 28 municipal hospitals, 200 municipal health centres, and 1,453 health posts [1]. These health facilities are run by 1,165 physicians (0.08 per 1,000 people), 18,485 nurses (1.19 per 1,000 people), 222 dentists (0.000 per 1,000 people), 919 pharmacists (0.002 per 1,000 people), 2,029 laboratory technicians (0.144 per 1,000 people), 294 other health workers (0.020 per 1000 people), and 256 health management and support staff (0.018 per 1,000 people) [2].

The total expenditure on health as a percentage of the GDP decreased from 3.5% in 1996 to 2.0% in 2005 [5]. General government expenditure on health constitutes 81.8% of the total expenditure on health. The remaining 18.2% consists of private expenditure on health; all of which comes from private households' out-of-pocket spending. The per capita total expenditure on health at an average exchange rate is US$37 of which 81.1% consists of government expenditure. In 2005, the total public expenditure in the health sector was US$447,245 million; out of which 40.2% was incurred at the primary health care level; 44.3% at central and provincial referral hospitals (i.e., second and third levels); 12.9% on administration; and 2.5% on training. About 47%, 36%, and 17% of the health sector expenditure was on personnel, goods and services, and investments respectively. Of the total expenditure on goods and services, 44.61% was on drugs and medical surgical material; 7.76% on transport; 6.26% on maintenance of facilities and equipment; 25.82% on hotel services; 1.56% on energy and water; 2.78% on office material; and 11.21% on other goods and services [1]. However, little is known about efficiency in the use of health sector resources.

Since Charnes, Cooper and Rhodes [6] proposed the use of the non-parametric technique of data envelopment analysis (DEA) to measure relative efficiencies of decision-making units (DMUs) in 1978, DEA has been widely used in the Americas, Western Europe, and Asia [7,8] to shed light on the efficiency of various aspects of national health systems. In Africa, the application of DEA in the health sector has been quite limited. So far, out of the 46 Member States in the WHO African Region, the approach has been applied to health facilities in only seven countries, that is, Ghana [9], Kenya [10, 11], Namibia [12], Seychelles [13], Sierra Leone [14], South Africa [15, 16,17], and Zambia [18]. Yet, the assessment of the efficiency ought to be more prevalent in low-income countries like Angola in order to maximise health services provision from the scarce health sector resources available.

Despite the fact that over 63% of the recurrent budget of the Ministry of Health is spent on the operations of the fixed healthcare facilities (health centres plus hospitals), to date no study has been conducted to assess the degree of efficiency in the Angolan health system. The purpose of this study was to contribute towards bridging this knowledge gap. There are a number of reasons as to why the Angolan Ministry of Health (and indeed all ministries of health in the WHO African Region) should be concerned with monitoring of hospital productivity: limited resources vis-à-vis unlimited health needs; increased productivity ought to be a key strategy of dealing with human resources crises (caused by attrition due to brain drain and premature HIV/AIDS deaths) facing the health systems; increased productivity results in improved quality of health care while productivity decrease results in waste of health-producing resources necessary for planning and implementing policies geared at productivity enhancement (an attribute of good health systems stewardship and governance); and demonstrated efforts to monitor and improve hospital performance can attract more domestic and external resources into the health sector.

METHODOLOGY AND DATA

Concept and Measurement of Technical Efficiency and Productivity of Hospitals

Health sectors are endowed with a limited supply of healthcare-producing resources such as human resources, pharmaceutical supplies, non-pharmaceutical supplies, clinical technologies, beds, building space, and ambulances among others. The population's health needs are unlimited (and thus insatiable), and thus resource scarcity limits the ability of health systems to meet all the needs. A fundamental economic problem is how to make the best use of the healthcare resources (i.e., avoid waste). In the context of municipal hospitals, technical efficiency means providing maximum health services out of available resources or minimising the use of available resources to produce a given level of health services. Although economic efficiency is a product of both technical/productive efficiency (producing health care without waste) with allocative efficiency (allocating health resources to their most highly valued uses), the absence of data on prices of inputs limits the focus of this study only to the measurement of technical efficiency.

Technical efficiency comprises both pure technical and scale efficiency components. Returns to scale tell us how output (e.g., hospital admissions) responds in the long run to changes in the scale or size of the firm (hospital in our case). In other words, suppose we consider a long-run situation in which all inputs are variable, and suppose a hospital increases the amount of all inputs by the same proportion, what would happen to output? There are three possibilities. First, output may increase by exactly the same proportion as the inputs; for example doubling of all inputs may lead to a doubling of output. This is the case of constant returns to scale (CRS). When a hospital is operating at CRS, technical efficiency is equal to scale efficiency. Second, output may increase by a larger proportion than each of the inputs; for example, a doubling of all inputs may lead to more than a doubling of output. This is the case of increasing returns to scale (IRS), also known as economies of scale, which may arise due to indivisibilities of some health inputs, greater specialisation, innovation (may be as a result of research and development), and/or increased performance of human resources for health (maybe due to increased motivation).

Lastly, output may increase by a smaller proportion than each of the inputs; for example, a doubling of all inputs may lead to less than the doubling of output. This is the case of decreasing returns to scale (DRS), also called diseconomies of scale, which may arise because of shortages of complementary inputs (e.g., medicines), low levels of staff motivation, and leadership problems (e.g., related to coordination and supervision). Data envelopment analysis is becoming a popular method of efficiency analysis in the non-profit sector [19-23]. It has the advantage of easily accommodating multiple inputs, multiple outputs production, and does not make behavioural assumptions (such as profit maximisation) about the decision-making units (hospitals).

DEA Conceptual Framework

The coverage of basic and effective health services is low; indicating that the majority of the population is not protected by basic health services. For example, there are only five doctors in the public sector per 100,000 inhabitants; only 20% of the population has access to essential drugs; only 34% of children aged 12-23 months are vaccinated with the third dose of DPT ; only 63% of children aged 12-23 months are vaccinated for polio; only 45% of child deliveries are attended by trained health personnel; only 66% of pregnant women attend one or more pre-natal consultations; and only 17% of women of reproductive age use any method of contraception [1]. This information clearly shows that there is a huge unmet demand for health services. Therefore, the authors thought that it would be immoral and unethical for the government to contemplate improving efficiency through input reduction vis-à-vis output increase.

This study assumes an output orientation; meaning that technical efficiency (TE) is taken to be the ability of a hospital to produce maximum output from a given level of inputs. Thus, the research question is, by how much could municipal hospitals expand their outputs without changing the quantity of the inputs used? The DEA model is as follows [6]:

$$Max \quad h_0 = \sum_{r=1}^{s} u_r y_{rj_0} + u_0 \tag{1}$$

Subject to:

$$\sum_{i=1}^{m} v_i x_{ij_0} = 1$$

$$\sum_{r=1}^{s} u_r y_{rj} - \sum v_i x_{ij} + u_0 \leq 0, \quad j = 1,...,n$$

$$u_r, \ v_i \geq 0$$

$$u_0 \underset{>}{\leq} 0$$

where

y_{rj} = amount of output r from hospital j

x_{ij} = amount of input i to hospital j

u_r = weight given to output r

v_i = weight given to input i

n = number of hospitals

s = number of outputs

m = number of inputs

The sign of u_0 determines the returns to scale:

$u_0 > 0$ means increasing returns to scale

$u_0 = 0$ indicates constant returns to scale

$u_0 < 0$ depicts decreasing returns to scale

Coelli et al. [23] expresses scale efficiency (SE) as the ratio of constant returns to scale technical efficiency (TE$_{CRS}$) to variable returns to scale technical efficiency (TE$_{VRS}$); that is, $SE = TE_{CRS}/TE_{VRS}$.

Malmquist Productivity Index (MPI)

We have used DEA-based Malmquist total factor productivity (TFP) index [22] to measure productivity change. Like DEA, the non-parametric Malmquist index does not require assumptions on the profit maximisation or cost minimisation and information on input and output prices. It allows the decomposition of productivity changes into technical efficiency change and technological change. Following Fare et al. [22] to define the output-oriented Malmquist index of productivity change for the municipal hospitals, we assume that for each time period t = 1,...,T the production technology S^t models the transformation of n inputs (i.e., physicians plus nurses, expenditures on supplies, beds), $x^t \in \Re_+^N$ into m outputs (outpatient department visits, inpatient department admissions), $y^t \in \Re_+^M$,

$$S^t = \left\{ \left(x^t, y^t\right) : x^t \text{ can produce } y^t \right\} \tag{2}$$

The output distance function for municipal hospitals is defined at t as the reciprocal of the maximum proportional expansion of the output vector y^t given inputs x^t [22]:

$$D_o^t\left(x^t, y^t\right) = \inf\left\{\Theta : \left(x^t, y^t/\Theta\right) \in S^t\right\}$$

$$= \sup\left\{\Theta : (x^t, y^t\Theta) \in S^t\right\}^{-1} \tag{3}$$

According to Fare et al. [22] the derivation of the Malmquist index calls for the definition of distance functions with respect to two different time periods such as:

$$D_o^t\left(x^{t+1}, y^{t+1}\right) = \inf\left\{\Theta : \left(x^{t+1}, y^{t+1}/\Theta\right) \in S^t\right\} \tag{4}$$

which measures the maximal proportional change in outputs required to make $\left(x^t, y^t\right)$ feasible in relation to the technology at t. Caves et al. [24] define the Malmquist productivity index (MPI) as:

$$M_o^t = \frac{D_o^t\left(x^{t+1}, y^{t+1}\right)}{D_o^t\left(x^t, y^t\right)} \tag{5}$$

Fare et al. [22] specified the output-oriented Malmquist productivity change index as the geometric mean of the productivity indices of two periods, and subsequently decomposed it into various sources of productivity change as follows:

$$M_o\left(y^{t+1}, x^{t+1}, y^t, x^t\right) = \left[\frac{D_0^t\left(x^{t+1}, y^{t+1}\right)}{D_0^t\left(x^t, y^t\right)} \times \frac{D_0^{t+1}\left(x^{t+1}, y^{t+1}\right)}{D_0^{t+1}\left(x^t, y^t\right)}\right]^{1/2}$$

$$= \left[\frac{D_0^{t+1}\left(x^{t+1}, y^{t+1}\right)}{D_0^t\left(x^t, y^t\right)}\right] \times \left[\frac{D_0^t\left(x^{t+1}, y^{t+1}\right)}{D_0^{t+1}\left(x^{t+1}, y^{t+1}\right)} \times \frac{D_0^t\left(x^t, y^t\right)}{D_0^{t+1}\left(x^t, y^t\right)}\right]^{1/2} \tag{6}$$

Efficiency change $= \left[\frac{D_0^{t+1}\left(x^{t+1}, y^{t+1}\right)}{D_0^t\left(x^t, y^t\right)}\right] \tag{7}$

Technical change $= \left[\frac{D_0^t\left(x^{t+1}, y^{t+1}\right)}{D_0^{t+1}\left(x^{t+1}, y^{t+1}\right)} \times \frac{D_0^t\left(x^t, y^t\right)}{D_0^{t+1}\left(x^t, y^t\right)}\right]^{1/2} \tag{8}$

The Malmquist productivity index attains a value greater than, equal to, or less than unity if a municipal hospital has experienced productivity growth, stagnation, or productivity decline net of the contribution of scale economies between periods t and $t + 1$. Malmquist productivity under variable returns to scale can be calculated in a similar manner but also has another part to overcome with scale efficiency change [24].

Data

One author (BC) visited the entire population of 28 municipal hospitals in Angola and reviewed their input and output records. Hospitals were assumed to utilise three inputs: doctors (physicians) plus nurses; expenditures on pharmaceutical and non-pharmaceutical supplies; and beds (a proxy of capital). The records kept at the hospitals suggested that they produced two intermediate outputs: outpatient department visits (including antenatal care visits) and inpatient department admissions. The choice of the inputs and outputs was influenced by the availability of data on these hospitals in public records. At the health-facility level, there was reasonably complete data for 2000, 2001, and 2002 only.

RESULTS AND DISCUSSION

Appendix 13.1 presents descriptive statistics of inputs and outputs. The quantity of outputs – number of outpatient plus antenatal visits and number of inpatient admissions – increased between 2000 and 2002. There was an increase in the total number of "doctors + nurses" input between 2000 and 2001; however, it remained constant between 2001 and 2002. Compared to the total expenditure on drugs and other supplies in 2000, in nominal terms, there was a 143.8% increase in 2001 and a 352.5% increase in 2002. Generally, the total number of beds remained fairly constant over the period under consideration.

Technical Efficiency

Appendix 13.2 reports the frequency (and percentage) distribution of technical and scale efficiency scores for the hospitals in our sample for 2000, 2001, and 2002. In 2002, 2001 and 2002 out of the 28 hospitals about 11 (39%), 12 (43%), and 10 (36%) hospitals respectively had a variable returns to scale technical efficiency of unity. Values of unity imply that the hospital is on the sample frontier (or technically efficient) in the associated year. Data envelopment analysis has revealed that 17 (61%), 16 (57%), and 18 (64%) of the hospitals were run inefficiently in 2000, 2001, and 2002 respectively and they needed to either reduce their inputs or increase their outputs in order to become efficient. The average technical efficiency scores were 66.2%, 65.8%, and 67.5% respectively during the years under consideration. This finding implies that if the hospitals were operating efficiently, they could have produced 33.8%, 34.2%, and 32.5% more output (outpatient visits and inpatient admissions) using their current levels of input endowment.

Generally, the Angolan hospitals' technical efficiency scores are lower than those reported in studies undertaken in other African countries. For example, Zere et al. [12] established the average technical efficiency of district hospitals in Namibia as ranging between 84.1% and 89.7% during the four-year period under investigation. Osei et al. [9] got an average technical efficiency score of 81.5% among the hospitals in Ghana. Kirigia et al. [11] estimated the average technical efficiency among public hospitals in Kenya to be 95.6%. Masiye et al. [25] obtained an average technical efficiency score of 55.9% for hospitals in Zambia. Kirigia et al. [16] found that the average technical efficiency score of hospitals in Kwazulu-Natal Province of South Africa was 90.6%. Zere et al. [17] computed the average technical efficiency scores to be 74%, 68%, and 70% for Level I, II, and III hospitals in Eastern, Northern, and Western Cape provinces of South Africa.

Scale Efficiency

In the period 2000 to 2002, out of the 28 hospitals:

1. Six (21%), five (18%), and eight (29%) hospitals manifested constant returns to scale. These hospitals were operating at their most productive scale sizes.

2. Twenty-one (75%), 9 (32%), and seventeen (61%) hospitals had increasing returns to scale (IRS). If a hospital is exhibiting IRS, it should expand its scale of operation in order to become scale efficient.

3. One (4%), fourteen (50%), and three (11%) hospitals had decreasing returns to scale (DRS). In order to operate at the most productive scale size, a hospital exhibiting DRS should scale down its scale of operation.

The average scale efficiency score in the sample was 83% in 2000, 81% in 2001, and 89% in 2002 implying that there was room for increasing total outputs by about 17% in 2000, 19% in 2001, and 11% in 2002.

Unlike the technical efficiency scores, the scale efficiency scores of the Angolan municipal hospitals are fairly similar to those of past studies undertaken in other African countries. For instance, Zere et al. [12] established the average scale efficiency of district hospitals in Namibia as ranging between 80.7% and 87.3%. Osei et al. [9] reported an average scale efficiency score of 89.1% among the hospitals in Ghana. Kirigia et al. [11] estimated the average scale efficiency among public hospitals in Kenya to be 96.8%. Kirigia et al. [16] found that the average scale efficiency score of hospitals in the Kwazulu-Natal Province of South Africa was 95.3%. Zere et al. [17] computed the average scale efficiency scores to be 88.9%, 78.9%, and 81.7% for Level I, II, and III hospitals in Eastern, Northern and Western Cape provinces of South Africa.

Scope for Output Increases and Implications for Policy

If the inefficient municipal hospitals in Angola were to operate as efficiently as their peers on the efficiency frontier, there would be scope for significant output increases or input savings. The total output increases and/or input reductions needed to make inefficient hospitals efficient are reported in Appendix 13.3. In 2002, for example, the inefficient hospitals combined would need to increase their total outpatient and antenatal visits by 590,267 (47.82%) and inpatient admissions by 87,061 (45.71%). Alternatively, those hospitals would need to reduce the number of nurses by 369 (6.55%); expenditure on drugs and other supplies by Kwanza 1,250,247 (60.77%); and the number of beds by 156 (8.82%).

Concerning hospitals with outputs falling short of the DEA targets, MoH policy makers could improve their efficiency by creating demand for the underutilised essential curative, promotive, and preventive services. This may require a combination of the following intervention strategies:

1. Use of health promotion approaches [26] to boost the target population's effective demand for specific promotive, preventive, curative, and rehabilitative health services.

2. Reduction of financial barriers to effective access to health services such as out-of-pocket expenses (e.g., user fees, consultancy fees, transport costs, diagnosis fees, drug costs, and bribes) and time costs (e.g., travel time, waiting/queuing time, diagnosis time, and treatment time) [27-29].

3. Improvement in responsiveness of health facilities to clients' (actual and potential patients) non-medical legitimate expectations [30].

4. Improvement in both technical and perceived quality of health services provided at the inefficient hospitals [31].

Alternatively, with regard to hospitals with excess inputs, policy makers could (if it is very difficult to reduce inefficiencies by inducing demand for care):

1. Transfer (instead of laying-off) excess technical staff to understaffed municipal health centres. Such a policy intervention should be preceded by an efficiency analysis of health centres to ensure that the excess human resources from hospitals are not transferred to lower-level facilities that are already operating inefficiently or experiencing decreasing returns to scale (which may deepen and propagate the existing inefficiencies). In addition, the country will need to have a clear transfer policy within the health human resource management policy to ensure that transfer is not regarded as discreditable. As indicated by Graham and Bennett [32], transfers can increase job satisfaction if *(a)* a transfer is regarded as a re-selection; *(b)* the need for a transfer is explained; or *(c)* an employee transferred to another health facility is given financial assistance from the ministry to cover relocation costs and refurnishing among others.

2. Excess expenditure on medicines and other supplies could instead be spent on health centres and health posts to strengthen the quality of services that these facilities provide. Once the technical quality of services is improved, it could potentially curtail unnecessary referrals from health centres and health posts facilities to hospitals.

3. Excess hospital beds could either be (*a*) transferred to public hospitals with shortage of beds; (*b*) sold to the private (or NGO) sector hospitals in need of beds; (*c*) opened for private practice while still in public hospitals; (*d*) transferred to health centre facilities in need of beds; or (*e*) auctioned in the open market for all types of use including non-health-related use [16].

Productivity Growth

Instead of presenting the disaggregated results for each hospital and year, we turn to a summary description of the average performance of each hospital over the three-year time period, that is, the Malmquist total factor productivity index. Since the Malmquist index is multiplicative, these averages are also multiplicative (i.e., they are geometric means). In the application of the Malmquist index to analyse the temporal differences in productivity, the year 2000 has been taken as the technology reference. The reader will recall that if the value of the Malmquist index or any of its components is less than 1, it denotes regress or deterioration in performance, whereas values greater than 1 denote improvement in the relevant performance.

The productivity change estimates are summarised below. Appendix 13.4 presents the Malmquist index summary of annual geometric means. In the last row (last column), we see that on average productivity increased by 4.5% over the 2000-2002 period for the hospitals in our sample. On average, that growth was due to improvements in efficiency rather than innovation. Whereas efficiency grew by 12.7%, technical change (innovation) regressed by 7.3% per annum. The efficiency change was attributable to a 5% positive change in pure technical efficiency and a 7.3% positive change in scale efficiency. In their productivity growth analysis of South African hospitals, Zere et al. [17] found that the total factor productivity had dropped by 12.1%, which was attributable to a 1.6% decline in efficiency and a 10.7% technological regress.

We now turn to an examination of the magnitude and sources of productivity change within each hospital. Appendix 13.5 provides a summary of the average annual values of the Malmquist productivity index and its components for each hospital (firm). About 17 (61%) out of 28 hospitals had improvements in productivity since their Malmquist indices were greater than unity. On the other hand, 11 (39%) of the hospitals had Malmquist indices of less than unity, implying deterioration in performance over time. None of the hospitals had a Malmquist index of unity, which would have signified stagnation.

Boa Entrada/cada, Cubal, and Muxima hospitals had the highest total factor productivity growth of 87.2%, 79.3%, and 74.6% respectively. From an analysis of the decomposition of the Malmquist TFP, productivity growth in the Boa Entrada/cada, Cubal, and Muxima hospitals seem to have been brought about mainly by improvements in efficiency (+84.8% and 135.9% respectively) rather than by a positive technological change. Contrastingly, Maternidade Caxito, Chinguar, and Ukuma hospitals displayed the greatest deterioration of 45.5%, 40.4%, and 34.5% respectively. The productivity decline was mainly due to a decrease in pure technical efficiency and, to a lesser extent, to technical regress.

Pure efficiency Change

As Fare et al. [22] posit, improvements in any of the components of the Malmquist index are associated with values greater than unity of those components and deterioration is associated with values less than unity. As indicated earlier, the first component of the MPI provides a measure of the contribution to productivity change of a change in technical efficiency between period t and $t+1$. Efficiency change is a product of pure efficiency change (PEFFCH) and scale efficiency change (SCH). The PEFFCH index is greater than, equal to, or less than unity if the relative technical efficiency of a hospital (firm) has increased, remained the same, or decreased between time periods t and $t+1$. The relative PEFFCH increased among 14 (50%) of the hospitals, remained the same among 8 (29%), and decreased in 6 (21%) of the hospitals. The Cubal hospital had a PEFFCH value of 2.413, the highest in the sample. If PEFFCH > SCH, then inefficiency is caused by scale inefficiency. Our study found the average PEFFCH was 1.050 while SCH was 1.073, which means that PEFFCH < SCH. This result showed that, on average, the main source of inefficiency was the inefficient (sub-optimal) use of inputs.

Scale Efficiency Change

The scale index attains a value greater than, equal to, or less than unity if a hospital's (firm's) scale of production contributes positively, not at all, or negatively to productivity change. Thirteen (46%) hospitals attained a scale index value of greater than unity implying that their scale of production contributed positively to productivity change. Six (21%) of the hospitals had a value equal to unity suggesting that the scale of production of those hospitals did not contribute at all to productivity change. Nine (32%) of the hospitals had a scale index of less than unity signifying that those hospitals' production contributed negatively to productivity change. The Muxima hospital had a SCH score of 2.022, which was the highest in the sample. The average SCH score was 1.073 implying that the scale of production on average contributed positively to efficiency change by 7.3%. Grifell-Tatje and Lovell [33, p. 368] expound that "a change in the scale of production contributes positively to productivity change if it is in the direction of technically optimal scale, while a change in the scale of production contributes negatively to productivity change if it is in the direction away from technically optimal scale".

Technical Change

The second component of the MPI provides a measure of the contribution to productivity change of whatever technical change occurs between periods t and $t+1$. This index attains a value of greater than, equal to, or less than unity if technical progress, stagnation or technical regress has occurred along a ray through a firm's data between periods t and $t+1$. About 11 (39%) of the hospitals experienced technical progress, none of the hospitals experienced technical stagnation, and 17 (61%) of the hospitals recorded technical regress. The average technical change score was 0.927; indicating a 7.3% technical deterioration.

Limitations of the Study and Suggestions for Further Research

Like other previous efficiency studies [9-18] in the WHO African Region, this study used intermediate outputs instead of indicators of the ultimate hospital care outcomes, such as quality-adjusted life years, due to non-availability of health facility-level data. We also assumed that all municipal hospitals are fairly homogeneous. We were not able to verify whether the hospitals had exactly the same standards in terms of type of services provided, severity of cases treated, quality of care provided, qualification and experience of staff, working schedules, functional building capacity and healthcare technology among other factors. This study did not take into account other inputs such as administrative costs and other outputs such as diagnostic services. In Angola, the patients delivering babies and those undergoing operations are usually admitted in hospitals, and thus, those two outputs are captured in the "number of admissions" output.

Since information on the prices of inputs was not available, it was not possible to estimate allocative efficiency, which would have enabled us to calculate the overall economic efficiency. Thus, the inefficiency estimates reported in this study should be considered as an underestimate of the level of waste existing within the health facilities. Generally, DEA has two main shortcomings: *(a)* being non-stochastic it does not capture random noise (e.g. effects of man-made disasters, natural disasters, strikes, etc.) and thus, it attributes any deviation from the frontier to inefficiency; and *(b)* being non-statistical it is not possible to undertake statistical tests of the hypothesis regarding the inefficiency and the structure of the production technology [19, 23].

There are various suggestions for future studies of this kind in the WHO African Region. For example:

1. Undertake a supplementary study to gather data on the prices of the various inputs (e.g., remunerations of doctors, nurses, beds) to facilitate an estimation of the allocative efficiency of municipal hospitals. If such an exercise were to be undertaken, researchers may also consider collecting data on quantities and prices of paramedical, administrative, and support staff to ensure that the analysis is more comprehensive than the study reported in this paper.

2. Analysis of both technical and allocative efficiency of health centres and health posts to inform the decisions by policy makers of where to transfer the excess inputs of inefficient hospitals in case it proves difficult to eradicate inefficiencies through creation of demand for hospital health services.

3. Application of DEA to test the hypothesis that private sector (including NGO) health facilities are more efficient than public facilities.

4. Study the feasibility of adapting national performance assessment frameworks currently being used in some developed countries to improve health facility performance [34]. In the process of undertaking such a study it would be important to explore the potential application of the strategies suggested by Goddard and Smith [35] for overcoming some of the adverse consequences (e.g., tunnel vision, sub-optimisation, measure fixation, myopia, complacency, misrepresentation, gaming, misinterpretation, and ossification) of performance-based management.

CONCLUSIONS

This study has *(a)* measured both the technical and scale efficiencies of 28 individual municipal hospitals; *(b)* identified the input reductions and/or output increases needed to make the inefficient health facilities efficient; and *(c)* estimated the magnitude and sources of productivity change within each hospital. The findings indicate that, on average, 61% of the hospitals were run inefficiently in 2000, 2001, and 2002. The inefficient hospitals combined would need to increase their total outpatient and antenatal visits by 47.82% and inpatient admissions by 45.71% in order to become efficient. Thus, there is enormous scope for treating additional 590,267 outpatient cases and 87,061 inpatient admissions per year without investing extra resources into the health sector from any source, public or private.

Alternatively, depending on the decision of policy makers, the quality of services in the primary healthcare facilities could be remarkably improved through transfer of the 369 excess nurses; Kwanza 1,250,247 excess expenditure on drugs and other supplies; and 156 excess beds to lower-level facilities currently experiencing shortages. Leveraging of efficiency savings to improve access and quality of health services will definitely be more equitable and politically less costly than levying of out-of-pocket payments for services.

There is evidence that 11 (39%) of the hospitals experienced total factor productivity deterioration over time during the three years. Such inefficiency is likely to hamper the government's efforts to improve access to and quality of care [19]. If relevant data were available, the Malmquist TFP type of analyses can be used to assess the effects of the key health sector reforms undertaken in the past on the efficiency of health facilities. The national and district health management information systems should be strengthened to routinely capture the input, input prices, and output data which could be used to monitor economic efficiency and productivity change among fixed health facilities such as health posts, health centres, and hospitals. The usefulness of such studies in aiding stewardship [36] or good governance of health systems in resource-constrained countries cannot be overemphasised.

ACKNOWLEDGEMENT

The authors are immensely grateful to Jehovah Jireh for His multifaceted support at all stages of preparing this manuscript; "Felix Masiye" (Harvard School of Public Health, USA) for the constructive comments; "Patricia Akweongo" (Navrongo Health Research Centre, Ghana) for follow-up on data collection; and to the anonymous reviewers of JMS for invaluable comments and suggestions. JMK and SB appreciate the enabling intellectual environment created by Dr Alimata J. Diarra-Nama in the Division of Health Systems and Services Development, WHO/AFRO. The data collection was funded by WHO/AFRO. The manuscript contains the analyses and views of the authors only and does not represent the decisions or stated policies of the institutions they work for.

REFERENCES

1. European Union and World Bank. *Angola public expenditure in the health sector*. Luanda; 2007.

2. World Health Organization. *The world health report 2006: working together for health*. Geneva: World Health Organization; 2006.

3. United Nations Development Programme. Human development report 2005: international cooperation at a crossroads: aid, trade and security in an unequal world. New York: Oxford University Press; 2005.

4. The World Bank. *World development indicators database*. Washington, D.C.; 2005. Available at: http://devdata.worldbank.org/

5. Government of Angola. Public financing of the social sectors in Angola. Luanda; 2002.

6. Charnes A, Cooper WW, Rhodes E. Measuring efficiency of decision-making units. *European Journal of Operational Research* 1978;2(6):429-444.

7. Chang H. Determinants of hospital efficiency: the case of central government-owned hospitals in Taiwan. *Omega International Journal of Management Science* 1998;26(2):307-317.

8. Wan TTH, Hsu N, Feng R, Ma A, Pan S, Chou M. Technical efficiency of nursing units in a tertiary care hospital in Taiwan. *Journal of Medical Systems* 2002;26(1):21-27.

9. Osei D, George M, d'Almeida S, George M, Kirigia JM, Mensah AO, Kainyu LH. Technical efficiency of public district hospitals and health centres in Ghana: a pilot study. *Cost Effectiveness and Resource Allocation* 2005;3:9. Available at: http://www.resource-allocation.com/content/3/1/9.

10. Kirigia JM, Emrouznejad A, Sambo LG, Munguti N, Liambila W. Using data envelopment analysis to measure the technical efficiency of public health centres in Kenya. *Journal of Medical Systems* 2004;28(2):155-166.

11. Kirigia JM, Emrouznejad A, Sambo LG. Measurement of technical efficiency of public hospitals in Kenya: using data envelopment analysis. *Journal of Medical Systems* 2002;26(1):39-45.

12. Zere AE, Mbeeli T, Shangula K, Mandlhate C, Mutirua K, Tjivambi B, Kapenambili W. Technical efficiency of district hospitals: evidence from Namibia using data envelopment analysis. *Cost Effectiveness and Resource Allocation* 2006; 4:5. Available at: http://www.resource-allocation.com/content/4/1/5.

13. Kirigia JM, Emrouznejad A, Vaz RG, Bastiene H, Padayachy J. A comparative assessment of performance and productivity of health centers in Seychelles. *International Journal of Productivity & Performance Management* 2008;57(1):72-92.

14. Renner Ade, Kirigia JM, Zere AE, Barry SP, Kirigia DG, Kamara C, Muthuri HK. Technical efficiency of peripheral health units in Pujehun District of Sierra Leone: a DEA application. *BMC Health Services Research* 2005;5:77. Available at: http://www.biomedcentral.com/1472-6963/5/77.

15. Kirigia JM, Sambo LG, Scheel H. Technical efficiency of public clinics in Kwazulu-Natal Province of South Africa. *East African Medical Journal* 2001;78(3 Suppl):S1-S13.

16. Kirigia JM, Sambo LG, Lambo E. Are public hospitals in Kwazulu-Natal Province of South Africa technically efficient? *African Journal of Health Sciences* 2000;7(3/4):24-31.

17. Zere EA, Addison T, McIntyre D. Hospital efficiency in sub-Saharan Africa: evidence from South Africa. *South African Journal of Economics* 2001;69(2):336-358.

18. Masiye F, Kirigia JM, Emrouznejad A, Sambo LG, Mounkaila A, Chimfwembe D, Okello D. Efficient management of health centres human resources in Zambia. *Journal of Medical Systems* 2006;30(6):473-81.

19. Kirigia JM, Asbu Z, Greene W, Emrouznejad A. Technical efficiency, efficiency change, technical progress and productivity growth in the national health systems of continental African countries. *Eastern Africa Social Science Research Review* 2007; 23(2):19-40.

20. Emrouznejad A, Parker B, Tavares G. Evaluation of research in efficiency and productivity: a survey and analysis of the first 30 years of scholarly literature in DEA. *Socio-Economic Planning Sciences* 2008;42:151-157.

21. Emrouznejad A, Podinovski V. *Data envelopment analysis and performance management.* Coventry: Warwick University; 2004.

22. Fare R, Grosskopf S, Norris M, Zhang Z. Productivity growth, technical progress, and efficiency change in industrialized countries. *The American Economic Review* 1994;84(1):66-83.

23. Coelli T, Rao DSP, Battese G. *An introduction to efficiency and productivity analysis.* Boston: Kluwer Academic Publishers; 1998.

24. Caves DW, Christensen LR, Diewert WE. The economic theory of index numbers and measurement of input, output and productivity. *Econometrica* 1982;50(6):1393-1414.

25. Masiye F, Ndulo M, Roos P, Odegaard K. A comparative analysis of hospitals in Zambia: a pilot study on efficiency measurement and monitoring. In: Seshamani V, Mwikisa CN, Odegaard K, editors. *Zambia's health reforms: selected papers 1995-2000.* Lund: Swedish Institute for Health Economics and University of Zambia, Department of Economics; 2002: 95-107.

26. World Health Organization Regional Office for Africa. *Health promotion: a strategy for the African Region.* Brazzaville:World Health Organization; 2003.

27. Mwabu G, Wang'ombe J. Health services pricing reforms in Kenya. *International Journal of Social Economics* 1997;24(1-3):282-293.

28. Kirigia JM, Preker A, Carrin G, Mwikisa C, Diarra-Nama AJ. An overview of health financing patterns and the way forward in the WHO African Region. *East African Medical Journal* 2006 83(8):S1-S28.

29. Jones AM, Kirigia JM. The determinants of the use of alternative methods of contraception among South African women. *Applied Economic Letters* 2000;7:501-504.

30. Murray CJL, Frenk J. A framework for assessing the performance of health systems. *Bulletin of the World Health Organization* 2000;78(6):717-731.

31. World Health Organization. The world health report 2000: health systems - improving performance. Geneva: World Health Organization; 2000.

32. Graham HT, Bennett R. *Human resources management.* London: Financial Times Pitman Publishing; 1998.

33. Grifell-Tatje E, Lovell CAK. The sources of productivity change in Spanish banking. *European Journal of Operational Research* 1997; 98(2):364-380.

34. Goddard M, Mannion R, Smith PC. Assessing the performance of NHS hospital trusts: the role of 'hard' and 'soft' information. *Health Policy* 1999;48:119-134.

35. Goddard M, Smith PC. Performance measurement in the new NHS. *Health Policy Matters* 2001;3:1-8.

36. Saltman RB, Ferrousier-Davis O. The concept of stewardship in health policy. *Bulletin of the World Health Organization* 2001;78(6):732-739.

Appendix 13.1   Descriptive statistics of inputs/outputs

	2000	2001	2002
Outputs			
OPD + ANC visits			
Total	1,224,474	1,260,296	1,234,454
Mean	43,731.2	45,010.57	44,087.64
Median	27,020	27,237.5	28,579.5
Standard deviation	54,506.1	51,808.19	52,450.36
Variance coefficient	1.246	1.15	1.19
Patient admissions			
Total	158,432	174,477	190,465
Mean	5,658.286	6,231.32	6,802.32
Median	1,697	1,995	2,938.5
Standard deviation	10,533.8	10,710.70	10,810.64
Variance coefficient	1.86	1.71	1.59
Inputs			
Doctors + nurses			
Total	5,410	5,633	5,633
Mean	193.214	201.18	201.18
Median	144.5	144.5	144.5
Standard deviation	179.740	204.44	204.44
Variance coefficient	0.930	1.016	1.016
Drugs + other supplies (in Kwanza)			
Total	454,631	1,108,596	2,057,287
Mean	16,236.821	39,592.71	73,474.54
Median	10,815.5	29,171.5	49,772.5
Standard deviation	19,773.038	39,819.65	65,922.38
Variance coefficient	1.218	1.0057	0.897
Beds			
Total	1,773	1,762	1,774
Mean	63.321	62.93	63.36
Median	61.5	58.5	58.5
Standard deviation	33.276	33.89	33.96
Variance coefficient	0.526	0.54	0.536

Appendix 13.2   Frequency distribution of technical and scale efficiency scores

	2000			2001			2002		
Category	**CRSTE**	**VRSTE**	**Scale**	**CRSTE**	**VRSTE**	**Scale**	**CRSTE**	**VRSTE**	**Scale**
<= 0.2425	7 (25)	5 (18)	1 (4)	6 (21)	4 (14)	1 (4)	4(14)	2 (7)	1 (4)
> 0.2425, <=0.4495	7 (25)	4 (14)	2 (7)	10 (36)	6 (21)	0 (0)	8 (29)	6 (21)	0 (0)
> 0.4495, <= 0.909	7 (25)	8 (29)	8 (29)	6 (21)	6 (21)	15 (54)	8 (29)	9 (32)	8 (29)
> 0.909, <= 0.999	1 (4)	0 (0)	11 (39)	1 (4)	0 (0)	7 (25)	0 (0)	1 (4)	11 (39)
> 0.999, <= 1	6 (21)	11 (39)	6 (21)	5 (18)	12 (43)	5 (18)	8 (29)	10 (36)	8 (29)

Note: CRSTE=technical efficiency from constant returns to scale (CRS) DEA;
        VRSTE= technical efficiency from variable returns to scale (VRS) DEA;
        Scale=scale efficiency = CRSTE / VRSTE;
        The figures in brackets are percentages calculated out of N=28.

*Appendix 13.3   Total output increases and/or input reductions needed to make
inefficient public hospitals efficient*

Variable	2000		2001		2002	
	Total actual values	Shortfall/ Excess	Total actual values	Shortfall/ Excess	Total actual values	Shortfall/ Excess
Outputs						
Outpatient + antenatal visits	1,224,474	897,004 (73.26%)	1,260,296	724,428 (57.48%)	1,234,454	590,267 (47.82%)
Inpatient admissions	158,432	82,636 (52.16%)	174,477	64,552 (37.00%)	190,465	87,061 (45.71%)
Inputs						
Doctors + nurses	5,410	619 (11.45%)	5,633	14 (0.24)	5,633	369 (6.55%)
Drugs and other supplies	454,631	168,662 (37.10%)	1,108,596	641,816 (57.89%)	2,057,287	1,250247 (60.77%)
Beds	1,773	459 (25.87%)	1,762	176 (9.97%)	1,774	156 (8.82%)

Appendix 13.4   Malmquist index summary of annual means

Year	Efficiency change	Technical change	Pure efficiency change	Scale efficiency change	Malmquist index
2001	1.046	1.037	1.023	1.022	1.086
2002	1.213	0.829	1.078	1.126	1.006
Mean	1.127	0.927	1.050	1.073	1.045

Note: A number <1 indicates productivity decline or deterioration; a number equal to 1 signifies
stagnation; a number >1 indicates growth.

Appendix 13.5 *Malmquist index of hospitals*

Hospital	Efficiency Change	Technical Change	Pure Efficiency change	Scale efficiency change	Malmquist Index
Cajueiros	1.000	0.909	1.000	1.000	0.909
Kilamba Kiaxi	1.000	0.777	1.000	1.000	0.777
Cacuaco	1.000	1.022	1.000	1.000	1.022
Samba	1.000	0.984	1.000	1.000	0.984
Maternidade Caxito	0.678	0.805	0.678	1.000	0.545
Caxito	1.101	1.049	1.093	1.008	1.155
Catete	0.771	1.033	0.503	1.533	0.796
Ambriz	1.612	0.774	1.000	1.612	1.247
Muxima	2.022	0.864	1.000	2.022	1.746
Porto Amboim	1.441	0.860	1.497	0.963	1.238
Gabela	0.817	0.916	0.854	0.957	0.748
Boa Entrada/cada	1.848	1.013	1.762	1.049	1.872
Kamakupa	1.349	1.052	1.257	1.073	1.420
Chinguar	0.679	0.879	0.625	1.086	0.596
Cacuso	1.442	1.009	1.367	1.055	1.454
Calandula	1.049	1.075	1.000	1.049	1.127
Lobito	1.162	0.705	1.043	1.114	0.819
Maternidade de Benguela	1.219	1.069	1.227	0.993	1.303
Pediatria de Benguela	1.000	1.077	1.000	1.000	1.077
Balombo	1.014	0.928	1.015	0.999	0.941
Cubal	2.359	0.760	2.413	0.978	1.793
Baia-Farta	1.159	0.887	1.158	1.001	1.028
Dombe Grande	1.082	0.909	1.071	1.010	0.984
Ganda	1.359	0.840	1.380	0.985	1.141
Chongoroi	1.225	0.831	1.230	0.996	1.018
Ukuma	0.657	0.997	0.663	0.991	0.655
Bailundo	0.978	1.054	0.987	0.990	1.030
Katchiungo	1.103	1.078	1.019	1.082	1.189
Mean	**1.127**	**0.927**	**1.050**	**1.073**	**1.045**

Note: All Malmquist index averages are geometric means

-14-

A Comparative Assessment of Performance and Productivity of Health Centres in Seychelles*

Joses M Kirigia, Ali Emrouznejad,
Rui G. Vaz, Henry Bastiene, Jude Padayachy

ABSTRACT

The purpose of this paper is to measure the technical and scale efficiency of health centres; to evaluate changes in productivity; and to highlight possible policy implications of the results for policy makers. Data envelopment analysis (DEA) is employed to assess the technical and scale efficiency and productivity change over a four-year period among 17 public health centres. During the period of study, the results suggested that the public health centres in Seychelles exhibited mean overall or technical efficiency of above 93 per cent. It was also found that the overall productivity increased by 2.4 per cent over 2001-2004.

Further research can be undertaken to gather data on the prices of the various inputs to facilitate an estimation of the allocative efficiency of clinics. If such an exercise were to be undertaken, researchers would also need to consider collecting data on quantities and prices of paramedical, administrative, and support staff to ensure that the analysis is more comprehensive than the study reported in this paper. Institutionalisation of efficiency monitoring would help to enhance further the already good health sector stewardship and governance.

Keywords: Community health centres, Productivity rates, Performance measures, Seychelles

* The original article appeared in *International Journal of Productivity and Performance Management* 2008;57(1):72-92. Reproduced with the permission of Emerald Group Publishing Ltd.

BACKGROUND

The Republic of Seychelles consists of an archipelago of 115 islands in the south-western Indian Ocean. It has a population of 82,474 people; 25% are 0-14 years, 66.9% are 15-64, and 7.9% are 65 years and above [1]. Seychelles has the highest human development index (HDI) in the African region. Human development index integrates life expectancy, educational attainment, and gross domestic product (GDP) per capita. The average life expectancy at birth is 72.7 years [2]. The maternal mortality rate is 21 per 100,000 live births, which is the lowest in the region [3]. Adult literacy rate is 91.9% compared with 60.5% for the African region. The country has the highest GDP per capita in the region estimated at $10,232 (purchasing power parity). For most of the population, wages and salaries are the most important sources of income (74%) and also pensions and social security benefits (16%) and self-employment (8%). However, in spite of significant social and economic progress approximately 6% of the population still lives below international poverty line; about 13% of the population does not have sustainable access to an improved water source and water-flushed toilets; 3% does not have access to electricity; 10% of homes have no television; and 29% do not have a fixed telephone line (Appendix 14.1).

The per capita total expenditure on health at average exchange rate is US$425 in Seychelles, which is nine times higher than that of the African Region. About 74% of that expenditure comes from government sources. Private spending constitutes only 26% of the total health expenditure with approximately 60% of it coming from household out-of-pocket expenditures [4]. The Seychelles three-tier healthcare system consists of 8 hospitals, 20 health centres, and community based integrated development activities. Each of the eight health regions has a hospital providing hospital-based medical care activities. Regarding distribution of health centres, five are in Central Mahe Region; two each in North Mahe and East Mahe; three each in South Mahe, West Mahe, and Praslin; and one each in La Digue and Silhouette [5]. Health centres serving population groups of 4,000 or more offer medical consultations, laboratory diagnosis and care; pharmaceutical services; maternal and child health including family planning; environmental and occupational health; health education; dental services; physiotherapy; social services; and counselling. Home-based care is also provided as required [5].

The dramatic improvement in health indicators has been achieved through intense health promotion and preventive care. Teams made up of a medical officer, nurses, dental and environmental health officers, dispensers, and physiotherapists provide ambulatory and peripatetic services on a daily or thrice weekly basis with coverage of over 90% of the population. The objective of government is to make health care available and accessible to all Seychelles citizens within the limits of the available resources. Article 29 of the country's 1993 Constitution reaffirms the right of citizens to free primary health care [5]. Any inefficiency depicts denial of health care for an additional citizen at zero extra cost. It also reduces the effectiveness of the health system in achieving the goals of health improvement, responsiveness to citizen's legitimate non-medical expectations, and fairness in healthcare financing [6]. To date no study in Seychelles has addressed the following questions:

1. Are health centres producing maximum outputs with the available inputs?

2. Are health centres operating at an optimal scale? Or are (dis)economies of scale prevalent (i.e. inefficiency due to largeness or smallness of health centre size)?

3. What is the trend of productivity over the years? What percentage of the observed productivity changes can be attributed to technical efficiency change and technological change/growth?

The aim of this study was to contribute towards bridging that knowledge gap. Its specific objectives were to measure the technical and scale efficiency of health centres in Seychelles; to evaluate changes in productivity over time with a view to analysing changes in efficiency and changes in technology; and to make the policy implications of the results explicit for policy makers and health centre managers.

METHODS

Concept and Measurement of Technical Efficiency and Productivity of Health Centres

A health system performs the functions of stewardship (oversight), health financing, creating resources/inputs (including human resources for health) for producing health, and delivering (providing) personal and non-personal services with a view to improving responsiveness to people's non-medical expectations, ensuring fair financial contribution to health systems and ultimately improving health status (health-related quality of life and/or length of life) [6]. A health system employs its scarce/limited resources (e.g., human resources, pharmaceutical supplies, non-pharmaceutical supplies, clinical technologies, beds, building space, ambulances) to produce promotive, preventive, curative, and rehabilitative services through the performance of the above-mentioned functions. A primary economic and public health problem is how to avoid wastage of health enhancing or maintaining scarce resources.

In the context of health centres, technical efficiency means providing maximum health services out of available resources or minimising the use of available resources to produce a given level of health services. Although economic efficiency is a product of both technical/productive efficiency (producing health care without waste) with allocative efficiency (allocating

-314-

health resources to their most highly valued uses), the absence of data on prices of inputs limits the focus of this study only to the measurement of technical efficiency.

Technical efficiency comprises both pure technical and scale efficiency components. Returns to scale/size tells us how output (e.g., PAP + MCH + FP + ANC + PNC + Immunisation + School health visits - PMFAPIS) responds in the long run to changes in the scale/size of the firm (health centre in our case). In other words, suppose we consider a long-run situation in which all inputs are variable and suppose a health centre increases the amount of all inputs by the same proportion, what would happen to output? There are three possibilities [7]:

1. Output may increase by exactly the same proportion as the inputs, for example, doubling of all inputs may lead to a doubling of output. This is the case of constant returns to scale (CRS). When a health centre is operating at CRS, technical efficiency is equal to scale efficiency.

2. Output may increase by a larger proportion than each of the inputs, for example, a doubling of all inputs may lead to more than a doubling of output. This is the case of increasing returns to scale (IRS) also known as economies of scale. Increasing returns to scale may arise due to indivisibilities of some health inputs, greater specialisation, innovation (may be as a result to research and development), and/or increased performance of human resources for health (may be due to increased motivation).

3. Output may increase by a smaller proportion than each of the inputs, for example, a doubling of all inputs may lead to less than doubling of output. This is the case of decreasing returns to scale (DRS) also called diseconomies of scale. Decreasing returns to scale may arise because of shortages of complementary inputs (e.g., medicines), low levels of staff motivation, and leadership problems (e.g., related to coordination and supervision).

Figure 14.1 illustrates the concept and measurement of technical efficiency [8,9]. It depicts a single input (number of nurses) and single output (number of PMFAPIS visits) production technology under CRS and VRS assumptions. Graphically, under the CRS assumption, the production frontier (0GCH) is a straight line. Contrastingly, the frontier (ABCD) under the VRS assumption is concave.

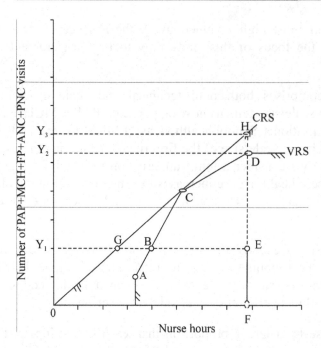

Figure 14.1   Technical efficiency

We shall use health centre *'E'* to demonstrate the estimation of overall technical efficiency and its decomposition into pure technical efficiency and scale efficiency. This health centre uses 0F nurse hours to produce $0Y_1$ number of PMFAPIS visits. Under a CRS technology, health centre E could have cared for a larger number of PMFAPIS visits ($0Y_3$) with the same number of nurse hours (0F). Likewise, under VRS technology, $0Y_2$ PMFAPIS visits could have been produced using the same number of nurse-hours, 0F.

The output-oriented technical efficiency of health centre E under constant returns to scale (TE_{CRS}) is:

$$TE_{CRS} = \frac{FE}{FH} \tag{1}$$

On the other hand, the output-oriented pure technical efficiency of health centre E under variable returns to scale (TE_{VRS}) is:

$$TE_{VRS} = \frac{FE}{FD} \tag{2}$$

Technical efficiency takes values between one (or 100%) and zero (or 0%). Technically efficient health centres have a technical efficiency score of one, whilst the inefficient ones have a score less than one. For illustration purpose, lets assume that the pure technical efficiency of health centre E is 90%. This implies that the health centre could have attended to 10% more PMFAPIS visits than it is currently attending to with the same number of nurse hours.

$$\text{Scale efficiency} = \frac{FH}{FD} = \frac{TE_{CRS}}{TE_{VRS}} \qquad (3)$$

The distances EH and ED represent technical inefficiencies under CRS and VRS assumptions respectively. Scale inefficiency equals the difference between the two, that is EH minus ED. Scale efficiency takes values between one (or 100%) and zero (or 0%). Scale efficient health centres have a score of one, whereas the inefficient ones have a score of less than one. For instance, if the scale efficiency score for health centre E is 95%, this implies inefficiency level of about 5% that is accounted for by inappropriate health centre size (inefficiently large or small).

Data Envelopment Analysis Conceptual Framework

The two approaches to the measurement of efficiency of decision-making units are: (*a*) parametric methods that include the estimation of production [10] and cost functions with a priori well-defined functional form and (*b*) construction of index numbers using non-parametric methods including data envelopment analysis (DEA) and Free Disposal Hall (FDH).

We choose to use DEA instead of stochastic frontier analysis methods to estimate technical and scale efficiency for the following reasons: DEA can handle multiple inputs and multiple output production scenario typical of health centres; it does not require an assumption of a functional form relating inputs to outputs; health centres are directly compared against a peer or combination of peers; and inputs and outputs can have very different units of measurement [11,12].

The DEA, a linear programming technique, was developed by Charnes *et al* [11] to facilitate measurement of efficiency when faced with production units (e.g. health centres) that employ multiple inputs to produce multiple outputs. The DEA technique has been widely and fruitfully applied to the evaluation of efficiency among primary health care decision-making units in Greece [13], Finland [14], the United Kingdom [15-17], and the United States of America [18]. However, applications of the methodology among primary healthcare facilities in the WHO African Region are few [19-23]. Prior to the study reported in this paper there had been no attempt to estimate efficiency of healthcare facilities, using either non-parametric or parametric methods, in Seychelles.

Under the assumption of variable returns to scale (VRS), DEA measures the technical efficiency (TE) of health centre z compared with n health centres in a peer group as follows [11]:

Objective function:

$$Max \quad TE_z = \sum_{r=1}^{s} u_r y_{rj_z} + u_z$$

(4)

Subject to constraint:

$$\sum_{i=1}^{m} v_i x_{ij_z} = 1$$

$$\sum_{r=1}^{s} u_r y_{rj} - \sum_{i=1}^{m} v_i x_{ij} + u_z \leq 0; \quad j = 1,...,n$$

$$u_r, \geq 0; \qquad r = 1,..., s,$$

$$v_i \geq 0; \qquad i = 1,...,m,$$

Where:

$y_{rj} (r = 1,...,s)$ = observed amount of rth output for j^{th} health centre

$x_{ij} (i = 1,...,m)$ = observed amount of ith input for j^{th} health centre

u_r = weight given to output r

v_i = weight given to input i

n = number of health centres

z = the health centre being evaluated in the set of $j=1,...,n$ centres

The weights u_r and v_i are not known a priori but are determined from the data by the above-mentioned model and assigned to each input and output in order to maximise the efficiency rating, TE_z of the health centre being evaluated. In order to generate efficiency scores for each health centre, the model was run 17 times; that is, as many times as the number of health centres. The relative efficiency score is bounded between 0 (completely inefficient) and 1 (100% technically efficient). Thus, any health centre whose

$TE_z < 1$ is technically inefficient compared to other health centres in the peer group.

Malmquist Productivity Index (MPI)

There are a number of reasons as to why the Seychelles Ministry of Health (and indeed all Ministries of Health in the African Region) ought to be concerned with monitoring of health centre productivity: limited resources vis-à-vis unlimited health needs; increased productivity ought to be a key strategy of dealing with shortages of human resources for health; increased productivity results into improved, effective access/utilisation of health services, while productivity decrease results into waste of health-producing resources; necessary for planning, implementing, monitoring and evaluating policies geared at productivity enhancement; an attribute of good health systems stewardship and governance; and demonstrated efforts to monitor and improve health centres' performance can attract more domestic and external resources into the health sector.

We have used DEA-based Malmquist total factor productivity (TFP) index [23,24] to measure productivity change. The Malmquist index does not require assumptions on the profit maximisation or cost minimisation or information on input and output prices. It allows the decomposition of productivity changes into technical efficiency change and technological change.

Fare et al [25] specified the output-oriented Malmquist productivity change index as the geometric mean of two periods productivity indices and subsequently decomposed it into various sources of productivity change as follows:

$$M_o\left(y^{t+1},x^{t+1},y^t,x^t\right) = \left[\frac{D_0^t\left(x^{t+1},y^{t+1}\right)}{D_0^t\left(x^t,y^t\right)}\times\frac{D_0^{t+1}\left(x^{t+1},y^{t+1}\right)}{D_0^{t+1}\left(x^t,y^t\right)}\right]^{1/2}$$

$$= \left[\frac{D_0^{t+1}\left(x^{t+1},y^{t+1}\right)}{D_0^t\left(x^t,y^t\right)}\right]\times\left[\frac{D_0^t\left(x^{t+1},y^{t+1}\right)}{D_0^{t+1}\left(x^{t+1},y^{t+1}\right)}\times\frac{D_0^t\left(x^t,y^t\right)}{D_0^{t+1}\left(x^t,y^t\right)}\right]^{1/2}$$

(5)

$$\text{Efficiency change} = \left[\frac{D_0^{t+1}\left(x^{t+1},y^{t+1}\right)}{D_0^t\left(x^t,y^t\right)}\right] \qquad (6)$$

$$\text{Technical change} = \left[\frac{D_0^t\left(x^{t+1},y^{t+1}\right)}{D_0^{t+1}\left(x^{t+1},y^{t+1}\right)}\times\frac{D_0^t\left(x^t,y^t\right)}{D_0^{t+1}\left(x^t,y^t\right)}\right]^{1/2} \qquad (7)$$

According to Grifell-Tatje and Lovell [26], Malmquist productivity index attains a value greater than, equal to, or less than unity if a firm (health centre) has experienced productivity growth, stagnation, or productivity decline net of the contribution of scale economies between periods t and $t + 1$.

Figure 14.2 illustrates decomposition of productivity growth for constant-returns-to-scale technology [25].

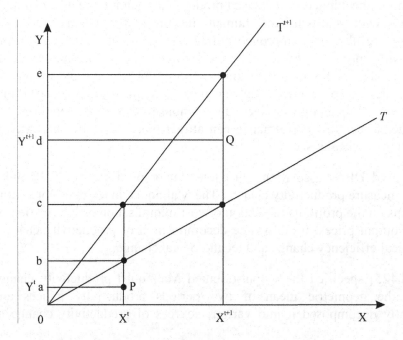

Figure 14.2   Output-based Malmquist productivity index

T^t and T^{t+1} represent the production technology in two periods, t and $t+1$. The health centre produces at point P in period t and at point Q in period $t + 1$. Using the last formula, the decomposition of the MPI from the above figure is given as:

$$\text{Efficiency change} = \frac{0d/0e}{0a/0b} \qquad (8)$$

That is, the efficiency change is the ratio of the Farrell technical efficiency in period $t +1$ to that in period t. The technical change is the geometric mean of the shift in technology evaluated at x^{t+1} and the shift in technology evaluated at x^t is as follows:

$$\text{Technical change} = \left[\frac{0d/0c}{0d/0e} \times \frac{0a/ob}{0a/0c} \right]^{\frac{1}{2}} \qquad (9)$$

Data

The data used in this study were obtained from Seychelles annual health statistics reports for 2001, 2002, 2003, and 2004. There are 17 health centres in Seychelles. This study covered the entire population of health centres in Seychelles. The report contained data for total number of hours worked by both doctors and nurses in a year. Thus, health centres were assumed to utilise two inputs: total number of doctor hours and total number of nurse hours. The report indicates that health centres produce 9 outputs: number of patients dressed, domiciliary cases treated, school health sessions, maternal and child health (MCH) visits, antenatal visits, postnatal visits, immunisations, pap smear visits, and family planning clinic visits. Given the small population of health centres, to increase degrees of freedom, the authors decided to combine the number of pap-smear (PAP) visits, family planning (FP) clinic visits, maternal and child health (MCH) visits, antenatal care (ANC) visits and post-natal care (PNC) visits, number of children immunised and those participating in school health programme into one variable, PMFAPIS. Thus, the DEA was estimated with three outputs: number of patients dressed, domiciliary cases treated, and PMFAPIS.

Output orientation was assumed since management of health centres has no control over inputs, especially its staffing. However, given their primary health care orientation, with a strong bias towards health promotion and disease prevention, they can influence the number of people seeking, for example, antenatal and postnatal care, family planning services, birthing services, immunisations, and schoool health education through their public health outreach work among communities. Thus, the output-oriented DEA model was used for the health centre analysis.

RESULTS

Technical and Scale Efficiency

The frequency distributions of technical and scale efficiency scores for the health centres in 2001, 2002, 2003, and 2004 are summarised in Appendix 14.2. In 2001, 2002, 2003 and 2004, out of the 17 health centres, about 10 (59 per cent), 8 (47 per cent), 9 (53 per cent), and 10 (59 per cent) centres respectively had a variable returns to scale technical efficiency score of 100 per cent. Values of 100 per cent imply that the health centre is technically efficient in the associated year. The individual health centres' technical and scale efficiency scores during the four years are presented in Appendices 14.3 and 14.4.

The yearly analysis has revealed that 7 (41 per cent), 9 (53 per cent), 8 (47 per cent), and 7 (41 per cent) of the health centres were run inefficiently in 2001, 2002, 2003, and 2004 respectively and needed to either increase their outputs (or reduce their inputs) in order to become efficient. The average VRS technical efficiency scores were 93 per cent, 92 per cent, 92 per cent, and 96 per cent respectively during the years under consideration. This finding implies that if the health centres were operating efficiently, they could have produced 7 per cent, 8 per cent, 8 per cent, and 4 per cent more output (number of patients dressed, domiciliary cases treated, maternal and child health visits, antenatal visits, postnatal visits, immunisations, pap smear visits, family planning clinic visits, and number participating in school health programme) respectively using their current levels of input endowment.

Scale Efficiency

In 2001, 2002, 2003, and 2004, out of the 17 health centres:

1. Five (29 per cent), six (35.3 per cent), seven (41.2 per cent), and seven (41.2 per cent) health centres respectively manifested constant returns to scale (CRS). These health centres were operating at their most productive scale sizes.

2. None (0 per cent), one (5.9 per cent), none (0 per cent), and two (11.8 per cent) health centres respectively had increasing returns to scale (IRS). If a health centre is exhibiting IRS, it should expand its scale of operation in order to become scale efficient [27, 28].

3. Eleven (70.6 per cent), ten (58.8 per cent), ten (58.8 per cent), and eight (47.1 per cent) health centres respectively had decreasing returns to scale (DRS). In order to operate at the most productive scale size, a health centre exhibiting DRS should scale down the size of its operation [27, 28].

The average scale efficiency score in the sample was 90 per cent in 2001, 93 per cent in 2002, 92 per cent in 2003, and 95 per cent in 2004 implying that there was room for increasing total outputs by about 10 per cent in 2001, 7 per cent in 2002, 8 per cent in 2003, and 5 per cent in 2004. This can be accomplished through appropriate adjustment in the size of the scale-inefficient health centres where feasible. However, due to indivisibility of physical facilities this may not be possible.

Scope for Output Increases and Implications for Policy

If the inefficient health centres in Seychelles were to operate as efficiently as their peers on the efficiency frontier, there would be scope for some output increases or input savings. Appendices 14.5 and 14.6 present the output increases and/or input reductions needed to make individual inefficient health centres efficient. The total output increases and/or input reductions needed to make inefficient health centres efficient are reported in Appendix 14.7. In 2004, for example, the inefficient health centres combined would need to increase the domiciliary care visits by 2,157 (17.6 per cent) and PFMAPIS visits by 2,937 (2.6 per cent) in order to become efficient.

Concerning health centres with outputs falling short of the DEA targets, MoH policy makers could improve their efficiency by creating demand for the under-utilised domiciliary care and pap smear tests, family planning services, maternal and child health services, antenatal care, postnatal care, immunisation, and school health. These are all essential components of primary health care [29]. This may require a combination of the following intervention strategies:

1. Use of health promotion approaches [30] to boost the target population's effective demand for domiciliary care and pap smear tests, family planning services, maternal and child health services, antenatal care, postnatal care, immunisation, and school health.

2. Reduction of financial barriers to effective access to health services such as out-of-pocket expenses (e.g., user fees and transport costs) and time costs (e.g., travel time, waiting/queueing time, diagnosis time, treatment time) [31,32]. The remaining monetary barriers could be eliminated if the countries were to pursue universal coverage policy through either introduction of a tax-funded national health service or national social health insurance [33,34].

Alternatively, if it is very difficult to reduce inefficiencies by inducing demand for services, policy makers could improve efficiency through transfer of excess nursing hours to health centres with a deficit.

Productivity Growth

In the application of the Malmquist productivity index to analyse the differences in productivity over time, the year 2001 has been taken as the technology reference. The reader will recall that if the value of the Malmquist index or any of its components is less than 1 it denotes regress or deterioration in performance, whereas values greater than 1 denote improvements in the relevant performance. Appendix 14.8 presents the Malmquist index summary of annual geometric means. In the last row (last column) we see that, on average, health centre productivity increased by 2.4 per cent over the four-year period. That growth was largely due to innovation. Whereas efficiency regressed by 15.7 per cent, technical change (innovation) improved by 21.5 per cent per annum.

We now turn to an examination of the magnitude and sources of productivity change within each health centre. Appendix 14.9 gives a summary of the average annual values of the Malmquist productivity index and its components for each health centre. About 5 (29.4 per cent) out of 17 health centres had improvements in productivity since they had Malmquist indexes greater than one. Silhouette, Anse Boileau, Anse Royale, Anse Aux Pins, and Beoliere health centres experienced total factor productivity growth of 49.4 per cent, 5.7 per cent, 4.6 per cent, 0.8 per cent, and 0.5 per cent respectively. In all five health centres productivity growth was entirely attributed to technical change (or innovation).

On the other hand, 11 (64.7 per cent) of the health centres had Malmquist indices of less than one indicating deterioration in performance over time. In all those health centres deterioration was brought about by efficiency regress except in Victorial where it emanated from technical regress. Only Takamaka health centre had a Malmquist index of exactly one, which signified stagnation.

Pure Efficiency Change

As indicated earlier, the first component of the MPI provides a measure of the contribution to productivity change of a change in technical efficiency between periods t and $t + 1$. Efficiency change is a product of pure efficiency change (PEFFCH) and scale efficiency change (SCH). As seen in Appendix 14.9, the average pure efficiency change (PEFFCH) was equal to one in all the health centres. This means that the relative technical efficiency of all the health centres remained the same between time period t and $t+1$.

Scale Efficiency Change

The scale efficiency change (SCH) index attains a value greater than, equal to, or less than unity if a health centre's scale of production contributes positively, not at all, or negatively to productivity change, [26]. None of the health centres attained a scale index of greater than unity. Two (11.8 per cent) of the health centres had a scale efficiency value equal to unity meaning that the scale of production of those centres did not contribute to productivity change. A total of 15 (88.2 per cent) of the health centres had a scale index of less than unity signifying that the production of those centres contributed negatively to productivity change. The average SCH score for the whole sample of health centres was 0.843 implying that the scale of production on average reduced efficiency change slightly by 15.7 per cent. Grifell-Tatje and Lovell [26] explain that such a change in the scale of production contributes negatively to productivity change if it is in the direction away from technically optimal scale.

Technical Change

The technical change component of the MPI provides a measure of the contribution to productivity change of whatever technical change occurs between periods t and $t+1$. About 16 (94 per cent) of the health centres experienced technical progress, none of the health centres experienced technical stagnation, and one (5.6 per cent) of the health centres recorded a small technical regress of 1.8 per cent. The average technical change score was 1.215; indicating a 21.5 per cent technical progress. This index attains a value of greater than unity if technical progress has occurred along a ray through a firm's (health centre) data between periods t and $t+1$.

Limitations of the study

Firstly, DEA does not capture random noise (e.g., epidemics and natural and man-made disasters) and thus it inadvertently attributes any deviation from the frontier to inefficiency [8,35]. Thus, by using DEA we may have overestimated the existing magnitudes of inefficiencies. Secondly, a number of key inputs were omitted from the study including pharmaceuticals, non-pharmaceutical supplies, and capital inputs (equipment, buildings, and vehicles). This was not deliberate. It is because the information on those variables was not available in the annual health statistics reports. Thirdly, it could be argued that the ultimate output of health centres is the aggregate improvement in health status of the beneficiaries of health centre services. Like other past efficiency studies [19-22] in the WHO African Region, this study used intermediate outputs instead of indicators of the ultimate health centres (e.g., quality-adjusted life years) due to non-availability of health facility-level data.

Fourthly, this study assumes that all clinics are fairly homogeneous. We were not able to verify whether the clinics had exactly the same standards in terms of type of services provided, severity of cases treated, quality of care provided, qualification and experience of staff, working schedules, functional building capacity, healthcare technology, etc. Lastly, since information on the prices of inputs was not available, it was not possible to estimate allocative efficiency, which would have enabled us to calculate the overall economic efficiency. Thus, the inefficiency estimates reported in this study should be considered as an underestimate of the level of waste existing within the clinics.

Suggestions for Further Research

We have four suggestions for further research within the Seychelles national health system. First, there is need to undertake a supplementary study to gather data on the prices of the various inputs (e.g., remunerations of doctors, nurses, beds) to facilitate an estimation of the allocative efficiency of clinics. If such an exercise were to be undertaken, researchers may also consider collecting data on quantities and prices of paramedical, administrative, and support staff to ensure that the analysis is more comprehensive than the study reported in this paper.

Second, it may be useful to study the feasibility of adapting national performance assessment frameworks currently being used in some developed countries to improve health facility performance [36]. In the process of undertaking such a study it would be important to explore the potential application of the strategies suggested by Goddard and Smith [37] for overcoming some of the adverse consequences (e.g., tunnel vision, sub-optimisation, measure fixation, myopia, complacency, misrepresentation, gaming, misinterpretation, and ossification) of performance-based management.

Third, it would be logical to apply DEA among the public hospitals and private sector (including NGO) health facilities to inform future health sector reforms. Evidence on hospital efficiency and productivity complemented with that on health centres will enable the health policy makers to have a complete picture on which to base decisions for improving performance of health facilities. Lastly, it might be worthwhile to explore the feasibility of the steps proposed in Renner et al [19] for institutionalising efficiency monitoring within the health information system of the Seychelles Ministry of Health.

CONCLUSION

This study has measured both the technical and scale efficiencies of 17 individual health centres; identified the input reductions and/or output increases needed to make the inefficient health centres efficient; and estimated the magnitude and sources of productivity change within each health centre. The findings indicate that seven, nine, eight, and seven of the health centres were run inefficiently in 2001, 2002, 2003, and 2004 respectively. In 2004, the inefficient health centres combined would need to increase the number of people domiciliary care by 2,157 (17.6%) and PFMAPIS by 2,937 (2.6%) in order to become efficient. Thus, there is some scope for providing the above-mentioned health services to additional persons without investing extra resources into the health sector from any source; public or private.

Alternatively, depending on the decision of policy makers the inefficiencies could be eliminated by shedding off 4,151 (2.7%) nursing hours. However, we would not recommend this course of action given their important role in provision of primary health care. There is evidence that 11 (64.7%) of the health centres experienced total factor productivity deterioration over time during the four years. If relevant data were available, the Malmquist TFP type of analyses can be used to assess the effects of the key health sector reforms undertaken in the past on the efficiency of health facilities. The national and district health management information systems should be strengthened to routinely capture the input, input prices, and output data which could be used to monitor economic efficiency and productivity change among fixed health facilities (e.g., health centres and hospitals).

The fifty-fifth session of the WHO Regional Committee for Africa called on "the WHO and the World Bank to support countries to institutionalise mechanisms for monitoring efficiency in the use of health sector resources" [38, p.135]. Institutionalisation of efficiency monitoring would help to enhance further the already good stewardship [39] and governance of the health sector in Seychelles.

ACKNOWLEDGEMENT

The data used in this study were obtained from the Seychelles Ministry of Health with the assistance of the WHO Country Office. Jehovah Adonai inspired the authors in undertaking the study and provided invaluable all round support at all the stages of the study. The article contains the views of the authors only and does not represent the opinions, decisions, or stated policies of the Seychelles Ministry of Health or the World Health Organization.

REFERENCES

1. Republic of Seychelles. *Health statistics.* Victoria: Government Printer; 2004.

2. United Nations Development Programme. *Human development index report 2005.* Oxford: Oxford University Press; 2005.

3. World Health Organization Regional Office for Africa. *Country cooperation strategy for Seychelles.* Brazzaville: World Health Organization; 2004.

4. World Health Organization. *World health report 2005: making every mother and child count.* Geneva: World Health Organization; 2005.

5. Republic of Seychelles. Health policy, strategy and organization in Seychelles - a sectoral review for constructive reform. Victoria: Government Printer; 2005.

6. World Health Organization. *The world health report 2000 – health systems: improving performance.* Geneva: World Health Organization; 2000.

7. Osei D, George M, d'Almeida S, Kirigia JM, Mensah AO, Kainyu LH. Technical efficiency of public district hospitals and health centres in Ghana: a pilot study. *Cost Effectiveness and Resource Allocation* 2005;3:9. Available at: http://www.resource-allocation.com/content/3/1/9

8. Zere EA, Addison T, McIntyre D. Hospital efficiency in sub-Saharan Africa: Evidence from South Africa. *South African Journal of Economics* 2000;69(2):336-358.

9. Fare R, Grosskopf S, Norris M, Zhang Z. Productivity growth, technical progress, and efficiency change in industrialized countries. *The American Economic Review* 1994;84(1):66-83.

10. Evans DB, Tandon A, Murray CJL, Lauer JA. Comparative efficiency of national health systems: cross national econometric analysis. *British Medical Journal* 2001;323:307-310.

11. Charnes A, Cooper WW, Rhodes E. Measuring the efficiency of decision-making units. *European Journal of Operational Research* 1978;2(6): 429-444.

12. Coelli T, Rao DSP, Battese G. *An introduction to efficiency and productivity analysis.* Boston, MA: Kluwer Academic Publishers; 1998.

13. Zavras AI, Tsakos G, Economou C, Kyriopoulos J. Using DEA to evaluate efficiency and formulate policy within a Greek national primary healthcare network. *Journal of Medical Systems* 2002;26(4):285-292.

14. Linna M, Nordblad A, Koivu M. Technical and cost-efficiency of oral health care provision in Finnish health centers. *Social Science and Medicine* 2002;56:343-353.

15. Hollingsworth B, Parkin D. The efficiency of the delivery of neonatal care in the UK. *Journal of Public Health Medicine* 2001; 23(1):47-50.

16. Salinas-Jimenez J, Smith P. Data envelopment analysis applied to quality in primary health care. *Annals of Operational Research* 1996;67:141-161.

17. Giuffrida A, Gravelle H. Measuring performance in primary care: econometric analysis and DEA. *Applied Economics* 2001;33:163-175.

18. Ozcan YA. Physician benchmarking: measuring variation in practice behavior in treatment of otitis media. *Health Care Management Science* 1998;1:5-17.

19. Renner A, Kirigia JM, Zere EA, Barry SP, Gatwiri DK, Kamara C, Muthuri LHK. Technical efficiency of peripheral health units in Pujehun district of Sierra Leone: a DEA application. *BMC Health Services Research* 2005; 5(77).Available at: http://www.biomedcentral.com/1472-6963/5/77

20. Kirigia JM, Emrouznejad A, Sambo LG, Munguti N, Liambila W. Using data envelopment analysis to measure the technical efficiency of public health centers in Kenya. *Journal of Medical Systems* 2004;28(2):155-166.

21. Kirigia JM, Sambo LG, Scheel H. Technical efficiency of public clinics in Kwazulu-Natal Province of South Africa. *East African Medical Journal* 2004;78(3 Suppl):S1-S13.

22. Masiye F, Kirigia JM, Emrouznejad A, Sambo LG, Mounkaila AB, Chimfwembe D, Okello D. Efficient Management of Health Centres Human Resources in Zambia. *Journal of Medical Systems* 2006;30:473–481.

23. Malmquist S. Index numbers and indifference curves. *Trabajos de Estatistica* 1953;4(1):209-242.

24. Caves DW, Christensen LR, Diewert WE. The economic theory of index numbers and measurement of input, output and productivity. *Econometrica* 1982;50(6):1393-1414.

25. Fare R, Grosskopf S, Norris M, Zhang Z. Productivity growth, technical progress, and efficiency change in industrialized countries. *The American Economic Review* 1994;84(1):66-83.

26. Grifell-Tatje E, Lovell CAK. The sources of productivity change in Spanish banking. *European Journal of Operational Research* 1997;98(2):364-380.

27. Chattopadhy S, Ray CS. Technical, scale, and size efficiency in nursing home care: a nonparametric analysis of Connecticut homes. *Health Economics* 1996;5:363-373.

28. Varian HR. *Intermediate microeconomics: a modern approach.* New Delhi: Affiliated East-West Press; 2003.

29. World Health Organization. Primary health care: report of the International Conference on Primary Health Care: Alma-Ata, USSR, 6-12 September 1978. Geneva: World Health Organization; 1978.

30. World Health Organization, Regional Office for Africa. *Health promotion: a strategy for the African Region.* Brazzaville: World Health Organization; 2003.

31. Mwabu G, Ainsworth M, Nyamete A. Quality of medical care and choice of medical treatment in Kenya: empirical analysis. *Journal of Human Resources* 1993;28(4):838-862.

32. Jones AM, Kirigia JM. The determinants of the use of alternative methods of contraception among South African women. *Applied Economic Letters* 2000;7:501-504.

33. Carrin G, James C. Social health insurance: key factors affecting the transition towards universal coverage. *International Social Security Review* 2005;58(1):45-64.

34. World Health Organization. *Sustainable health financing, universal coverage and Social health insurance.* World Health Assembly resolution WHA58.33. Geneva: World Health Organization; 2005.

35. Coelli TJ. *A guide to DEAP version 2.1: a data envelopment analysis [computer] program,* Centre for Efficiency and Productivity Analysis (CEPA) Working Paper 96/08. Department of Econometrics; University of New England, Armidale, NSW Australia; 1996.

36. Goddard M, Mannion R, Smith PC. Assessing the performance of NHS hospital trusts: the role of 'hard' and 'soft' information. *Health Policy* 1999; 48:119-134.

37. Goddard M, Smith PC. Performance measurement in the new NHS. *Health Policy Matters* 2001;**3**:1-8.

38. World Health Organization Regional Office for Africa. *Fifty-fifth session of the WHO Regional Committee for Africa: final report*. Brazzaville; 2005.

39. Saltman RB, Ferrousier-Davis O. The concept of stewardship in health policy. *Bulletin of the World Health Organization* 2001;78(6):732-739.

Appendix 14.1 *Socio-economic, national health accounts, and health indicators for 2002*

Indicator	Seychelles	African Region
Human development index	0.853	0.465
GDP per capita (PPP$)	10,232	1,856
Total health expenditure as a % of GDP	5.2	5.3
Per capita total expenditure on health at average exchange rate (US$)	425	47.1
Per capita government expenditure on health at average exchange rate (US$)	316.0	27.4
Government health expenditure as a % total health expenditure	74.3	51.3
Private health expenditure as a % of total health expenditure	25.7	48.7
Government health expenditure as a % of total government expenditure	6.6	9.3
External expenditure on health as a % of total health expenditure	7.5	19.9
Social security expenditure as a % of government expenditure on health	5	5.2
Out-of-pocket spending as a % of private expenditure on health	60.4	79.7
Private plan expenditure as a % of private expenditure on health	0	8.0
Total population	81,000	14,943,000
Adult literacy rate (%)	91.9	60.5
Combined gross enrolment ratio for primary, secondary and tertiary schools	85	50
Annual population growth rate (%)	1	2
Dependency ratio (per 100)	46	87
Percentage of population aged 60+ years	9.1	5
Total fertility rate	1.8	5
Life expectancy at birth (years)	72.7	46.1
Infant mortality rate (per 1,000)	11.8	104
Probability of dying (per 1,000) under age 5 years	15	147
Probability of dying (per 1,000) between ages 15 and 60 years (males)	235	503
Probability of dying (per 1,000) between ages 15 and 60 years (females)	92	434
Maternal mortality rate (per 100,000 live births)	21	807
Newborns immunised with BCG 2003 (%)	99	82
1-year-olds immunised with 3 doses of DTP 2003 (%)	99	71
Children under 2 years immunised with 1 dose of measles 2003 (%)	99	70
Adult illiteracy rate (% aged 15 and above)	8.1	40.5
Population without sustainable access to an improved water source (%)	13	34.7
Children underweight for age (% under age 5)	6	23.6
Physicians (per 100,000 people)	132	18
Births attended by skilled health personnel (%)		53

Sources: WHO [4] and UNDP [2]

Appendix 14.2   Frequency distribution of technical and scale efficiency scores

Efficiency score bracket	2001			2002			2003			2004		
	CRS	VRS	Scale	CRS	VRS	Scale	CRS	VRS	Scale	CRS	VRS	Scale
51-60	1	0	0	0	0	0	1	0	0	0	0	0
61-70	2	1	0	3	0	0	2	1	0	0	0	0
71-80	5	1	4	2	2	0	5	2	2	5	2	2
81-90	2	4	4	5	4	6	2	2	5	1	1	1
91-99	2	1	4	1	3	5	0	3	3	4	4	7
100	5	10	5	6	8	6	7	9	7	7	10	7
Total	17	17	17	17	17	17	17	17	17	17	17	17

Appendix 14.3   Health centres' technical and scale efficiency scores during 2001-2002

Health centre	Efficiency summary results for 2001				Efficiency summary results for 2002			
	CRSTE	VRSTE	Scale	Returns to scale	CRSTE	VRSTE	Scale	Returns to scale
Victoria	1	1	1	CRS	1	1	1	CRS
English River	0.8	1	0.8	DRS	1	1	1	CRS
Mont Fleuri	0.837	0.92	0.909	DRS	0.735	0.805	0.913	DRS
Beau Vallon	0.694	0.868	0.8	DRS	0.844	0.912	0.925	DRS
Glacis	0.736	0.834	0.882	DRS	0.773	0.873	0.885	DRS
Les Mamelles	0.942	1	0.942	DRS	1	1	1	CRS
Anse Aux Pins	0.752	1	0.752	DRS	0.843	0.982	0.859	DRS
Anse Royale	0.586	0.788	0.744	DRS	0.626	0.756	0.828	DRS
Baie Lazare	1	1	1	CRS	0.877	0.822	0.994	IRS
Takamaka	0.871	1	0.871	DRS	0.93	1	0.93	DRS
Beoliere	0.946	1	0.946	DRS	0.84	1	0.84	DRS
Port Glaud	1	1	1	CRS	1	1	1	CRS
Anse Boileau	0.791	0.898	0.881	DRS	0.816	0.926	0.881	CRS
Baie Ste Anne	0.709	0.841	0.843	DRS	0.7	0.814	0.859	DRS
Grand Anse	1	1	1	CRS	1	1	1	CRS
La Digue	0.635	0.701	0.906	DRS	0.702	0.742	0.946	DRS
Silhouette	1	1	1	CRS	1	1	1	CRS
Median	0.84	1	0.91		0.84	0.98	0.93	
Mean	0.84	0.93	0.90		0.86	0.92	0.93	
Std	0.141	0.095	0.088		0.126	0.094	0.065	

Appendix 14.4   Health centres' technical and scale efficiency scores during 2003-2004

Health centre	Efficiency summary results for 2003				Efficiency summary results for 2004			
	CRSTE	VRSTE	Scale	Returns to scale	CRSTE	VRSTE	Scale	Returns to scale
Victoria	1	1	1	CRS	1	1	1	CRS
English River	0.790	1	0.790	DRS	0.846	1	0.846	DRS
Mont Fleuri	0.794	0.842	0.943	DRS	0.803	0.863	0.93	DRS
Beau Vallon	0.847	0.926	0.915	CRS	1	1	1	CRS
Glacis	0.694	0.753	0.921	DRS	0.729	0.748	0.974	DRS
Les Mamelles	1	1	1	CRS	1	1	1	CRS
Anse Aux Pins	0.883	1	0.883	DRS	0.958	1	0.958	DRS
Anse Royale	0.566	0.683	0.83	DRS	0.747	0.964	0.775	DRS
Baie Lazare	1	1	1	CRS	1	1	1	CRS
Takamaka	0.721	0.918	0.785	DRS	0.744	0.964	0.787	DRS
Beoliere	1	1	1	CRS	1	1	1	CRS
Port Glaud	1	1	1	CRS	0.974	0.982	0.992	IRS
Anse Boileau	0.792	0.945	0.838	DRS	0.963	1	0.963	DRS
Baie Ste Anne	0.616	0.759	0.812	DRS	0.759	0.759	0.999	IRS
Grand Anse	1	1	1	CRS	0.960	0.987	0.973	DRS
La Digue	0.721	0.845	0.853	DRS	1	1	1	CRS
Silhouette	1	1	1	CRS	1	1	1	CRS
Median	**0.85**	**1**	**0.92**		**0.96**	**1**	**0.99**	
Mean	**0.85**	**0.92**	**0.92**		**0.91**	**0.96**	**0.95**	
STD	**0.150**	**0.106**	**0.84**		**0.110**	**0.084**	**0.076**	

Appendix 14.5   Output (input) increases (reductions) needed to make individual inefficient health centres efficient during 2001-2002

Health centre	2001					2002				
	Outputs			Inputs		Outputs			Inputs	
	O1	O2	O3	I1	I2	O1	O2	O3	I1	I2
Victoria	0	0	0	0	0	0	0	0	0	0
English River	0	0	0	0	0	0	0	0	0	0
Mont Fleuri	0	187	0	0	1,229	0	0	117	0	5,400
Beau Vallon	0	0	0	4,354	0	0	0	0	1,665	0
Glacis	0	0	1,392	0	1,597	0	0	1,312	0	2,599
Les Mamelles	0	0	0	0	0	0	0	0	0	0
Anse Aux Pins	0	0	0	0	0	0	32	1,753	0	5,291
Anse Royale	0	0	347	0	8,624	82	0	0	3,652	4,541
Baie Lazare	0	0	0	0	0	0	115	0	0	0
Takamaka	0	0	0	0	0	0	0	0	0	0
Beoliere	0	0	0	0	0	0	0	0	0	0
Port Glaud	0	0	0	0	0	0	0	0	0	0
Anse Boileau	0	0	437	0	587	0	341	851	0	1,100
Baie Ste Anne	0	0	0	386	0	0	65	496	1,549	0
Grand Anse	0	0	0	0	0	0	0	0	0	0

.../cont.

Appendix 14.5 (cont.)

Health centre	2001					2002				
	Outputs			Inputs		Outputs			Inputs	
	O1	O2	O3	I1	I2	O1	O2	O3	I1	I2
La Digue	0	214	446	0	1,635	0	0	513	0	1,105
Silhouette	0	0	0	0	0	0	0	0	0	0
Total	0	401	2,620	4,740	13,672	82	553	5,040	6,866	20,035
Median	0	0	0	0	0	0	0	0	0	0
Mean	0	24	150	279	804	5	33	296	404	1,179
Std	0	67	357	1,054	2,099	20	85	533	992	1,990

Appendix 14.6   Output (input) increases (reductions) needed to make individual inefficient health centres efficient during 2003-2004

Health centre	2003					2004				
	Outputs			Inputs		Outputs			Inputs	
	O1	O2	O3	I1	I2	O1	O2	O3	I1	I2
Victoria	0	0	0	0	0	0	0	0	0	0
English River	0	0	0	0	0	0	0	0	0	0
Mont Fleuri	708	323	0	0	3,442	0	299	0	0	2,029
Beau Vallon	0	0	0	790	0	0	0	0	0	0
Glacis	0	0	2,159	0	880	0	0	183	0	0
Les Mamelles	0	0	0	0	0	0	0	0	0	0
Anse Aux Pins	0	0	0	0	0	0	0	0	0	0
Anse Royale	0	632	0	0	3,053	0	713	2,754	0	0
Baie Lazare	0	0	0	0	0	0	0	0	0	0
Takamaka	0	145	0	0	4,857	0	176	0	0	2,123
Beoliere	0	0	0	0	0	0	0	0	0	0
Port Glaud	0	0	0	0	0	0	138	0	0	0
Anse Boileau	0	252	2,027	0	1,066	0	0	0	0	0
Baie Ste Anne	0	504	0	0	0	703	0	0	0	0
Grand Anse	0	0	0	0	0	129	0	0	0	0
La Digue	0	181	1493	0	2	0	0	0	0	0
Silhouette	0	0	0	0	0	0	0	0	0	0
Total	708	2,038	5,679	790	13,300	0	2,157	2,937	0	4,151
Median	0	0	0	0	0	0	0	0	0	0
Mean	42	120	334	46	782	0	127	173	0	244
Std	172	199	754	192	1,506	0	235	667	0	690

Appendix 14.7   Output (input) increases (reductions) needed to make inefficient health centres efficient

Variable	Total Actual values (2001)	Shortfall/excess (2001)	Total actual values (2002)	Shortfall/excess (2002)	Total actual values (2003)	Shortfall/Excess (2003)	Total actual values (2004)	Shortfall/excess (2004)
Dressing	93,445	0	86,739	82	84,291	708	79,461	0
Domiciliary care	10,532	401	8,190	553	10,637	2,038	12,245	2,157
Pap + FP + MCH + ANC + Post + Immunised + School Health Sessions	115,718	2,620	113,402	5,040	115,993	5,679	114,739	2,937
Doctor hours	267,848	4,740	278,504	6,866	280,951	790	288,590	0
Nurse hours	121,730	13,672	126,380	20,035	136,120	13,300	154,128	4,151

Appendix 14.8   Malmquist index summary of annual means (output oriented)

Year	Efficiency change [A=(C x D)]	Technical change [B]	Pure efficiency change [C]	Scale efficiency change [D=(A/C)]	Malmquist index of total factor productivity change [E=A x B]
2002	0.706	1.552	1	0.706	1.095
2003	1.346	0.707	1	1.346	0.952
2004	0.63	1.633	1	0.63	1.029
Mean	**0.843**	**1.215**	**1**	**0.843**	**1.024**

Appendix 14.9   Malmquist index summary of firm means

Decision-making unit	Efficiency change [A=(C x D)]	Technical change [B]	Pure efficiency change [C]	Scale efficiency change [D=(A/C)]	Malmquist index of total factor productivity change [E=A x B)]
Victoria	1	0.982	1	1	0.982
English River	0.643	1.406	1	0.643	0.904
Mont Fleuri	0.84	1.139	1	0.84	0.956
Beau Vallon	0.878	1.132	1	0.878	0.993
Glacis	0.845	1.147	1	0.845	0.97
Les Mamelles	0.822	1.128	1	0.822	0.927
Anse Aux Pins	0.889	1.13	1	0.889	1.005
Anse Royale	0.901	1.161	1	0.901	1.046
Baie Lazare	0.815	1.174	1	0.815	0.957
Takamaka	0.822	1.217	1	0.822	1.000
Beoliere	0.893	1.128	1	0.893	1.008
Port Glaud	0.748	1.178	1	0.748	0.881
Anse Boileau	0.931	1.136	1	0.931	1.057
Baie Ste Anne	0.77	1.291	1	0.77	0.994
Grand Anse	0.799	1.136	1	0.799	0.904
La Digue	0.812	1.143	1	0.812	0.928
Silhouette	1	2.494	1	1	2.494
Mean	**0.843**	**1.215**	**1**	**0.843**	**1.024**

Note: All Malmquist index averages are geometric means

-15-

Productivity Changes in Benin Zone Hospitals:

A nonparametric Malmquist approach[*]

Joses M. Kirigia, Luis G. Sambo, Omar Mensah,
Chris Mwikisa Eyob Asbu, Patrick Makoudode and Athanase Hounnankan

ABSTRACT

Background: To date no study in Benin has attempted to determine whether hospitals in the country are technically efficient and whether there has been productivity growth in the hospital sector as a result of the various health sector reforms undertaken in the recent past. The objectives of this study were to measure the technical and scale efficiency of hospitals in Benin and to assess the changes in productivity over five years (2003-2007) with a view to analysing the source of change.

Methods: DEAP software was used to analyse the technical efficiency and productivity growth among a sample of 23 zonal hospitals in the Republic of Benin over a period of five years from 2003 to 2007.

Results: The yearly analysis revealed that 20 (87 per cent), 20 (87 per cent), 14 (61 per cent), 12 (52 per cent), and 8 (35 per cent) of the hospitals were run inefficiently in 2003, 2004, 2005, 2006, and 2007 respectively and they needed to either increase their outputs (or reduce their inputs) in order to become efficient. The average variable returns to scale technical efficiency scores were 63 per cent, 64 per cent, 78 per cent, 78 per cent, and 86 per cent respectively during the years under consideration. On average, the productivity of hospitals decreased by 5.3 per cent over the five-year period. The productivity decline was largely attributed to technical regress. Whereas the relative efficiency of the hospitals being assessed

[*] The original article appeared in *African Journal of Health Economics* 2011;3:1-13. Reproduced with the permission of West African Health Economics Network (WAHEN).

increased by 25.3 per cent, technical change (innovation) regressed by 24.4 per cent per annum.

Conclusion: There is some scope for providing outpatient curative and preventive care and inpatient care to extra patients without additional investment into the above-mentioned health services. This would entail leveraging of health promotion approaches and lowering of financial barriers to access to boost the consumption of underutilised health services, especially health promotion and disease prevention services.

INTRODUCTION

The Republic of Benin has a surface area of 112,622 km^2 and is situated on the west coast of Africa. It has a population of 8,439,000 people; 46% of whom live in urban areas [1]. The human development index for Benin is 0.459, which gives the country a rank of 161 out of 179 countries with data (UNDP 2008). The human poverty index value of 44.5% for Benin ranks 125 among 135 developing countries for which the index has been calculated [2]. The average life expectancy is 57 years. As shown in Appendix 15.1, the health indicators for Benin are higher than the WHO African Region averages [3].

The per capita total expenditure on health at average exchange rate was US$26 in Benin [4], which was two times lower than that of the region and US$8 lower than the US$34 per capita recommended by the WHO Commission for Macroeconomics and Health [5]. Approximately 50.2 per cent of total expenditure on health came from government sources. Private spending on health constituted 49.8 per cent of the total health expenditure with about 94.9 per cent of it coming from household out-of-pocket expenditures. Such high out-of-pocket expenditures constitute a barrier to efficient health service utilisation.

The country has a total health workforce of 10,275 (1.485 density per 1,000). The workforce consists of 311 physicians (0.045 density per 1,000); 5,789 nurses (0.84 density per 1,000); 12 dentists (0.002 density per 1,000); 11 pharmacists (0.002 density per 1,000); 178 public and environmental health workers (0.03 density per 1000); 88 community health workers (0.01 density per 1,000); 477 laboratory technicians (0.07 density per 1,000); 128 other health workers (0.02 density per 1,000); and 3,281 health management and support workers (0.47 density per 1,000) [6]. The overall health workforce density of Benin is lower than the regional average health workforce density of 2.626 per 1,000. Benin is one of the 57 countries in the world experiencing a health workforce crisis. This implies that there is great need in Benin to utilise efficiently the available health workforce.

The Benin health system consists of three levels. Firstly, there is the central level organised around the Ministry of Health headquarters whose mandate is to develop policies and norms and standards, mobilise resources, and oversee the overall management of the system. Secondly, the intermediate level includes six regional directorates of public health whose mission is to translate national health policy into action and provide supervisory support to the peripheral level. Finally, the peripheral level is organised in 34 operational public health zones. Each zone covers a population of 100,000 to 200,000 inhabitants. Each zone has a hospital, health centres, and village health posts/units. There are approximately 491 public health centres; 34 zone public hospitals; 5 department/provincial hospitals; 5 specialised public hospitals; 34 religious mission clinics; and 1,409 private-for-profit clinics [7].

Given the scarcity of health systems inputs, there is dire need to ensure that all resources are optimally used in providing health services to the greatest number of people possible. Unfortunately, to date no study in Benin has addressed the following questions:

1. Are hospitals producing maximum outputs with the available inputs?

2. Are hospitals operating at an optimal scale? Or are (dis)economies of scale rampant (i.e., inefficiency due to largeness or smallness of hospital size)?

3. What is the trend of productivity over the years? What percentage of the observed productivity changes are due to technical efficiency change and technological change?

This study was meant to contribute to bridging that knowledge gap. Its specific objectives were to measure the technical and scale efficiency of hospitals in Benin; to assess the changes in productivity over five years (2003-2007) with a view to analysing changes in efficiency and changes in technology; and to discuss possible implications for policy.

METHOD AND DATA

Concept and Measurement of Technical Efficiency and Productivity of Hospitals

The overall goals/outcomes of any health system are to "improve health and health equity in ways that are responsive (to clients' non-medical expectations), financially fair, and make the best, or most efficient, use of available   resources" [8, p.2]. The route to achieving health outcomes is through realising greater access and coverage for effective health services or interventions. The extent to which a health system realises its goals depends on the effectiveness (quality and safety) with which it performs the functions of leadership and governance; service delivery; health workforce development; medicines, vaccines and technologies; health information; and health financing [9,10]. A health system decision-making unit (e.g., hospital, health centre, health post) utilises scarce inputs (e.g., health workforce, medicines, vaccines, non-pharmaceutical supplies, equipment, infrastructure and information) to deliver health services to the catchment population. Given their scarcity, it is a moral, economic, and public health imperative that all health systems inputs should be put to optimal use to deliver effective health services to as many people as is technically feasible. In a nutshell, this means that all inputs should be put into economically efficient use.

Economic efficiency is a product of technical efficiency and allocative efficiency. Due to dearth of data on health system input prices, the study reported in this paper was limited to measurement of hospital technical efficiency comprising of both pure technical and scale efficiency components. A hospital can manifest either constant returns to scale (CRS), increasing returns to scale (IRS), or decreasing returns to scale (DRS). Returns to scale inform health decision-makers what happens if, for example, they increase all hospital inputs by the same proportion. This could result in three scenarios: (*a*) CRS -doubling of all inputs results in doubling of outputs; (*b*) IRS - doubling of all inputs may lead to more than a doubling of output; and (*c*) doubling of all inputs leads to less than doubling of output. The implications for policy depend on which scenario prevails.

Figure 15.1 shows a production function where a hospital employs medical doctor hours to provide inpatient health services. It portrays two production frontiers. The first production frontier, which is a straight line 0GCH, assumes CRS. The second frontier, depicted by a concave line ABCD, assumes VRS. For example, if a hospital is producing at point *'E'* using 0F medical doctor hours to attend to $0Y_1$ number of admissions, it is technically inefficient assuming either CRS or VRS. Under CRS technology, hospital E could have cared for a larger number of admissions $(0Y_3)$ with the same number of medical doctor hours (0F). If there are CRS, technical efficiency $\left(TE_{CRS}\right)$ of hospital E is given by the ratio $TE_{CRS} = {}^{FE}\!/\!_{FH}$. Similarly, under VRS technology, hospital E could have attended to $0Y_2$ admissions employing the same number of medical doctor-hours, 0F. Pure technical efficiency $\left(TE_{VRS}\right)$ assuming VRS is measured as $TE_{VRS} = {}^{FE}\!/\!_{FD}$.

A technically efficient hospital has a technical efficiency score of one (or 100%), whereas the inefficient ones have a score less than one (or less than 100%). For example, supposing that the pure technical efficiency of hospital E was 75%. This implies that the hospital could have attended to 25% more admissions than it is currently attending to with the same number of doctor hours. Alternatively, hospital E could reduce medical doctor hours by 25% and still attend to its current number of admissions.

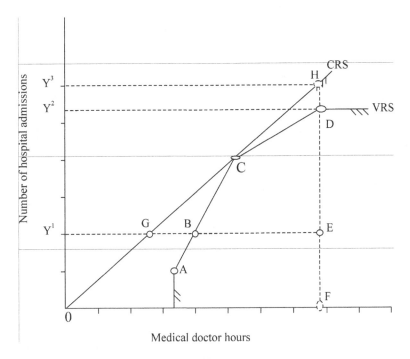

Figure 15.1 Hospital technical efficiency

In Figure 15.1, scale inefficiency is the difference between EH (technical efficiency under CRS) and ED (technical efficiency under VRS). Practically, scale efficiency (SE) is calculated as the ratio of technical efficiency under CRS and technical efficiency under VRS. Thus, $SE = {}^{FH}\!/_{FD} = {}^{TE_{CRS}}\!/_{TE_{VRS}}$ or $SE = {}^{Y_1 G}\!/_{Y_1 B} = {}^{TE_{CRS}}\!/_{TE_{VRS}}$. Scale efficiency compares the average product of the hospital at point 'E' to average product at the technically optimal point 'C'. This comparison tells us if the hospital has scale inefficiency due to being too small (in the IRS portion of the production function, e.g. E) or too large (in the decreasing returns to scale portion of the production function, e.g., D).

Scale efficient hospitals have a score of one (or 100%), whilst the inefficient ones have a score of less than one (or less than 100%). For example, if the scale efficiency score for hospital E was 85%, it means that about 15% of inefficiency is accounted for by unsuitable hospital size (inefficiently large or small). Since in Figure 15.1 a hospital producing at E is operating in the IRS portion of the production function, it implies that the hospital is too large and there is scope for downsizing by 15% while attending to its current level of admissions.

Data Envelopment Analysis Conceptual Framework

Efficiency analysts usually have a choice of employing either econometric [11] or mathematical programming methods, such as data envelopment analysis (DEA) [12], to estimate technical and scale efficiency. In this study, we chose to use DEA due to its capability of estimating efficiency of hospitals that typically use multiple inputs to produce multiple outputs. Data envelopment analysis method has widely been used in measurement of technical efficiency of hospitals in Asia [13-17], Europe [18-34], and North America [35-37]. However, applications of DEA among hospitals in the WHO African Region are few [38-43]. This is the first study to attempt measurement of hospital efficiency and productivity in the Republic of Benin. Under the assumption of variable returns to scale (VRS), DEA measures the technical efficiency (TE) of hospital z compared with n hospitals in a peer group as follows [11]:

Objective function:

$$\text{Max TE}_z = \sum_{r=1}^{s} u_r y_{rj_z} + u_z \tag{4}$$

Subject to constraints:

$$\sum_{i=1}^{m} v_i x_{ij_z} = 1$$

$$\sum_{r=1}^{s} u_r y_{rj} - \sum_{i=1}^{m} v_i x_{ij} + u_z \leq 0; \qquad j = 1,...,n$$

$$u_r, \geq 0; \qquad r = 1,..., s,$$

$$v_i \geq 0; \qquad i = 1,...,m,$$

Where

$y_{rj}(r = 1,...,s)$ =actual amount of rth output for j^{th} hospital

$x_{ij}(i = 1,...,m)$ = actual amount of ith input for j^{th} hospital

u_r = weight given by DEA to output r

v_i = weight given by DEA to input i

n = number of hospitals in the sample

z = the hospital being assessed in the set of j=1,…,n hospitals

The above DEA model determined weights u_r and v_i from the data and assigned them to each input and output so as to maximise the efficiency rating (TE_z) of the hospital being evaluated. The above model was run 23 times to obtain the efficiency scores for each hospital in the sample. The relative hospital efficiency scores are bounded between 0% (completely inefficient) and 100% (technically efficient). Therefore, any hospital that scores 100% is deemed technically efficient and any hospital with a technical efficiency score of less than 100% is deemed technically inefficient.

Malmquist Productivity Index (MPI)

Productivity is the relationship between the output of a hospital and the health system inputs that have gone into producing that output. Productivity is the ratio of actual health service produced per unit of health input consumed [44]:

$$\text{Productivity} = \frac{\text{Actual hospital output}}{\text{Hospital inputs consumed}}.$$

Productivity measurement is usually in terms of the level and trends over time in the productivity. The productivity ratio refers to the productivity at a specific point in time expressed as health service output units delivered per unit of health system input used. Productivity trend ratios are commonly converted into either output-oriented or input-oriented index measures of change in productivity. The output-oriented indices define the index as a measurement of increased outputs derived from the inputs' net growth. These indices shed light on the question: How much more output has been produced, using a given level of inputs and the present state of technology, relative to what could have been produced under a given reference technology using the same level of inputs? Input-oriented indices measure change in productivity by examining the reduction in input use, which is feasible given the need to produce a given level of output under a reference technology [45].

One can use either Fisher index [46], Tormqvist index [47], or Malmquist index [48] to measure productivity change. However, in the current study we opted to use the input-based Malmquist productivity index because of its positive attributes, namely, (*a*) it requires information only on hospital inputs and outputs quantities and not their prices; (*b*) it does not impose behavioural assumptions (e.g., profit maximisation, cost minimisation, revenue maximisation) in its construction, which would be inappropriate especially for public hospitals whose objective is not to maximise profits but to maximise provision of quality health services; (*c*) it can be calculated using non-parametric techniques, which impose properties of monotonicity and convexity, but do not impose functional structure on the production technology as does econometric methods; (*d*) it accommodates a typical hospital multiple inputs and outputs; and (*e*) it decomposes into constituent sources of productivity change, that is, pure technical efficiency change, technical change, and scale change [49].

In this study, we were confronted with the problem of comparing the input of a hospital at two different points in time $(t, t+1)$ in terms of the maximum factor by which the input in $t+1$ period could be reduced such that the hospital could still produce the health service output levels observed for the other time period t. Suppose hospitals $s = 1, 2, ..., n$ utilise the health system input vector $x \equiv (x_1, ..., x_N)$ to produce the health service output vector $y \equiv (y_1, y_2, ..., y_M)$. The hospital production function can be specified as $y_1 = F^s(\hat{y}, x)$, $s = t, t+1$ [50]. It represents the maximum amount of the first health service output that hospital s can produce using the vector of inputs x given that the vector of "other" outputs $\hat{y}$ must also be produced.

Following the footsteps of Shepard [51], Fare and Grosskopf [52] define the input distance function as $D_i^t(y^t, x^t) = \sup\{\lambda > 0 : (x^t/\lambda) \in L^t(y^t)\}$. In order to define the input based Malmquist productivity index, two mixed period distance functions are required, namely, $D_i^{t+1}(y^t, x^t)$ and $D_i^t(y^{t+1}, x^{t+1})$. Using the period t benchmark technology, Fare and Grosskopf [52] employed the two distance functions to define the input-based Malmquist index $M_{ic}(y^t, x^t, y^{t+1}, x^{t+1})$:

$$M_i^{t+1}(y^{t+1}, x^{t+1}, y^t, x^t) = \left[\frac{D_i^t(y^{t+1}, x^{t+1})}{D_i^t(y^t, x^t)} \times \frac{D_i^{t+1}(y^{t+1}, x^{t+1})}{D_i^{t+1}(y^t, x^t)} \right]^{1/2}.$$

Ray and Desli [53] decomposed the above-mentioned input-based Malmquist productivity index as follows:

$$M_{ic}(y^t, x^t, y^{t+1}, x^{t+1}) = TE\Delta(y^t, x^t, y^{t+1}, x^{t+1}) \times T\Delta(y^t, x^t, y^{t+1}, x^{t+1})$$
$$\times S\Delta(y^t, x^t, y^{t+1}, x^{t+1})$$

Where:

Technical efficiency change $TE\Delta(y^t, x^t, y^{t+1}, x^{t+1}) = \left[\frac{D_i^{t+1}(y^{t+1}, x^{t+1})}{D_i^t(y^t, x^t)} \right],$

Technical change $TA\left(y^t,x^t,y^{t+1},x^{t+1}\right)=\left[\dfrac{D_i^t\left(y^{t+1},x^{t+1}\right)}{D_i^{t+1}\left(y^{t+1},x^{t+1}\right)}\times\dfrac{D_i^t\left(y^t,x^t\right)}{D_i^{t+1}\left(y^t,x^t\right)}\right]^{\frac{1}{2}},$

"scale change factor" $SA\left(y^t,x^t,y^{t+1},x^{t+1}\right)$

$$=\left\{\left[\dfrac{D_{ic}^t\left(y^{t+1},x^{t+1}\right)}{D_i^t\left(y^{t+1},x^{t+1}\right)}\div\dfrac{D_{ic}^t\left(y^t,x^t\right)}{D_i^t\left(y^t,x^t\right)}\right]\times\left[\dfrac{D_{ic}^{t+1}\left(y^{t+1},x^{t+1}\right)}{D_i^{t+1}\left(y^{t+1},x^{t+1}\right)}\div\dfrac{D_{ic}^{t+1}\left(y^t,x^t\right)}{D_i^{t+1}\left(y^t,x^t\right)}\right]\right\}^{\frac{1}{2}}$$

The subscript "c" on an input distance function implies that it is defined relative to a constant returns to scale technology; and subscript "i" refers to input-based Malmquist index. $TEA\left(y^t,x^t,y^{t+1},x^{t+1}\right)$ measures the contribution to productivity change of a change in pure technical efficiency between periods t and $t+1$; $TA\left(y^t,x^t,y^{t+1},x^{t+1}\right)$ measures the contribution to productivity change of technical change (shift in technology) between periods t and $t+1$ along a ray through a particular hospital's period $t+1$ data; and $SA\left(y^t,x^t,y^{t+1},x^{t+1}\right)$ is the change in scale efficiency and scale technology between times t and $t+1$. The latter provides a measure of the contribution of scale economies to hospital productivity change.

According to Grifell-Tatje and Lovell [49], $M_{ic}\left(y^t,x^t,y^{t+1},x^{t+1}\right)$ attains a value greater than, equal to, or less than one depending on whether the hospital in question experienced productivity growth, stagnation, or productivity decline between periods t and $t+1$ from the perspective of period t technology. $TEA\left(y^t,x^t,y^{t+1},x^{t+1}\right)$ is greater than, equal to, or less than unity depending on whether the relative efficiency of the hospital being assessed increased, remained the same, or decreased between periods t and $t+1$. $TA\left(y^t,x^t,y^{t+1},x^{t+1}\right)$ attains a value greater than, equal to, or less than one depending on whether the hospital being appraised had technical progress, stagnation, or technical regress. $SA\left(y^t,x^t,y^{t+1},x^{t+1}\right)$ attains a value greater than, equal to, or less than one depending on whether a change in a specific hospital's scale of production contributes positively, not at all, or negatively to productivity change.

Data

The sample consisted of 30 hospitals. However, complete inputs and outputs data were available for only 23 of those hospitals; that is, 68% of the 34 total number of zone hospitals in Benin. Thus, the final analysis was based on the latter group of hospitals. One of the researchers visited all the hospitals in the sample. At each of the hospitals he met with the medical officer in charge, explained the purpose of the study, and was given access to the relevant inputs and outputs records. He complemented the hard data from the hospital records with interactive interviews with the people in charge of different hospital departments. The inputs and outputs data were collected for 2003, 2004, 2005, 2006, and 2007.

The DEA was estimated with five inputs: total number of doctor/physician hours; total number of nurse and midwives hours; total number of hours of laboratory, X-ray, anaesthetists, paramedics, and assistants; non-salary running costs; and number of beds (a proxy of capital inputs). There were two outputs; outpatients visits and number of hospital admissions. The study reported in this paper used the DEA software developed by Coelli 54] to measure the yearly technical efficiency, yearly scale efficiency, and distance functions that compose the Malmquist index and its components.

RESULTS

Technical and Scale Efficiency

Appendix 15.2 presents the median, mean, and standard deviations for the outputs and inputs of hospitals in Benin. Appendix 15.3 summariss the frequency distributions of technical and scale efficiency scores for hospitals in year 2003, 2004, 2005, 2006 and 2007. In 2003, 2004, 2005, 2006, and 2007, out of the 23 hospitals, approximately three (13 per cent), three (13 per cent), nine (39 per cent), eleven (48 per cent), and fifteen (65 per cent) hospitals respectively had a variable returns to scale technical efficiency score of 100 per cent. Hospitals with values of 100 per cent are deemed technically efficient in the associated year.

The individual hospital's technical and scale efficiency scores during the five years are presented in Appendix 15.4. The yearly analysis has revealed that 20 (87 per cent), 20 (87 per cent), 14 (61 per cent), 12 (52 per cent), and 8 (35 per cent) of the hospitals were run inefficiently in 2003, 2004, 2005, 2006, and 2007 respectively and they needed to either increase their outputs (or reduce their inputs) in order to become efficient. The average VRS technical efficiency scores were 63 per cent, 64 per cent, 78 per cent, 78 per cent, and 86 per cent respectively during the years under consideration. This finding implies that if the hospitals were operating efficiently they could have produced 37 per cent, 36 per cent, 22 per cent, 22 per cent, and 14 per cent more output (number of outpatient visits and admissions) using their current levels of input endowment. Alternatively, the hospitals could produce their current levels of health service output with 37 per cent, 36 per cent, 22 per cent, 22 per cent, and 14 per cent less of their existing health system input endowment.

In 2003, 2004, 2005, 2006, and 2007, out of the 23 hospitals, four (17 per cent), two (9 per cent), two (9 per cent), three (13 per cent), and eight (35 per cent) hospitals respectively displayed constant returns to scale (CRS). These hospitals were operating at their most productive scale sizes. Eighteen (78 per cent), twenty (87 per cent), sixteen (70 per cent), eighteen (78 per cent), and thirteen (57 per cent) hospitals had increasing returns to scale (IRS) during the five years respectively. If a hospital displays IRS, it should expand its scale of operation in order to become scale efficient (Chattopadhy and Ray, 1996; Varian, 2003). Three (13 per cent), one (4 per cent), five (22 per cent), two (9 per cent), and four (17 per cent) hospitals manifested decreasing returns to scale (DRS). In order to operate at the most productive scale size, a hospital exhibiting DRS should scale down its operation. The average scale efficiency score in the sample was 51 per cent in 2003, 46 per cent in 2004, 52 per cent in 2005, 59 per cent in 2006, and 77 per cent in 2007 implying that there was room for increasing total outputs by about 49 per cent in 2003, 54 per cent in 2004, 48 per cent in 2005, 41 per cent in 2006, and 23 per cent in 2007. This can be accomplished through appropriate adjustment at the size of the scale-inefficient hospitals where feasible. However, due to indivisibility of physical facilities this may not be possible.

Scope for Output Increases and Implications for Policy

The inefficient hospitals in Benin could operate as efficiently as their peers on the efficiency frontier either by increasing their outputs or reducing utilisation of their inputs. Appendix 15.5 presents the output increases and/or input reductions needed to make individual inefficient hospitals efficient. The total output increases and/or input reductions needed to make inefficient hospitals efficient are reported in Appendix 15.6. In 2007, for example, the inefficient hospitals combined would need to increase the outpatients visits by 260,066 (70 per cent) and the number of admissions by 13,786 (12.4 per cent) in order to become efficient.

Concerning hospitals with outputs falling short of the DEA targets, MoH policy makers could improve their efficiency by creating demand for the underutilised outreach health promotion and outpatient services, for example, family planning services, antenatal and postnatal care, hospital deliveries, child growth monitoring, immunisation, HIV/AIDS education, insecticide-treated bed nets, antimalaria treatment for fever, potable drinking water, and clean sanitation (see Appendix 15.1). Demand for underutilised preventive and curative services can be boosted through use of health promotion methods, for example, health education; behaviour change communication; social marketing; information, education, and communication (IEC); social mobilisation; advocacy; and lobbying [55]; and through implementation of either tax-funded health services or national social health insurance [56,57,58] which dramatically lower financial barriers to health services access when needed.

Alternatively, if it is very difficult to reduce inefficiencies by inducing demand for services, policy makers could improve efficiency through transfer of human resources for health and of beds to primary health level health facilities experiencing shortages. Savings of non-salary running costs could be invested in strengthening of primary level health facilities and community health outreach activities. Those health service levels are critically important in the quest to achieve the health-related United Nations Millennium Development Goals [59].

Productivity Growth

In the application of the Malmquist productivity index to analyse the differences in productivity over time, the year 2003 has been taken as the technology reference. We should remember that the Malmquist productivity index or any of its components attains a value greater than, equal to, or less than one depending on whether a hospital in question experienced productivity growth, stagnation, or productivity decline between periods t and $t+1$. Appendix 15.7 portrays the Malmquist productivity index summary of annual geometric means. In the last row (last column), we see that, on average, the productivity of hospitals decreased by 5.3 per cent over the five-year period. That productivity decline was largely attributed to technical regress. Whereas the relative efficiency of hospitals being assessed increased by 25.3 per cent, technical change (innovation) regressed by 24.4 per cent per annum.

It is prudent now to examine the magnitude and sources of productivity change within each hospital. Appendix 15.8 provides a summary of the average annual values of the Malmquist productivity index and its components for individual hospitals. Ten (43.5 per cent) out of 23 hospitals experienced productivity growth given that they had Malmquist productivity indicess greater than one. HZ Bembereke, HZ Kandi, HZ ST Jean de Dieu Tanguiéta, CHD Natitingou, HZ Abomey Calavi, CHD Borgou, HZ St Jean de Boko, HZ Sourou Sero, HZ ST Martin De Papane, and HZ Sakete hospitals experienced total factor productivity growth of 0.5%, 3.7%, 0.7%, 0.9%, 1.1%, 3.8%, 1.1%, 3.8%, 4.3%, and 1.1% respectively. In all ten hospitals productivity growth was entirely due to improvement in relative technical efficiency.

In contrast, the Malmquist productivity indices for 13 (56.5 per cent) hospitals were less than one, signifying productivity decline over time. More specifically, the 13 hospitals registered total factor productivity decline ranging from 1.5% in HZ Banikora hospital to 26.3% in HZ Bassila. In all the thirteen hospitals, productivity decline was totally due to technical regress, that is, lack of innovation. None of the hospitals had Malmquist productivity index of exactly one, which would have signified stagnation. The average total factor productivity (TFP) score for the entire sample was 0.951 (STDEV=0.085), which signifies that on average hospitals experienced productivity decline between periods t and $t+1$ of 4.9 per cent.

Efficiency Change and Pure Efficiency Change

The first component, efficiency change (EFFCH), of the MPI measures the contribution to productivity change of a change in technical efficiency between periods t and $t+1$. Efficiency change is a product of pure efficiency change (PECH) and scale efficiency change (SECH) [49]. HZ Dassa-Zou and HZ Bassila hospitals had EFFCH score of one, which means that their relative efficiency remained the same. All the remaining 21 hospitals registered EFFCH scores ranging from a minimum of 1.045 (4.5% increase in HZ Save Hospital) to a maximum of 1.438 (43.8% increase in HZ Sakete Hospital) between periods t and $t+1$. The increase in EFFCH was as follows: 0% in two hospitals; between 1% and 9% in two hospitals between 20% in three hospitals; 21% to 30% in six hospitals; 31% to 40% in six hospitals; and over 40% in 4 hospitals. The average EFFCH score for the entire sample was 1.260 (STDEV=0.134) signifying that EFFCH contributed positively to total factor productivity change by 26%.

Pure Efficiency Change

The reader will recall that pure efficiency change (PECH) measures the contribution to productivity change of a change in pure technical efficiency between periods t and $t+1$. As portrayed in Appendix 15.8, the average pure efficiency change (PECH) was less than one in three hospitals implying that the relative efficiency of those hospitals decreased (by 0.4%) between period t and $t+1$. The PECH score was equal to one in three hospitals, which means that their relative technical efficiency remained the same between time period t and $t+1$. In the remaining 17 hospitals, The PECH score ranged from a minimum of 1.027 (i.e., increase of 2.7% in HZ Save hospital) to a maximum of 1.433 (i.e., increase of 43.3% in both HZ Come and HZ Pobe hospitals). The contribution of PECH to total factor productivity change among the 17 hospitals was distributed as follows: 1 to 10% in 12 hospitals; 11 to 20% in one hospital; 21 to 30% in one hospital; and over 30% in three hospitals. The average PECH score was 1.099 (STDEV=0.134), which means that pure PECH contributed a 9.9% change in the total factor productivity change.

Scale Efficiency Change

Scale efficiency change (SECH) is a measure of the contribution of scale economies to productivity change between times t and $t+1$. The reader will remember that SECH attains a value greater than, equal to, or less than one depending on whether a change in a specific hospital's scale of production contributes positively, not at all, or negatively to productivity change [49]. Three hospitals (HZ Come, HZ Pobe, and HZ ST Martin De Papane) had a SECH index value of less than one signifying that the three hospitals' production scale contributed negatively to total factor productivity change. The HZ Dassa-Zou and HZ Bassila hospitals had a SECH value equal to one, which means that their scale of production did not contribute to total factor productivity change. The remaining 18 (78.3 per cent) hospitals had a SECH index greater than one implying that those hospitals' scale of production contributed positively to productivity change. The percentage contribution to productivity change of those 18 hospitals was distributed as follows: 1 to 10% in five hospitals; 11 to 20% in three hospitals; 21 to 30% in six hospitals; and above 30% in four hospitals. The average SECH score for the whole sample of hospitals was 1.158, implying that the scale of production on average contributed positively to productivity change by 15.8 per cent.

Technical Change

The technical change (TECHCH) component of MPI measures the contribution to productivity change of technical change (shift in technology) between periods t and $t+1$ along a ray through a particular hospital's period $t+1$ data. Let us keep in mind that TECHCH attains a value greater than, equal to, or less than one depending on whether the hospital being appraised had technical progress, stagnation, or technical regress. All the 23 hospitals had a TECHCH score of less than one signifying that all hospitals experienced technical regress. There was wide variation in the magnitude of technical regress: 16 to 20% in five hospitals; 21 to 25% in nine hospitals; 26 to 30% in eight hospitals; and over 30% in one hospital (HZ Alplahoue). The average technical change score was 0.757 (STDEV=0.047) indicating a 24.3 per cent technical regress between periods t and $t+1$.

Limitations of the study

First, DEA does not capture random noise (e.g., epidemics, natural, and man-made disasters), and thus, it inadvertently attributes any deviation from the frontier to inefficiency [42,59,60]. Thus, by using DEA we may have overestimated the existing magnitudes of inefficiencies. Second, it would be argued that the ultimate output of hospitals is the aggregate change in health status of the patients who received hospital outpatient and inpatient services. However, due to paucity of data on health status indices such as quality-adjusted life years [61] or health disability indicators such as disability-adjusted life years [62], this study used intermediate outputs, that is, number of outpatient visits and number of hospital admissions. Finally, unavailability of health system inputs prices hampered estimation of allocative efficiency and hence calculation of total economic efficiency of hospitals. Thus, the technical efficiency estimates reported in this paper should be viewed as an underestimation of the actual levels of waste prevailing in hospitals of Benin.

CONCLUSIONS

This study has quantified both the technical and scale efficiency of 23 hospitals in Benin; identified the input reductions and/or output increases needed to make inefficient hospitals efficient; and magnitudes and sources of total factor productivity in each hospital. The analysis revealed that 20 (87%), 20 (87%), 14 (61%), 12 (52%), and 8 (35%) of the hospitals were run inefficiently in 2003, 2004, 2005, 2006, and 2007 respectively. In 2007, all the hospitals manifesting variable returns to scale technical inefficiency would need to increase the number of outpatient visits by 260,066 and inpatient admissions by 13,786 so as to become technically efficient. Therefore, there is some scope for providing outpatient curative and preventive care and inpatient care to extra patients without additional investment into the abovementioned health services. This would entail leveraging of health promotion approaches and lowering of financial barriers to access to boost the consumption of underutilised health services, especially health promotion and disease prevention services.

Alternatively, depending on the decision of policy makers, the hospital inefficiencies could be ameliorated by transferring 55,823 doctors/physician hours; 15,781 hours of other staff (nurses, midwives, laboratory technicians, radiologists, anaesthetist, paramedical assistants); and US$1,584,069 of non-salary running funds to peripheral health facilities and community health programmes. Overall, the mean Malmquist total factor productivity index declined by 4.9 per cent between 2003 and 2007. The decline was fully explained by technical regress of 24.3 per cent. The decline in Malmquist index would have been higher were it not for the 26 per cent increase in average technical efficiency. In their health financing strategy for the African Region [63], the Fifty-Sixth WHO Regional Committee for Africa recommended that member countries should institutionalise efficiency monitoring within national health management information systems (NHIS). Therefore, NHIS capacities ought to be enhanced to routinely capture the input, input prices, and output data which could be used to monitor economic efficiency and productivity change among hospitals and lower level facilities.

REFERENCES

1. World Health Organization Regional Office for Africa. *Benin country health system fact sheet 2006*. Brazzaville: World Health Organization; 2006.

2. United Nations Development Programme. *Human development report 2009*. New York: UN; 2009.

3. World Health Organization. *World health statistics 2009*. Geneva: World Health Organization; 2009.

4. World Health Organization. *National health accounts*. Geneva: World Health Organization; 2009.

5. World Health Organization. Macroeconomics and Health: investing in health for economic development. Report of the Commission on Macroeconomics and Health. Geneva: World Health Organization; 2001.

6. World Health Organization. *World health report 2006*. Geneva: World Health Organization; 2006.

7. Republic of Benin. *Health profile of Benin*. Cotonou: Government Printer; 2009.

8. World Health Organization. *Strengthening health systems to improve health outcomes: WHO's framework for action*. Geneva: World Health Organization; 2007.

9. Murray CJL, Frenk J. A framework for assessing the performance of health systems. *Bulletin of the World Health Organization* 2000; 78 (6):717-731.

10. World Health Organization: *World health report 2000 – health systems: improving performance*. Geneva: World Health Organization; 2000.

11. Aigner DF, Lovell CAK, Schmidt P. Formulation and estimation of stochastic production function models. *Journal of Econometrics* 1977; 6: 21-37.

12. Charnes A, Cooper WW, Rhodes E. Measuring the efficiency of decision-making units. *European Journal of Operational Research* 1978;2(6):429-444.

13. Chang H, Cheng M-A, Das S. Hospital ownership and operating efficiency: evidence from Taiwan. *European Journal of Operational Research* 2004;159(2):513-527.

14. Chang H. Determinants of hospital efficiency: the case of central government-owned hospitals in Taiwan. *Omega* 1998;26(2): 307-317.

15. Chen A, Hwang Y, Shao B. Measurement and sources of overall and input inefficiencies: evidence and implications in hospital services. *European Journal of Operational Research* 2005;161(2): 447-468.

16. Hu J-L, Huang Y-F. Technical efficiencies in large hospitals: a managerial perspective. *International Journal of Management* 2004;21(4):506-513.

17. Watchorariroj B, Tang J. The effects of size and information technology on hospital efficiency. *Journal of High Technology Management Research* 2004;15(1):1-16.

18. Barbetta GP, Turati G, Zago AM. Behavioural differences between public and public not-for-profit hospitals in the Italian National Health Service. *Health Economics* 2007;16(1):75-96.

19. Biorn E, Hagen TP, Iversen T, Magnussen J. The effect of activity-based financing on hospital efficiency: a panel data analysis of DEA efficiency scores 1992-2000. *Health Care Management Science* 2003;6(4):271-283.

20. Fare R, Grosskopf S, Lindgren B, Bjorn RP. Productivity changes in Swedish pharmacies 1980-1989: a non-parametric Malmquist approach. *Journal of Productivity Analysis* 1992;3(1-2): 85-101.

21. Gannon B. Testing for variation in technical efficiency of hospitals in Ireland. *The Economic and Social Review* 2005;36(3):273-294.

22. Gannon B. Total factor productivity growth of hospitals in Ireland: a nonparametric approach. *Applied Economics Letters* 2008;15(2):131-135.

23. Giokas DI. Greek hospitals: how well their resources are used. *Omega* 2001;29(1):73-83.

24. Hofmarcher MM, Paterson I, Riedel M. Measuring hospital efficiency in Austria – a DEA approach. *Health Care Management Science* 2002;5(1):7-14.

25. Kontodimopoulos N, Bellali T, Labiris G, Niakas D. Investigating sources of inefficiency in residential mental health facilities. *Journal of Medical Systems* 2006;30(3):169-176.

26. Linna M. Health care financing reform and the productivity change in Finnish hospitals. *Journal of Health Care Finance* 2000;23(3):83-100.

27. Lyroudi K, Glaveli N, Koulakiotis A, Angelidis N. The productive performance of public hospital clinics in Greece: a case study. *Health Services Management Research* 2006;19(2):67-72.

28. Maniadakis N, Thanassoulis E. Assessing productivity changes in UK hospitals reflecting technology and input prices. *Applied Economics* 32(12):1575-1589.

29. Martinussen PE, Midttun L. Day surgery and hospital efficiency: empirical analysis of the Norwegian hospitals 1999-2001. *Health Policy* 2004;68(2):183-196.

30. McCallion G, Glass JC, Jackson RB, Kerr Christine A, McKillop DG. Investigating productivity change and hospital size: a nonparametric frontier approach. *Applied Economics* 2000;32(2):161-174.

31. Pilyavsky A, Staat M. Health care in the CIS countries: the case of hospitals in Ukraine. *European Journal of Health Economics* 2006;7(3):189-195.

32. Staat M. Efficiency of hospitals in Germany: a DEA-bootstrap approach. *Applied Economics* 2006;38(29-30):2255-2263.

33. Steinmann L, Zweifel P. On the (in)efficiency of Swiss hospitals. *Applied Economics* 35(3):361-370.

34. Steinmann L, Dittrich G, Karman A, Zweifel P. Measuring and comparing the (in)efficiency of German and Swiss hospitals. *European Journal of Health Economics* 2004;5(3):216-226.

35. Brown H, Shelton III, Pagan JA. Managed care and the scale efficiency of US hospitals. *International Journal of Health Care Finance and Economics* 2006;6(4):278-289.

36. Ferrier GD, Rosko MD, Valdmanis VG. Analysis of uncompensated hospital care using a DEA model of output congestion. *Health Care Management Science* 2006;9(2):181-188.

37. Harrison JP, Coppola MN, Wakefield M. Efficiency of federal hospitals in the United States. *Journal of Medical Systems* 2004;28(5):411-422.

38. Kirigia JM, Lambo E, Sambo LG. Are public hospitals in Kwazulu-Natal Province of South Africa technically efficient? *African Journal of Health Sciences* 2000;7(3-4): 25-32.

39. Kirigia JM, Emrouznejad A, Sambo LG. Measurement of technical efficiency of public hospitals in Kenya: using data envelopment analysis. *Journal of Medical Systems* 2002;26(1):39-45.

40. Osei D, George M, d'Almeida S, Kirigia JM, Mensah AO, Kainyu LH. Technical efficiency of public district hospitals and health centres in Ghana: a pilot study. *Cost Effectiveness and Resource Allocation* 2005, 3:9. Available at: http://www.resource-allocation.com/content/3/1/9

41. Kirigia JM, Emrouznejad A, Cassoma B, Asbu EZ, Barry S. A performance assessment method for hospitals: the case of municipal hospitals in Angola. *Journal of Medical Systems* 2008;32(6):509-519.

42. Zere E, McIntyre D, Addison T. Technical efficiency and productivity of public sector hospitals in three South African provinces. *South Africa Journal of Economics* 2001;69(2):336-358.

43. Zere E, Mbeeli T, Shangula K, Mandlhate C, Mutirua K, Tjivambi B, Kapenambili W. Tehnical efficiency of district hospitals: evidence from Namibia using data envelopment analysis. *Cost Effectiveness and Resource Allocation* 2006;4:5.

44. Soniat EJ, Raaum RB. *Government productivity measurement as an analytical tool. Handbook for productivity measurement and improvement.* Oregon: Productivity Press; 1993.

45. Kirikal L. Productivity, the Malmquist Index and the empirical study of banks in Estonia. Tallin: TUT Press; 2005.

46. Fisher I. *The making of index numbers.* Boston: Houghton-Mifflin; 1922.

47. Tormqvist. The bank of Finland's consumption price index. *Bank of Finland Monthly Bulletin* 1936;10:1-8.

48. Malmquist S. Index numbers and indifference surfaces. *Trabajos de Estadistica* 1953;4:209-232.

49. Grifell-Tatje E, Lovell CAK. The sources of productivity change in Spanish banking. *European Journal of Operational Research* 1997;98(2):364-380.

50. Caves DW, Christensen LR, Diewert WE. The economic theory of index numbers and measurement of input, output and productivity. *Econometrica* 1982;50:1393-1414.

51. Shepard RW. *Theory of cost and production functions*. Princeton: Princeton University Press; 1970.

52. Fare R, Grosskopf S. Malmquist productivity indexes and Fisher ideal indexes. *The Economic Journal* 1992;102:158-160.

53. Ray SC, Desli E. Productivity growth, technical progress, and efficiency change in industrialized countries: comment. *American Economic Review* 1997; 87(5):1033-1039.

54. Coelli T. *A guide to DEAP, version 2.1: a data envelopment analysis [computer] program*, Centre for Efficiency and Productivity Analysis (CEPA) Working Paper 96/08. Department of Econometrics, University of New England; Armidale, NSW Australia;1996.

55. Nyamwaya D. Health promotion: a tool for fostering comprehensive health development agendas in the African Region. *African Health Monitor* 2008;6(1):26-29.

56. Carrin G, James C. Social health insurance: key factors affecting the transition towards universal coverage. *International Social Security Review* 2005;58(1):45-64.

57. Carrin G, James C, Adelhardt M, Doetinchem O, Eriki P, Hassan M, Hombergh H, Kirigia J, Koemm K, Korte R, Krech R, Lankers C, Lente J, Maina T, Malonza K, Mathauer I, Mboya TO, Muchiri S, Mumani Z, Nganda B, Nyikal J, Onsongo J, Rakuom C, Schramm B, Scheil-Adlung X, Stierle F, Whitaker D, Zipperer M. Health financing reform in Kenya – assessing the social health insurance proposal. *South African Medical Journal* 2007;97(2):130-135.

58. Carrin G, Doetinchem O, Kirigia J, Mathauer I, Musango L. Social health insurance: how feasible is its expansion in the African Region? *DevIssues* 2008;10(2):7-9.

59. Emrouznejad A, Podinovski. *Data envelopment analysis and performance management*. Aston: Aston University; 2004.

60. Emrouznejad A, Parker BR, Tavare G. Evaluation of research in efficiency and productivity: a survey and analysis of the first 30 years of scholarly literature in DEA. *Socio-Economic Planning Sciences* 2008;42(3):151-157.

61. Kirigia JM. (ed.). *Economic evaluation of public health problems in sub-Saharan Africa*. Nairobi: University of Nairobi Press; 2009.

62. Murray CJ. Quantifying the burden of disease: the technical basis for disability-adjusted life years. *Bulletin of the World Health Organization* 1994;72:429-445.

63. World Health Organization Regional Office for Africa: *Health financing: a strategy for the African Region.* Brazzaville: World Health Organization; 2006.

Appendix 15.1   *Comparison of health indicators and health services coverage of Benin with averages for the WHO African Region*

Variable	Benin	WHO African Region average
Total expenditure on health as % of gross domestic product	4.7	5.5
General government expenditure on health as a % of total expenditure on health	50.2	47.1
Private expenditure on health as a % of total expenditure on health	49.8	52.9
General government expenditure on health as a % of total government expenditure	10.657	8.7
External resources for health as a % of total expenditure on health	21	10.7
Out-of-pocket expenditure as a % of private expenditure on health	94.9	49.8
Private prepaid plans as a % of private expenditure on health	5.1	39.6
Per capita total expenditure on health at average exchange rate (US$)	26	58
Per capita total expenditure on health (PPP int.$)	61	111
Per capita government expenditure on health at average exchange rate (US$)	13	27
Per capita government expenditure on health (PPP int.$)	31	52
Health indicators		
Life expectancy (2007)	57	52
Healthy life expectancy (HALE) at birth in years (2007)	50	45
Neonatal mortality rate (per 1,000 live births)	36	40
Infant mortality rate (probability of dying between birth and age 1 per 1,000 live births) 2007	78	88
Under-5 mortality rate (probability of dying by age 5 per 1,000 live births)	123	145
Adult mortality rate (probability of dying between 15 and 60 years per 1,000 population)	289	401
Maternal mortality ratio (per 100,000 births)	840	900
Malaria mortality rate per 100,000 population	146	104
Prevalence of HIV among adults =>15 years per 100,000 population	1,161	4,735
Adolescent fertility rate (per 1,000 girls aged 15-19)	114	117
Health services coverage		
Measles immunisation coverage among 1-year-olds (%)	61	74
Births attended by skilled health personnel (%)	78	46
Contraceptive prevalence (%)	18.6	24.1
Antenatal care coverage (%); at least 1 visit	84	73
Antenatal care coverage (%); at least 4 visits	61	45
Unmet need for family planning services (%)	27.2	24.4
Proportion of males aged 15-24 years with comprehensive correct knowledge of HIV/AIDS (%)	30	–
Proportion of females aged 15-24 years with comprehensive correct knowledge of HIV/AIDS (%)	16	23
Antiretroviral therapy cover among people with advanced HIV infection (%)	49	30
Children aged <5 years sleeping under insecticide-treated bed nets (%)	20	14
Children aged <5 years who received any antimalarial treatment for fever (%)	54	36
Access to improved drinking water sources (%)	65	59
Access to improved sanitation (%)	30	33

Source: WHO [3]

Appendix 15.2   Descriptive statistics of outputs and inputs of Benin hospitals

Year	OPDvisits	Admissions	Doctors	Other staff[a]	Non-salary running costs	Beds
2003						
Median	12,264	4,263	15,360	122,888	114,983,765	94
Mean	15,144	5,104	24,361	233,143	164,324,479	117
STDEV	12,116	3,779	21,285	314,540	179,151,042	70
2004						
Median	11,267	3,566	13,440	132,480	111,327,784	99
Mean	14,857	4,703	23,259	184,736	158,108,000	131
STDEV	13,687	4,024	18,894	178,493	189,188,762	119
2005						
Median	9,687	3,910	11,520	170,861	89,664,513	110
Mean	14,254	4,720	23,016	209,522	147,156,316	123
STDEV	11,699	3,696	17,143	188,338	157,853,061	70
2006						
Median	10,638	3,977	11,520	192,023	66,063,011	121
Mean	14,329	4,989	22,735	224,444	162,717,778	124
STDEV	10,897	3,457	18,289	203,536	167,019,614	71
2007						
Median	10,123	3,346	13,728	205,855	56,453,980	103
Mean	16,130	4,832	23,138	232,401	139,482,785	122
STDEV	14,935	3,526	18,380	197,547	141,994,607	73

[a]Nurses, midvives, laboratory technicians, radiologists, anaesthetists, and paramedical assistants

Appendix 15.3   Frequency distribution of technical and scale efficiency scores

Efficiency score	2003			2004			2005			2006			2007		
	CRS	VRS	Scale	CRS	VRS	Scale	CRS	VRS	Scale	CRS	VRS	Scale	CRS	VRS	Scale
<10	3	0	0	5	0	0	0	0	0	0	0	0	0	0	0
10-20	5	0	4	4	0	5	6	0	0	4	0	0	0	0	0
21-30	9	3	1	10	2	4	2	0	5	3	0	0	1	0	0
31-40	1	0	5	1	1	2	7	0	5	8	2	8	3	0	0
41-50	1	4	5	0	4	6	2	0	1	1	0	6	2	0	3
51-60	1	3	0	0	3	0	3	8	7	1	7	1	5	6	1
61-70	0	3	2	0	3	0	0	2	1	2	0	1	5	0	7
71-80	1	5	0	1	5	1	0	2	0	1	2	2	1	2	4
81-90	0	2	1	0	2	1	1	1	2	0	0	0	0	0	0
91-99	0	0	1	0	0	2	0	1	0	0	1	2	0	0	0
100	2	3	4	2	3	2	2	9	2	3	11	3	6	15	8
Total	**23**	**23**	**23**	**23**	**23**	**23**	**23**	**23**	**23**	**23**	**23**	**23**	**23**	**23**	**23**

Appendix 15.4   Hospitals' technical and scale efficiency during 2003-2007

Firm	Efficiency 2003				Efficiency 2004			
	CRSTE	VRSTE	Scale	Returns to scale	CRSTE	VRSTE	Scale	Returns to scale
HZ Bembereke	0.232	1	0.232	DRS	0.167	1	0.167	DRS
HZ Kandi	0.131	0.773	0.17	IRS	0.081	0.773	0.105	IRS
HZ Banikoara	0.133	0.421	0.315	IRS	0.09	0.426	0.211	IRS
HZ Kouande	0.339	0.773	0.438	IRS	0.374	0.773	0.485	IRS
HZ ST Jean de Dieu Tanguiéta	0.244	0.773	0.315	IRS	0.162	0.773	0.21	IRS
CHD Natitingou	0.185	0.421	0.438	IRS	0.207	0.426	0.487	IRS
HZ Abomey Calavi	0.092	0.543	0.17	IRS	0.054	0.515	0.105	IRS
HZ Ouidah	0.295	0.797	0.37	IRS	0.162	0.773	0.21	IRS
CHD Borgou	0.185	0.421	0.438	IRS	0.207	0.426	0.487	IRS
HZ St Jean de Boko	0.092	0.543	0.17	IRS	0.054	0.515	0.105	IRS
HZ Sourou Sero	0.185	0.421	0.438	IRS	0.207	0.426	0.487	IRS
HZ ST Martin De Papane	0.271	0.288	0.941	IRS	0.237	0.305	0.777	IRS
HZ Save	0.543	0.898	0.605	IRS	0.291	0.903	0.322	IRS
HZ Dassa-Zounme	1	1	1	CRS	1	1	1	CRS
HZ Klouekanmey	0.713	0.847	0.842	IRS	0.735	0.813	0.904	IRS
HZ Aplahoue	0.277	0.633	0.438	IRS	0.186	0.692	0.269	IRS
HZ Bassila	1	1	1	CRS	1	1	1	CRS
HZ Ordre de Malte Djougou	0.481	0.75	0.641	IRS	0.285	0.762	0.374	IRS
CHD Lokossa	0.209	0.619	0.338	IRS	0.292	0.697	0.419	IRS
HZ Come	0.236	0.237	0.996	DRS	0.243	0.268	0.905	IRS
HZ Adjohoun	0.209	0.619	0.338	IRS	0.292	0.697	0.419	IRS
HZ Pobe	0.236	0.237	0.996	DRS	0.243	0.268	0.905	IRS
HZ Sakete	0.092	0.543	0.17	IRS	0.054	0.515	0.105	IRS
Median	**0.236**	**0.619**	**0.438**		**0.207**	**0.697**	**0.419**	
Mean	**0.321**	**0.633**	**0.513**		**0.288**	**0.641**	**0.455**	
Std	**0.261**	**0.239**	**0.301**		**0.265**	**0.234**	**0.311**	

.../cont.

Appendix 15.4 (cont.)

Firm	Efficiency 2005				Efficiency 2006			
	CRSTE	VRSTE	Scale	Returns to scale	CRSTE	VRSTE	Scale	Returns to scale
HZ Bembereke	0.482	1	0.482	DRS	0.372	1	0.372	DRS
HZ Kandi	0.354	1	0.354	IRS	0.535	1	0.535	IRS
HZ Banikoara	0.153	0.546	0.281	IRS	0.184	0.546	0.338	IRS
HZ Kouande	0.599	1	0.599	IRS	0.774	1	0.774	IRS
HZ ST Jean de Dieu Tanguiéta	0.281	1	0.281	IRS	0.403	1	0.403	IRS
CHD Natitingou	0.325	0.546	0.595	IRS	0.27	0.546	0.495	IRS
HZ Abomey Calavi	0.189	0.538	0.35	IRS	0.204	0.529	0.386	IRS
HZ Ouidah	0.281	1	0.281	IRS	0.403	1	0.403	IRS
CHD Borgou	0.325	0.546	0.595	IRS	0.27	0.546	0.495	IRS
HZ St Jean de Boko	0.189	0.538	0.35	IRS	0.204	0.529	0.386	IRS
HZ Sourou Sero	0.325	0.546	0.595	IRS	0.27	0.546	0.495	IRS
HZ ST Martin De Papane	0.475	0.572	0.83	DRS	0.47	1	0.47	DRS
HZ Save	0.38	1	0.38	IRS	0.384	1	0.384	IRS
HZ Dassa-Zounme	1	1	1	CRS	1	1	1	CRS
HZ Klouekanmey	0.853	1	0.853	DRS	1	1	1	CRS
HZ Aplahoue	0.556	0.809	0.686	IRS	0.684	0.952	0.718	IRS
HZ Bassila	1	1	1	CRS	1	1	1	CRS
HZ Ordre de Malte Djougou	0.515	0.907	0.568	IRS	0.698	1	0.698	IRS
CHD Lokossa	0.181	0.761	0.238	IRS	0.313	0.763	0.41	IRS
HZ Come	0.365	0.672	0.543	DRS	0.309	0.315	0.979	IRS
HZ Adjohoun	0.181	0.761	0.238	IRS	0.313	0.763	0.41	IRS
HZ Pobe	0.365	0.672	0.543	DRS	0.309	0.315	0.979	IRS
HZ Sakete	0.189	0.538	0.35	IRS	0.204	0.529	0.386	IRS
Median	**0.354**	**0.761**	**0.543**		**0.372**	**0.952**	**0.495**	
Mean	**0.416**	**0.781**	**0.522**		**0.46**	**0.777**	**0.588**	
Std	**0.248**	**0.204**	**0.232**		**0.268**	**0.253**	**0.246**	

…/cont.

Appendix 15.4 (cont.)

Firm	Efficiency 2007			
	CRSTE	VRSTE	Scale	Returns to scale
HZ Bembereke	0.638	1	0.638	DRS
HZ Kandi	0.556	1	0.556	IRS
HZ Banikoara	0.256	0.546	0.469	IRS
HZ Kouande	1	1	1	CRS
HZ ST Jean de Dieu Tanguiéta	0.699	1	0.699	IRS
CHD Natitingou	0.469	1	0.469	IRS
HZ Abomey Calavi	0.393	0.534	0.736	IRS
HZ Ouidah	0.469	1	0.469	IRS
CHD Borgou	0.551	0.552	0.997	IRS
HZ St Jean de Boko	0.393	0.534	0.736	IRS
HZ Sourou Sero	0.551	0.552	0.997	IRS
HZ ST Martin De Papane	0.759	1	0.759	DRS
HZ Save	0.648	1	0.648	IRS
HZ Dassa-Zounme	1	1	1	CRS
HZ Klouekanmey	1	1	1	CRS
HZ Aplahoue	1	1	1	CRS
HZ Bassila	1	1	1	CRS
HZ Ordre de Malte Djougou	1	1	1	CRS
CHD Lokossa	0.521	0.742	0.703	IRS
HZ Come	0.696	1	0.696	DRS
HZ Adjohoun	0.521	0.742	0.703	IRS
HZ Pobe	0.696	1	0.696	DRS
HZ Sakete	0.393	0.534	0.736	IRS
Median	**0.638**	**1.000**	**0.736**	
Mean	**0.661**	**0.858**	**0.77**	
Std	**0.237**	**0.205**	**0.191**	

Appendix 15.5 Output (input) increases (reductions) needed to make individual inefficient hospitals efficient

Decision-making unit (hospital)	Output and input shortages/slacks 2003						Output and input shortages 2004					
	Outputs		Inputs				Outputs		Inputs			
	1	2	1	2	3	4	1	2	1	2	3	4
HZ Bembereke	-	-	-	-	-	-	-	-	-	-	-	-
HZ Kandi	39,943	8,076	611	36,975	12,607,959	-	52,247	8,606	611	15,855	15,189,312	-
HZ Banikoara	28,951	7,755	14,989	34,595	304,926,659	-	42,301	7,813	12,096	-	303,163,684	-
HZ Kouande	31,945	5,463	611	36,975	12,607,959	-	45,176	4,956	611	15,855	15,189,312	-
HZ St Jean de Dieu Tanguiéta	28,951	7,755	611	36,975	12,607,959	-	43,248	7,868	611	15,855	15,189,312	-
CHD Natitingou	31,945	5,463	14,989	34,595	313,780,864	-	44,229	4,901	12,096	-	312,017,889	-
HZ Abomey Calavi	39,943	8,076	3,730	27,740	64,251,373	-	52,247	8,606	4,683	12,228	5,618,640	-
HZ Ouidah	25,446	7,781	-	40,425	11,187,716	-	43,248	7,868	611	15,855	15,189,312	-
CHD Borgou	31,945	5,463	14,989	34,595	304,926,659	-	44,229	4,901	12,096	-	303,163,684	-
HZ St Jean de Boko	39,943	8,076	3,730	27,740	64,251,373	-	52,247	8,606	4,683	12,228	5,618,640	-
HZ Sourou sero	31,945	5,463	14,989	34,595	304,926,659	-	44,229	4,901	12,096	-	303,163,684	-
HZ St Martin De Papane	2,510	1,762	849	342,697	515,979,676	-	15,501	2,148	2,717	1,812	494,038,221	-
HZ Save	3,673	7,566	-	707	16,099,453	-	9,274	5,789	1,007	-	-	25
HZ Dassa-Zounme	-	-	-	-	-	-	-	-	-	-	-	-
HZ Klouekanmey		3,840	-	50,606	76,174,571	22		921		39,141	86,026,874	18
HZ Aplahoue	37,274	5,479	-	10,365	8,171,260	-	40,712	6,702	1,013			1
HZ Bassila	-	-	-	-	-	-	-	-	-	-	-	-
HZ Ordre de Malte Djougou	1,164	5,324	-	560	45,863,754	4	1,621	4,447	1,536	-	36,158,183	6
CHD Lokossa	25,694	6,502	2,907	-	25,300,744	-	22,180	4,817	3,561	-	53,137,255	-
HZ Come	29,903	-	800	-	38,642,662	-	24,876	715	2,321	-	21,512,749	-
HZ Adjohoun	25,694	6,502	2,907	-	25,300,744	-	22,180	4,817	3,561	-	53,137,255	-
HZ Pobe	29,903	-	800	-	38,642,662	-	24,876	715	2,321	-	21,512,749	-
HZ Sakete	39,943	8,076	3,730	27,740	64,251,373	-	52,247	8,606	4,683	12,228	5,618,640	-
Total	526,716	114,421	81,239	777,886	2,260,502,078	26	676,868	108,705	82,912	141,055	2,064,645,397	50
Mean	22,901	4,975	3,532	33,821	98,282,699	1	29,429	4,726	3,605	6,133	89,767,191	2
STDEV	15,440	3,089	5,533	69,620	142,534,135	5	19,825	3,127	4,272	9,826	142,719,449	6
Median	28,951	5,463	800	27,740	38,642,662	26	40,712	4,901	2,321	-	15,189,312	-

Appendix 15.6   Output (input) increases (reductions) needed to make inefficient hospitals efficient

	Outpatient visits	Admissions	Doctors hours	Other staff[a] hours	Non-salary running costs (CFA)	Beds
2003						
Total actual values	348,308	117,382	560,294	5,362,296	3,779,463,009	2,687
Shortfall/excess	526,716	114,421	81,239	777,886	2,260,502,078	26
2004						
Total actual values	341,707	108,172	534,966	4,248,939	3,636,483,989	3,010
Shortfall/excess	676,868	108,705	82,912	141,055	2,064,645,397	50
2005						
Total actual values	327,832	108,561	529,374	4,819,017	3,384,595,267	2,836
Shortfall/excess	202,455	25,414	98,908	92,230	1,881,004,350	100
2006						
Total actual values	329,566	114,744	522,908	5,162,219	3,742,508,898	2,846
Shortfall/excess	110,329	15,133	85,616	121,014	1,326,425,061	14
2007						
Total actual values	370,995	111,126	532,164	5,345,215	3,208,104,047	2,806
Shortfall/excess	260,066	13,786	55,823	15,781	792,034,581	–

[a]Nurses, midwives, laboratory technicians, radiologists, anaesthetists, and paramedical assistants

Appendix 15.7   Malmquist index summary of annual means

Year	Efficiency change	Technical change	Pure efficiency change	Scale efficiency change	Total factor productivity change
2	0.83	0.955	1.021	0.813	0.793
3	1.714	0.624	1.266	1.353	1.069
4	1.111	0.909	0.968	1.147	1.011
5	1.558	0.602	1.137	1.370	0.938
Mean	**1.253**	**0.756**	**1.092**	**1.147**	**0.947**

Appendix 15.8 Malmquist index summary of firm geometric means

Firm	Efficiency change	Technical change	Pure efficiency change	Scale efficiency change	Total factor productivity change
HZ Bembereke	1.287	0.780	1	1.287	1.005
HZ Kandi	1.435	0.723	1.067	1.345	1.037
HZ Banikoara	1.178	0.836	1.067	1.104	0.985
HZ Kouande	1.311	0.723	1.067	1.229	0.947
HZ ST Jean de Dieu Tanguiéta	1.302	0.774	1.067	1.22	1.007
CHD Natitingou	1.262	0.799	1.241	1.017	1.009
HZ Abomey Calavi	1.438	0.703	0.996	1.443	1.011
HZ Ouidah	1.123	0.786	1.059	1.061	0.883
CHD Borgou	1.314	0.79	1.07	1.228	1.038
HZ St Jean de Boko	1.438	0.703	0.996	1.443	1.011
HZ Sourou Sero	1.314	0.79	1.07	1.228	1.038
HZ ST Martin De Papane	1.294	0.806	1.365	0.948	1.043
HZ Save	1.045	0.828	1.027	1.017	0.866
HZ Dassa-Zounme	1	0.754	1	1	0.754
HZ Klouekanmey	1.088	0.834	1.042	1.044	0.908
HZ Aplahoue	1.378	0.665	1.121	1.23	0.917
HZ Bassila	1	0.737	1	1	0.737
HZ Ordre de Malte Djougou	1.201	0.756	1.075	1.118	0.907
CHD Lokossa	1.256	0.717	1.046	1.201	0.901
HZ Come	1.31	0.747	1.433	0.914	0.978
HZ Adjohoun	1.256	0.717	1.046	1.201	0.901
HZ Pobe	1.31	0.747	1.433	0.914	0.978
HZ Sakete	1.438	0.703	0.996	1.443	1.011
Median	**1.294**	**0.754**	**1.067**	**1.201**	**0.978**
Mean	**1.260**	**0.757**	**1.099**	**1.158**	**0.951**
STDEV	**0.134**	**0.047**	**0.134**	**0.166**	**0.085**

-16-

Assessment of Productivity of Hospitals in Botswana: *A DEA Application**

*Naomi Tlotlego, Justice Nonvignon,
Luis G. Sambo, Eyob Z. Asbu, Joses M. Kirigia*

ABSTRACT

Background: The Botswana national health policy states that the Ministry of Health shall from time to time review and revise its organisation and management structures to respond to new developments and challenges in order to achieve and sustain a high level of efficiency in the provision of health care. Even though the government clearly views assuring efficiency in the health sector as one of its leadership and governance responsibilities, to date no study has been undertaken to measure the technical efficiency of hospitals which consume the majority of health sector resources. The specific objectives of this study were to quantify the technical and scale efficiency of hospitals in Botswana and to evaluate changes in productivity over a three-year period in order to analyse changes in efficiency and technology use.

Methods: The DEAP software was used to analyse technical efficiency along with the DEA-based Malmquist productivity index which was applied to a sample of 21 non-teaching hospitals in the Republic of Botswana over a period of three years (2006 to 2008).

Results: The analysis revealed that 16 (76.2%), 16 (76.2%) and 13 (61.9%) of the 21 hospitals were run inefficiently in 2006, 2007, and 2008 with average variable returns to scale (VRS) technical efficiency scores of 70.4 per cent, 74.2 per cent and 76.3 per cent respectively. On average, the Malmquist total factor productivity (MTFP)

---

* The original article appeared in *International Archives of Medicine* 2010;3(27):1-20. Reproduced with the permission of BioMed Central Ltd.

decreased by 1.5 per cent. Whilst hospital efficiency increased by 3.1 per cent, technical change (innovation) regressed by 4.5 per cent. Efficiency change was thus attributed to an improvement in pure efficiency of 4.2 per cent and a decline in scale efficiency of 1 per cent. The MTFP change was highest in 2008 (MTFP=1.008) and lowest in 2007 (MTFP=0.963).

Conclusions: The results indicate significant inefficiencies within the sample for the years under study. In 2008, taken together, the inefficient hospitals would have had to increase the number of outpatient visits by 117,627 (18%) and inpatient days by 49,415 (13%) in order to reach full efficiency. Alternatively, inefficiencies could have been reduced by transferring 264 clinical staff and 39 beds to health clinics, health posts, and mobile posts. The transfer of excess clinical staff to those facilities which are closest to the communities may also contribute to accelerating progress towards the Millennium Development Goals related to child and maternal health.

Nine (57.1%) of the 21 hospitals experienced MTFP deterioration during the three years. We found the sources of inefficiencies to be either adverse change in pure efficiency, scale efficiency, and/or technical efficiency. In line with the report *Health financing: A strategy for the African Region*, which was adopted by the fifty-sixth WHO Regional Committee for Africa, it might be helpful for Botswana to consider institutionalising efficiency monitoring of health facilities within health management information systems.

BACKGROUND

Botswana is situated in Southern Africa and has a population of 1.921 million people – 61.1 per cent of whom live in urban areas [1]. In 2008, the country generated total gross national income (GNI) of US$12,754 million and GNI per capita of US$6,640. In 2007, the country had a human development index (HDI) of 0.694, which was higher than the average HDI for Africa that stood at 0.547. Adult literacy stood at 82.9 per cent and combined gross enrolment in education was 70.6 per cent – higher than Africa's averages of 63.3 per cent and 55.9 per cent respectively [2].

As can be seen in Appendix 16.1, health MDG indicators for Botswana are generally better than those for the African Region as a whole. The country also has a higher density of physicians, nursing and midwifery personnel, other health service providers, and hospital beds than the average for the region while health service coverage for indicators such as care of women during pregnancy and childbirth, reproductive health services, immunisation to prevent common childhood infections, and treatment for HIV and tuberculosis is also above regional averages. However, the prevalence of HIV among adults, at 22,757 per 100,000 of the population, is five times higher than the average for the region [3], while the neonatal mortality rate, adult mortality rate, HIV/AIDS-specific mortality rate, TB among HIV-positive people, and incidence and prevalence of tuberculosis are all significantly higher than regional averages.

In 2008, Botswana spent 5.6 per cent of its gross domestic product (GDP) on health, which translated to a per capita total expenditure on health at purchasing power parity (PPP) of int$762 [4]. About 74.3 per cent of total expenditure on health came from general government spending (i.e., approximately int$568 per person) with the remainder coming from private spending. The latter comprises 27.35 per cent of out-of-pocket spending by households and 5.2 per cent from private prepaid plans. Botswana received only 5.7 per cent of total expenditure on health from external sources.

In 2008, Botswana's under-five mortality rate stood at 40 per 1,000 live births, maternal mortality stood at 380 per 100,000 live births, and life expectancy was 56 years [3]. This compares with under-five mortality of 37 per 1,000 live births, maternal mortality of 180 per 100,000 live births, and life expectancy of 71 years in Algeria where total per capita expenditure on health is just int$338 (roughly half of Botswana's). Cape Verde also did more with less with a per capita total expenditure on health of int$148, delivering an under-five mortality rate of 32 per 1,000 live births, maternal mortality of 210 per 100,000 live births, and life expectancy of 70 years. Meanwhile Mauritius, with total per capita expenditure on health of int$502, achieved an under-five mortality rate of 17 per 1,000 live births, maternal mortality of 15 per 100,000 live births, and life expectancy of 73 years. Algeria, Cape Verde, and Mauritius all deliver better health outcomes in these areas at lower levels of per capita expenditure than Botswana.

Even though the majority of health sector resources in Botswana are spent on hospitals, to date no study has been attempted to address the following questions:

1. Are hospitals producing the maximum outputs with the available inputs?

2. Are hospitals operating at optimal scale?

3. What is the trend of hospital productivity?

4. What percentage of observed productivity changes can be attributed to technical efficiency change and technological change/growth?

The specific objectives of this study were to measure the technical and scale efficiency of hospitals in Botswana and to evaluate changes in productivity over a three-year period in order to analyse changes in efficiency and changes in technology. Finally, the study sought to highlight possible implications for government policy.

One of the policy statements under the leadership and governance rubric in Botswana's national health policy [5, p.18] reads: "The MOH shall from time to time review and revise its organisation and management structures to respond to new developments and challenges in order to gain and maintain high efficiency in the provision of health care". The government clearly views assuring efficiency in the health sector as one of its key leadership and governance responsibilities. This study provides evidence that might help Botswana's policy makers achieve their stated goals.

Prior Research on Hospital Productivity

After an extensive literature search, Emrouznejad *et al.* [6] identified more than 4,000 research articles published in journals or book chapters applying data envelopment analysis (DEA) to measure efficiency and productivity around the world. They found that banking, education (including higher education), health care, and hospital efficiency were the most popular application areas. O'Neill *et al* [7] did a systematic review of 79 DEA-based hospital efficiency studies published from 1984 to 2004 from 12 countries around the world. In the African Region, DEA has only been applied to analyse the efficiency of hospitals in Angola [8], Benin [9], Ghana [10], Kenya [11], Namibia [12], South Africa [13,14], Uganda [15], and Zambia [16]. The literature reviews by both Emrouznejad *et al* [6] and O'Neill *et al* [7] have shown that many studies have applied DEA to estimate efficiency of hospitals but that only a few addressed productivity growth.

In this section, we review a few recent studies that have used Malmquist DEA to decompose productivity of hospitals. Zere et al [14] used Malmquist DEA to assess changes in productivity from 1992/93 to 1997/98 in 10 acute care hospitals in the Western Cape Province of South Africa. The hospitals were assumed to use recurrent expenditures and beds to produce outpatient visits and inpatient days. The mean Malmquist total factor productivity change (MTFP) score was 0.879, efficiency change (EFFCH) score was 0.984, and technical change (TECH) score was 0.893. The decrease in Western Cape Province hospitals' productivity was attributed to 1.6% regress in efficiency and 10.7% decline in technological innovation.

Ouellete and Vierstraete [17] evaluated productivity changes of emergency units of 15 hospitals in Montreal Canada for 1997-98 and 1998-99 using Malmquist DEA. The inputs used included non-physician hours worked, expenditure on furniture and equipment, number of stretchers, and full-time equivalent number of physicians. The output was number of cases. The study found that overall mean MTFP was 0.92, EFFCH was 0.94 and TECH was

1.05. The 8% decrease in productivity was primarily attributed to a decrease in efficiency.

Barros *et al* [18] assessed productivity change of 51 hospitals in Portugal using both the Luenberger indicators and the Malmquist index during the years 1997 to 2004. The inputs included number of beds, number of full-time equivalent personnel, and total variable costs. The outputs included case flows (number of persons that leave the hospital), length of stay, number of consultations, and number of emergency cases. The Luenberger indicator was 0.008, EFFCH was -0.001, and TECH was 0.009. On the other hand, the MTFP was 1.042, EFFCH was 1.036, and TECH was 0.995. The Malmquist DEA results imply that on average productivity of the hospitals under consideration grew mainly due to improvement in efficiency.

Gannon [19] applied Malmquist DEA on samples of 6 regional, 8 general, and 22 country hospitals in Ireland for the period 1995 to 1998. The inputs used were number of beds and full-time equivalent (FTE) people employed. The outputs included number of discharges and deaths, outpatient attendances, and day cases. The study revealed that regional hospitals had MTFP of 1.028, EFFCH of 0.994, and TECH of 1.034. The general hospitals had EFFCH equal to 0.999, TECH equal to 1.013, and MTFP equal to 1.012. The country hospitals had EFFCH of 1.005, TECH of 0.992, and MTFP of 0.997. Therefore, on average the productivity of both regional and general hospitals improved while that of county hospitals declined between 1995 and 1998.

Dash [20] applied Malmquist DEA to study productivity of 29 district headquarters hospitals in India during the years 2002 to 2007. The inputs included number of beds, number of nursing staff, and number of physicians (surgeons). The outputs were number of inpatients, number of outpatients, number of surgeries undertaken, emergency cases handled, medico-legal cases, and deliveries. The hospitals had an MTFP value of 1.2358, EFFCH of 1.15, and TECH of 1.07. Therefore, the 23.6% hospital productivity growth was explained by a 15% improvement in efficiency combined with a 7% increase in innovation.

Ng [21] employed Malmquist DEA to assess productivity of 12 coastal hospitals and 17 inland hospitals in China from 2002 to 2005. The study used three inputs (i.e., number of doctors and nurses, other health staff, and beds and two outputs (i.e., number of outpatient visits and inpatient stays). The coastal hospitals had an MTFP score of 1.1307, a TECH score of 1.1467, and an EFFCH score of 0.9860. The latter was attributed to a 1.41% increase in SECH and a 2.77% regress in pure efficiency change. Contrastingly, inland hospitals' MTFP was 0.9853, which was explained by both a TECH score of 1.0851 and an EFFCH score of 0.9080. The 9.2% efficiency regress was attributed to deterioration in both scale efficiency change (SECH) of 3.57% and pure technical efficiency change (PECH) of 5.83%.

Kirigia *et al* [8] estimated the performance of 28 municipal hospitals in Angola using Malmquist DEA during the period 2000-2002. The inputs included number of physicians plus nurses, number of beds, and expenditures on pharmaceutical and non-pharmaceutical supplies. The hospitals were assumed to produce two outputs, namely, number of OPD visits and inpatient admissions. The municipal hospitals productivity grew by 4.5% (MTFP=1.045). That growth was attributed to an average efficiency improvement of 12.7% (EFFCH=1.127) and a technological regress of 7.3% (TECH=0.927). The improvement in EFFCH was due to a 5% increase in PECH (PECH=1.050) and a 7.3% increase in SECH (SECH=1.073).

Dimas *et al* [22] used Malmquist DEA to examine the efficiency and productivity of 22 Greek public general hospitals for the period 2003-2005. The inputs employed included number of beds, total personnel salary, and total expenditure on medicines, supplies, and other materials. The outputs included number of patient-days, number of patients in the outpatient department, and number of emergency cases. In 2003/2004 the MTFP was 1.02; depicting a 2% productivity growth which was attributed to a 5% increase in innovation (TECH=1.05) and a 1% decline in efficiency (EFFCH= 0.99). The latter was due to PECH of 0.97 and SECH of 1.02. In 2003/2005 hospital productivity declined by 5% (MTFP=0.95) due to decrease in efficiency of 4% (EFFCH=0.96) tempered by a 2% increase in innovation (TECH=1.02). The efficiency regress was attributed to PECH of 0.98 and SECH of 0.99.

Karagiannis and Velentzas [23] applied Malmquist DEA to estimate productivity changes after the inclusion of quality variables for a panel of eight Greek public hospitals during the period 2002-2007. The inputs included number of beds, number of doctors, and number of nursing and other personnel. The output used was number of inpatient days. The authors did estimations of the model excluding (Model A) and including (Model B) the quality variable. According to the conventional Malmquist productivity index (Model A), productivity decreased with an average of 1.2% during the period 2002-2007 (MTFP=0.988). There occurred a technical regress of 0.4% (TECH=0.996) and an efficiency deterioration of 0.9% (EFFCH=0.991). The latter resulted from a 1.3% (PECH=0.987) deterioration in PECH tempered with a 0.4% (SECH=1.004) increase in SECH. According to the quality adjusted Malmquist productivity index (Model B), productivity regressed by 1.4% (MTFP=0.986) due to a 0.3% regress in innovation (TECH=0.997) and a 1.2% decrease in efficiency (EFFCH=0.988). There was a 0.2% (QCH=1.002) increase in overall productivity due to improvement in quality.

Lobo *et al* [24] evaluated the performance and productivity change among 30 Brazilian Federal University hospitals during the years 2003 to 2006 using Malmquist DEA. The inputs used included labour force (physicians and full-time equivalent non-physicians), operational expenses (not including payroll), beds, and service-mix, whilst the outputs included number of, admissions, inpatient surgeries, and outpatient visits. The university hospitals productivity growth of 20.9% (MTFP=1.20859) was attributed solely to increase of 36.5% in innovation (TECH=1.36542) tempered with a 10.3% decrease in efficiency (EFFCH= 0.89716).

Chang *et al* [25] examined the impact of Taiwan Quality Indicator Project (TQIP) participation on 31 regional hospitals productivity over the periods 1998-2002 and 1998-2004 using Malmquist DEA. The inputs utilised included number of physicians, nurses, supporting ancillary services personnel, and patient beds. The hospitals were assumed to produce a number of outpatient visits, ambulatory and emergency room visits, patient days, and net inpatient mortalities. In 1998-2002 the MTFP was 0.7877, quality change (QC) was 0.8645, EFFCH was 0.9712, and TECH was 0.9520. In 1998-2004 MTFP was 0.8748, QCH was 0.8939, EFFCH was 0.9792, and TECH was 0.9873.

METHODS

A health system includes all organisations, institutions, and activities whose primary purpose is to promote, restore, or maintain people's health; that is both length of life and health-related quality of life [26]. One of the pivotal health system institutions is the hospital which combines limited health system inputs (e.g., health workforce, medical products, non-medical supplies, clinical technologies, beds, building space, and ambulances) to produce preventive, curative, and rehabilitative services.

In the context of hospitals, technical efficiency means making the best use of given quantities of health system inputs and existing technology. Allocative efficiency, on the other hand, relates to the optimal allocation of health system inputs. Economic efficiency is a product of both technical efficiency and allocative efficiency [27]. Our study focuses on the measurement of technical efficiency using data envelopment analysis (DEA).

Data Envelopment Analysis

As a linear programming method, DEA is designed to measure the relative efficiencies of a set of decision-making units (DMU) such as hospitals [6,7]. The DEA technique measures the efficiency of a DMU relative to the efficiency of its peer group with a notional "production frontier" representing optimal efficiency. All DMUs lie on or below the "production frontier". The DEA technique solves as many linear programming problems as the number of the DMUs in the study sample [28].

The efficiency of a hypothetical hospital producing one health service output from one health system input would be obtained by dividing the quantity of that output by the quantity of the input. However, "real world" hospitals use multiple inputs (e.g., health workforce, medicines, non-medical supplies, and capital inputs) to produce multiple outputs (e.g., preventive, curative, and rehabilitative services). In such a scenario, the efficiency of a hospital needs to be expressed as the weighted sum of health service outputs divided by the weighted sum of health system inputs.

According to Charness et al [28], the efficiency (E) of a target hospital from the set "j" can then be obtained by solving the following fractional programming model:

$$\text{Max} \quad E_0 = \sum_{R=1}^{s} U_r Y_{r0} \Big/ \sum_{I=1}^{m} V_i X_{i0} \tag{1}$$

Subject to: $E_j \leq 1, \quad j = 1, ..., n$

$u_r, v_r \geq 0$

where Y_{rj} is the amount of health service output r $(r = 1,..., s)$ from hospital j; X_{ij} is the amount of health system input i $(i = 1,..., m)$ in j^{th} hospital; u_r is the weight given to health service output r; v_i is a weight given to health system input i; and n is the number of hospitals in the sample. Charness et al [28] converted model (1) into the following constant returns to scale (CRS) linear programming model:

$$\text{Max} \quad E_0 = \sum u_r y_{rj0} = 1 \tag{2}$$

$$\text{Subject to:} \quad \sum_{r=1}^{s} v_i x_{ij0} = 1$$

$$\sum_{i=1}^{m} u_r y_{rj} - \sum v_i x_{ij} \leq 0, \quad j = 1,..., N.$$

The latter constraint means that all DMUs are either on or below the frontier. Model (2) implies that increases in the amount of health system inputs will be matched by increases in outputs, for example, the doubling of inputs leads to a doubling of outputs. This CRS model assumes that hospitals are operating at an optimal scale of production, and hence, technical efficiency is equal to scale efficiency.

However, in reality a hospital can manifest either CRS, increasing returns to scale (IRS), or decreasing returns to scale (DRS). In an IRS (or economies of scale) scenario, increases in the amount of health system inputs will result in a proportionately greater increase in outputs, for example, a doubling of all inputs will lead to more than a doubling of outputs. Where a hospital is experiencing DRS (diseconomies of scale), a doubling of inputs would lead to less than a doubling of outputs. In order to allow for the variability of returns to scale, the linear programming problem (3) was estimated for each hospital in the sample [29]:

$$\text{Max } E_0 = \sum u_r y_{rj0} + U_0 \tag{3}$$

$$\text{Subject to: } \sum_{r=1}^{s} v_i x_{ij0} = 1$$

$$\sum_{i=1}^{m} u_r y_{rj} - \sum v_i x_{ij} + U_0 \le 0, \quad j = 1,...,N$$

$$U_r, V_i \ge 0.$$

The relative efficiency score (E) lies between 0 (totally inefficient) and 1 (optimal technical efficiency).

Malmquist Productivity Index

Productivity is a measure of the relationship between the outputs of a hospital and the health system inputs that have gone into producing those outputs. An increase in productivity occurs when output per health worker hour is raised and/or there is use of more and/or better health technology. In general, a productivity index is defined as the ratio of an output quantity index to an input quantity index; that is:

$$P_t = \frac{Y_t}{X_t} \tag{4}$$

Where P_t is a productivity index; time period $t = 0,...,T$; Y_t is an output quantity index; and X_t is an input quantity index. Each index represents accumulated growth from period 0 to period t. In a real hospital, X_t comprises more than one input and Y_t more than one output. Because hospital outputs and inputs are heterogeneous, it is not possible to add all outputs to form an output quantity index or to add all inputs to form an input quantity index. Disaggregated data on the quantities of outputs and inputs need weighting to form output and input quantity indices [30].

We opted to use the DEA-based Malmquist productivity index (MPI) to study efficiency and productivity changes over a period of time for a number of reasons: it requires information solely on quantities of inputs and outputs and not on their prices; it does not require the imposition of functional form on the structure of production technology; it easily accommodates multiple hospital inputs and outputs; and it can be broken down into the constituent sources of productivity change–efficiency changes and technological changes [31]. An increase in the efficiency level can be interpreted as a move by the hospital to "catch-up" with the efficiency frontier. Improvement in hospital's health technology shifts the efficiency frontier upward [27].

Malmquist DEA is applied to panel data to calculate indices of changes in total factor productivity (TFP), technology, technical efficiency, and scale efficiency. The MPI takes a value of more than one for productivity growth, a value of one for stagnation, and a value of less than one for productivity decline. The output-oriented MPI is defined as the geometric mean of two periods' productivity indices subsequently broken down into various sources of productivity change [32]:

$$M_0(y^{t+1}, x^{t+1}, y^t, x^t) =$$

$$\underbrace{\left[\frac{D_0^{t+1}(x^{t+1}, y^{t+1})}{D_0^t(x^t, y^t)} \right]}_{EFFCH} \times \underbrace{\left[\frac{D_0^t(x^{t+1}, y^{t+1})}{D_0^{t+1}(x^{t+1}, y^{t+1})} \times \frac{D_0^t(x^t, y^t)}{D_0^{t+1}(x^t, y^t)} \right]^{\frac{1}{2}}}_{TECH} \qquad (5)$$

where D represents the distance function; M_o is the output-oriented Malmquist productivity index; EFFCH is change in relative hospital efficiency (i.e., the change in the gap between observed production and maximum feasible production) between years t and $t+1$; and TECH is a measure of the technical change in the hospital production technology, that is, it measures the shift in technology use between years t and $t+1$.

Efficiency change (EFFCH) estimated under the assumption of CRS can be broken down to allow identification of change in scale efficiency, that is the productivity change resulting from a scale change that brings the hospital closer to or farther away from the optimal scale of output as identified by VRS technology [32]:

$$\left[\frac{D_0^{t+1}(x^{t+1}, y^{t+1})_{CRS}}{\underbrace{D_0^t(x^t, y^t)_{CRS}}_{CRS\ EFFCH}} \right] =$$

$$\underbrace{\frac{D_0^{t+1}(x^{t+1}, y^{t+1})_{VRS}}{D_0^t(x^t, y^t)_{VRS}}}_{Pure\ EFFCH} \times \underbrace{\left[\frac{D_0^{t+1}(x^t, y^t)_{VRS}}{D_0^t(x^t, y^t)_{CRS}} \times \frac{D_0^{t+1}(x^{t+1}, y^{t+1})_{CRS}}{D_0^{t+1}(x^{t+1}, y^{t+1})_{VRS}} \right]}_{Scale\ EFFCH} \qquad (6)$$

where CRS (or VRS) signify a gap measured under the assumption of constant (or variable) returns to scale. Pure EFFCH (the first term on the right) measures change in technical efficiency under the assumption of a VRS technology. Scale EFFCH (the bracketed term on the right) in a given period captures the deviations between the VRS technology and the CRS technology at observed inputs (i.e., it measures changes in efficiency due to movement toward or away from the point of optimal hospital scale).

The M_0 attains a value greater than, equal to, or less than one if a hospital has experienced productivity growth, stagnation, or productivity decline net of the contribution of scale economies between periods t and $t+1$. EFFCH is greater than one, equal to, or less than one if a hospital is moving closer to, unchanging, or diverging from the production frontier. TECH is greater than, equal to, or less than one when the technological best practice is improving, unchanged, or deteriorating respectively [33].

Data

Botswana's health system consists of three referral hospitals under the Ministry of Health (MOH), seven district hospitals also under the MOH, two mission district hospitals (fully funded by government), three mine hospitals, two private hospitals, seventeen primary hospitals under MOH control, and an array of private general practitioners. There are also 104 health clinics with beds, 173 health clinics without beds, 349 health posts, and 856 mobile posts under the Ministry of Local Government. Both district and primary hospitals refer patients to the three referral hospitals; Princess Marina in Gaborone, Nyangabgwe Hospital in Francistown, and Lobatse Mental Hospital [34]. District and primary hospitals were the focus of this study. A simple random sample of 21 (67.7 per cent) hospitals was drawn from the 31 district and primary hospitals and included Kanye and Bamalete mission hospitals as well as the Delta private hospital.

The data used in this study cover the period from 2006 to 2008 and were collected through visits to all the 21 primary and secondary hospitals in

Botswana in 2009 by JN and NT using the WHO/AFRO hospital efficiency questionnaire [35]. The study is based on two inputs as follows: (a) the number of clinical staff (physicians, nursing and midwifery personnel, and dentistry personnel, other technical health service providers); and (b) the number of hospital beds as a proxy of capital inputs. Due to the absence of disaggregated data, we omitted the cost of medical products (medicines, vaccines, and technologies) and non-medical supplies.

According to English et al [36], beyond offering outpatient and inpatient medical and surgical services, district hospitals also play important roles in health-related information, communication, coordination, and training including integration with other local health-related services such as water and sanitation; training of health workers; supervision and monitoring of health workers in the peripheral health centres; and managing health information systems. Although we were cognisant of the latter four services, it was not possible to factor them in due to the limited scope of our study. This study used only two outputs: (a) number of outpatient department visits, and (b) number of inpatient days. The choice of inputs and outputs was based on the published hospital efficiency literature in the African Region [12,14]. We were not able to verify whether all the hospitals had exactly the same standards in terms of type of services provided, quality of care provided, qualification and experience of staff, working schedules, functional building capacity, and hospital technology among others. The DEAP computer program [37] was used in the estimation of the yearly hospital efficiencies and the Malmquist productivity indices.

RESULTS AND DISCUSSION

Technical Efficiency

Appendix 16.2 presents individual hospital's technical and scale efficiency scores during the three years. In 2006, 2007, and 2008 out of the 21 hospitals five (24%), five (24%), and eight (38%) hospitals registered a variable returns to scale technical efficiency (VRSTE) score of 100 per cent, respectively. Therefore, 16 (76%), 16 (76%), and 13 (62%) of the hospitals can be said to have been run inefficiently over the same time period.

Average VRSTE scores of Botswana stood at 70.4 per cent, 74.2 per cent, and 76.3 per cent. This finding implies that if run efficiently, the hospitals could have produced 29.6 per cent, 25.8 per cent, and 23.7 per cent more output (number of outpatient department visits and number of inpatient days) for the same volume of inputs. These average VRSTE scores were higher than those of Angola (65.8%–67.5%) [8], Ghana (61%) [10] and Zambia (67%) [16]. However, they were fairly similar to those obtained in Benin (63.3%–85.8%) [9], Kenya (84%) [11], Namibia (62.7%–74.3%) [12], and Eastern, Northern, and Western Cape Provinces of South Africa (82%–82.8%) [14]. Technical efficiency scores for Kwazulu-Natal Province of South Africa (90.6%) [13] and Uganda (90.2%–97.3%) [15] were significantly higher than those of Botswana.

Scale Efficiency

In 2006, 2007, and 2008, out of the 21 hospitals:

1. Two (9.5%), three (14.3%), and three (14.3%) hospitals respectively showed constant returns to scale (CRS). Among these hospitals, the doubling of health system inputs led to a doubling of health service outputs. In other words, the size of these hospitals did not affect productivity. The average and marginal productivity of these hospitals remained constant whether the hospital was small or large [38]. In short, they were operating at their most productive scale.

2. Three (14.3%), nine (42.9%), and eight (38.1%) hospitals manifested increasing returns to scale (IRS). This may have arisen because the larger scale of a particular operation allowed health managers and workers to specialise in their tasks and make use of more sophisticated health technologies [38]. Hospitals manifesting IRS ought to expand their scale of operation in order to become scale efficient.

3. Sixteen (76.2%), nine (42.9%), and ten (47.6%) hospitals experienced decreasing returns to scale (DRS) which may be associated with the problems of coordinating tasks and maintaining lines of communication between management and workers [38]. The hospitals experiencing DRS need to reduce their scale of operation in order to operate at the most productive scale size [39].

The average scale efficiency score was 79.2 per cent in 2006, 84.7 per cent in 2007, and 78.9 per cent in 2008 indicating that there was scope to increase total hospital outputs by approximately 20.9 per cent in 2006, 15.3 per cent in 2007, and 21.1 per cent in 2008. Where technically and politically feasible, this can be achieved through the appropriate reduction in the size of the scale-inefficient hospitals. These average scale efficiency scores were within the range of those for Angola (81%–89%) [8], Benin (41.9%–73.6%) [9], Ghana (81%) [10], Namibia (73.2%–83.7%) [12], South Africa (Eastern, Northern and Western Cape Provinces) (82.5%–90%) [14] and Zambia (80%) [16]. However, the average scale efficiency scores for Botswana were lower than those of Kenya (90%) [11], Kwazulu-Natal Province of South Africa (95.3%) [13], and Uganda (97.5%) [15].

Scope for Output Increases (input reductions) and Implications for Policy

Appendix 16.3 shows the output (input) increases (reductions) needed to make individual inefficient hospitals efficient during the three years. Appendix 16.4 reports the total output increases and/or input reductions needed to make inefficient hospitals efficient. In 2008, for example, the inefficient hospitals combined would need to increase outpatient visits by 117,627 (18%) and inpatient days by 49,415 (13%) so as to become efficient. Alternatively, the inefficient hospitals could become efficient by reducing the number of clinical staff by 264 (9%) and number of beds by 39 (2%).

With regard to hospitals whose outputs fall short of the DEA targets, MOH policy makers in Botswana could improve efficiency by improving access and utilisation of under-utilised neonatal, infant, and maternal health services, some of which are mentioned in Appendix 16.1. This may require a multi-pronged strategy involving, firstly, use of health promotion strategies and techniques such as advocacy; social mobilisation; social marketing; information, education and communication (IEC); regulation and legislation; partnerships and alliances with public, private, non-governmental organisations, and civil society; and inter-sectoral action to address determinants of health to improve the use of under-utilised health services [40]. Secondly, ensuring universal access to health services through pooled pre-paid contributions collected on the basis of ability to pay through either tax-based funding or social health insurance, or a mix of both [41–43]. This would be in line with Botswana's national health policy statement that [5, p.23]: "The Government shall ensure availability of financial resources for a prepaid package of essential health interventions to all people living in Botswana so that the services are available to the client free of charge".

Alternatively, if it is not feasible to attenuate inefficiencies through the improved utilisation of hospital health services, policy makers could achieve the same objective through the transfer of excess clinical staff and beds to health clinics, health posts, and mobile health posts. This course of action would need to be guided by an efficiency analysis of these lower level health facilities.

Productivity Growth

The year 2006 has been taken as the technology reference when using the Malmquist total factor productivity (MTFP) index to analyse differences in productivity over time and it is worth remembering that according to the index, a value of less than one denotes deterioration in performance, values greater than one denote improvements in performance, and a value of one signifies no change.

Appendix 16.5 presents the Malmquist index summary of annual geometric means. In the last row (last column), we observe that, on average MTFP decreased slightly by 1.5 per cent [i.e. $(1-0.985) \times 100$] over the 2006-2008 period for the sample. On average, the deterioration in MTFP was due to technical change rather than efficiency change. Whereas the efficiency of the hospitals increased by 3.5 per cent, technical change (innovation) regressed by 4.5 per cent. The efficiency change was attributed to an increase in pure efficiency of 4.2 per cent and a decline in scale efficiency of 1 per cent. The MTFP change was highest in 2008 (MTFP=1.008) and lowest in 2007 (MTFP=0.963). The Botswana district hospitals average MTFP score of 0.985 was comparable to those obtained in Montreal, Canada, of 0.92 [17], China inland of 0.9853 [21], Greece of 0.986-0.988 [23], Ireland County of 0.977 [19], South Africa of 0.879 [14]; and Taiwan of 0.7877 [25]. Unlike Botswana, hospitals in a number of countries had an average MTFP score greater than one signifying productivity growth. Angola municipal hospitals had 1.045 [8]; Brazilian Federal University hospitals had 1.209 [24]; China coastal hospitals had 1.1307 [21]; India district hospitals had 1.2358 [20]; Ireland regional hospitals had 1.028 [19]; and Portugal hospitals had 1.042 [18].

Appendix 16.6 provides a summary of the annual geometric mean values of the MPI and its components for each hospital. Nine (42.9%) out of 21 hospitals had MPI scores greater than one indicating growth in productivity. Rakops (7.4%), Letlhakane (1.2%), Kanye (1.8%), Maun (1.9%), Phikwe (1.5%), Mahalpye (7.5%), Delta (8.2%), Bamalete (22.4%), and Deborah (22.4%) hospitals registered MTFP growth of 7.4 per cent, 1.2 per cent, 1.8 per cent, 1.9 per cent, 1.8 per cent, 7.5 per cent, 8.2 per cent, 22.4 per cent and 4.5 per cent respectively. The productivity growth in Letlhakane, Phikwe, and Mahalpye hospitals was attributed to technological innovation only. Meanwhile, productivity growth in hospital performance in the Kanye, Maun, Delta, Bamalete, and Deborah hospitals was due to improvements in efficiency only. It was only in Rakops hospital where total factor productivity growth was fully explained by both improvements in efficiency and technological innovation.

Conversely, 12 (57.1 per cent) of the hospitals had Malmquist index scores of less than one indicating deterioration in productivity over time. Productivity regression in the Palapye hospital was solely due to a decline in efficiency. In Masunga, Mmadinare, Sefhare, Gweta, and Athlone hospitals productivity regression was attributed to both decline in efficiency and innovation whilst in Bobonong, Thebephatwa, Orapa, Scottish, Sekgoma, and Jwaneng hospitals productivity regression was due solely to deterioration in technological innovation.

Pure Efficiency Change

As shown in Appendix 16.6, ten hospitals had an average pure efficiency change (PECH) score of greater than one. Hospitals registering a pure technical efficiency increase included Phikwe (3.7%), Rakops (4.2%), Athlone (7.3%), Bamalete (7.7%), Mahalapye (8.2%), Sekgoma (15.6%), Thebephatswa (17.6%), Deborah (18.5%), Scottish (32%) and Maun (33.7%).

Bobonong, Delta, Kanye, and Letlhakane hospitals registered a PECH score of one indicating no change in efficiency at those hospitals between 2006 and 2008. On the other hand, a decline in PECH occurred at Palapye (18.3%), Jwaneng (7.4%), Mmadinare (6.8%), Masunga (6%), Sefhare (5.8%), Gweta (1%), and Orapa (0.3%). The average PECH score for the entire sample was 1.042, implying that PECH reduced efficiency change by 4.2 per cent.

Scale Efficiency Change

Scale efficiency change (SECH) is expressed as a value of less than, equal to, or greater than one if a hospital's scale of production contributes negatively, not at all, or positively to productivity change [20]. The scale of production of the hospitals contributed positively to TFP change in Gweta (0.2%), Mmadinare (0.7%), Sefhare (1%), Masunga (5.4%), Kanye (8.6%), Orapa (15.5%), Bamaleta (16.2%), Jwaneng (28.2%) and Delta (32.5%).

Bobonong and Letlhakane hospitals had a scale index value of one which means that those hospitals' scale of production did not contribute to MTFP change. On the other hand, the SECH score for 10 hospitals was less than one. This indicates that the scale of production in Maun (23.2%), Mahalapye (22.2%), Sekgoma (18.4%), Athlone (11.5%), Deborah (9.3%), Phikwe (9.1%), Palapye (8.3%), Thebephatswa (6.3%) and Rakops (0.3%) hospitals contributed negatively to productivity change. The average SECH score for the entire sample was 0.99 indicating that the scale of production on average reduced efficiency change by 1 per cent.

Technical Change

Sixteen hospitals (76.2%) registered technical change (TECH) of less than one indicating a decline in technical innovation. The lack of technological innovation led to a decrease in TPF change in Mmadinare (18.4%), Delta (18.4%), Jwaneng (18.4%), Thebephatswa (18.2%), Orapa (15.5%), Gweta (8.8%), Scottish (8.4%), Kanye (6.3%), Sefhare (5.2%), Masunga (5%), Athlone (3.1%), Deborah (3%), Sekgoma (2.5), Bamalete (2.2%), Maun (0.7%) and Bobonong (0.3%). Letlhakane, Rakops, Phikwe, Palapye and Mahalapye registered technological growth or progress between the periods t and $t + 1$ of 1.2%, 3.4%, 7.1 per cent, 19.8% and 21.7% respectively.

The technological progress shown by certain hospitals suggests that they applied an advance in scientific knowledge in the form of inventions or innovations with regard to both physical and human capital that allowed a greater output, and probably quality of health services, with health system input prices held constant. The advances may have resulted from the application of improved health technologies to health service production processes, but they may also have resulted from increases in health workforce motivation or skill and from improvements in health services organisation.

Technological progress (or regression) depends on a number of factors including the availability of appropriate health technology (i.e., ecologically relevant and versatile for easy adaptation/application requiring a minimum of new skills) plus complementary inputs and institutional changes; the existence of channels of communication between health policy makers and hospital management teams; access to new appropriate technologies at affordable prices; availability of training facilities/opportunities to enable relevant health workforce to acquire new skills to take full advantage of a new technological possibility; and the availability of funds to finance the needed health technology investments [44].

CONCLUSION

This study has measured the technical and scale efficiency of 21 hospitals in Botswana; quantified the output (input) increases (reductions) necessary to make inefficient hospitals efficient; and estimated the magnitude and sources of total factor productivity change within each hospital. The results indicate that 16 (76.2%), 16 (76.2%), and 13 (61.9%) of the 21 hospitals were run inefficiently in 2006, 2007, and 2008 respectively. In 2008, the inefficient hospitals, taken together, would need to increase the number of outpatient visits by 117,627 (18%) and inpatient days by 49,415 (13%) in order to become efficient. There is scope for providing more child and maternal health services to additional persons by using the existing health system inputs more efficiently (i.e., without waste).

Alternatively, inefficiencies could be reduced by transferring 264 clinical staff and 39 beds to primary health level facilities. The transfer of excess clinical staff to those facilities which are closest to the communities may go a long way in reducing infant, child, and maternal deaths in line with the MDGs targets.

Nine (57.1 per cent) of the 21 hospitals experienced MTFP deterioration during the three years. We found the sources of inefficiencies to be either adverse changes in pure efficiency, scale efficiency, and/or technical efficiency. In line with the "Health financing: A strategy for the African Region" [42], which was adopted by the fifty-sixth WHO Regional Committee for Africa, Botswana needs to consider institutionalising efficiency monitoring of health facilities within health management information systems (HMIS). Renner *et al* [45] propose a number of steps that could be followed by countries that decide to institutionalise health facility efficiency monitoring within HMIS.

ACKNOWLEDGEMENT

We are grateful to Ministry of Health in Botswana for having authorised the study to be undertaken and for inputs during the dissemination workshops. We are also thankful to the WHO Country Office in Botswana for follow-up and facilitation. We are indebted to the University of Botswana for hosting the dissemination workshop. The fieldwork was funded by WHO. We do acknowledge the editorial support provided by Gary Humphreys. The article contains the perceptions and views of the authors only and does not represent decisions or the stated policies of University of Botswana, University of Ghana, or World Health Organization.

REFERENCES

1. World Bank. *World development indicators database.* http://data.worldbank.org/data-catalog. Accessed 19 April, 2010.

2. UNDP. *Human development report 2009.* Oxford: Oxford University Press; 2009.

3. World Health Organization. *World health statistics 2009.* Geneva: World Health Organization; 2009.

4. World Health Organization. *National health accounts.* Geneva: World Health Organization; 2010.

5. Republic of Botswana. National Health Policy - Towards a healthier Botswana. Gaborone; 2010.

6. Emrouznejad A, Parker BR, Tavares G. Evaluation of research in efficiency and productivity: a survey and analysis of the first 30 years of scholarly literature in DEA. *Socio-Economic Planning Sciences* 2008; 42:151–157.

7. O'Neil L, Rauner M, Heidenberger K, Kraus M. A cross-national comparison and taxonomy of DEA-based hospital efficiency studies. *Socio-Economic Planning Sciences* 2008;42:158-189.

8. Kirigia JM, Emrouznejad A, Cassoma B, Asbu EZ, Barry S. A performance assessment method for hospitals: the case of municipal hospitals in Angola. *Journal of Medical Systems* 2008;32(6):509-519.

9. Kirigia JM, Mensah AO, Mwikisa CN, Asbu EZ, Emrouznejad A, Makoudode P, Hounnankan A. Technical efficiency of zone hospitals in Benin. *The African Health Monitor* 2010;12:30-39.

10. Osei D, George M, d'Almeida S, Kirigia JM, Mensah AO, Kainyu LH. Technical efficiency of public district hospitals and health centres in Ghana: a

pilot study. *Cost Effectiveness and Resource Allocation* 2005; 3:9. Available at: http://www.resource-allocation.com/content/3/1/9.

11. Kirigia JM, Emrouznejad A, Sambo LG. Measurement of technical efficiency of public hospitals in Kenya: using data envelopment analysis. *Journal of Medical Systems* 2002;26(1):39-45.

12. Zere E, Mbeeli T, Shangula K, Mandlhate C, Mutirua K, Tjivambi B, Kapenambili W. Technical efficiency of district hospitals: evidence from Namibia using data envelopment analysis. *Cost Effectiveness and Resource Allocation* 2006;4:5. Available at: http://www.resource-allocation.com/content/4/1/5.

13. Kirigia JM, Lambo E, Sambo LG. Are public hospitals in Kwazulu-Natal Province of South Africa technically efficient? *African Journal of Health Sciences* 2000;7(3-4): 25-32.

14. Zere E, McIntyre D, Addison T. Technical efficiency and productivity of public sector hospitals in three South African provinces. *South African Journal of Economics* 2001;69(2):336-358.

15. Yawe BL, Kavuma SN. Technical efficiency in the presence of desirable and undesirable outputs: a case study of selected district referral hospitals in Uganda. *Health Policy and Development* 2008;6(1):37-53.

16. Masiye F. Investigating health system performance: an application of data envelopment analysis to Zambian hospitals. *BMC Health Services Research* 2007;7:58. Available at: http://www.biomedcentral.com/1472-6963/7/58.

17. Ouellete P, Vierstraete V. Technological change and efficiency in the presence of quasi-fixed inputs: a DEA application to the hospital sector. *European Journal of Operational Research* 2004;154(3):755-763.

18. Barros CP, Menezes AG, Peypoch N, Solonandrasana B, Vieira JV. An analysis of hospital efficiency and productivity growth using the Luenberger indicator. *Health Care Management Science* 2007;11(4):373-381.

19. Gannon B. Total factor productivity growth of hospitals in Ireland: a nonparametric approach. *Applied Economics Letters* 2008; 15(2):131 – 135.

20. Dash U. *Evaluating the comparative performance of district headquarters hospitals, 2002-07: a non-parametric Malmquist approach.* IGIDR Proceedings/Project Reports Series PP-062-26. Mumbai: Indira Gandhi Institute of Development Research (IGIDR); 2009.

21. Ng YC. The productive efficiency of the health care sector of China. *The Review of Regional Studies* 2008;38(3):381–393.

22. Dimas G, Goula A, Soulis S. Productive performance and its components in Greek public hospitals. *International Journal of Operations Research* 2010. DOI: 10.1007/s12351-010-0082-2.

23. Karagiannis R, Velentzas K. Productivity and quality changes in Greek public hospitals. *International Journal of Operations Research* 2010. Doi 10.1007/s12351-010-00800-4.

24. Lobo MSC, Ozcan YA, Silva ACM, Lins MPE, Fiszman R. Financing reform and productivity change in Brazilian teaching hospitals: Malmquist approach. *Central European Journal of Operations Research* 2010;18(2):141-152.

25. Chang S-H, Hsiao H-C, Huang L-H, Chang H. Taiwan quality indicator project and hospital productivity growth. *Omega* 2011;39:14-22.

26. World Health Organization. Everybody's business - strengthening health systems to improve health outcomes: WHO's framework for action. Geneva: World Health Organization; 2007.

27. Coelli TJ, Rao DSP, O'Donnell CJ, Battese GE. *An introduction to productivity and efficiency analysis.* New York: Springer Science; 1998.

28. Charnes A, Cooper WW, Rhodes E. Measuring the efficiency of decision-making units. *European Journal of Operational Research* 1978;2(6):429–444.

29. Banker RD, Charnes A, Cooper WW. Some models for estimating technical and scale inefficiencies in data envelopment analysis. *Management Science* 1984;30(9):1078-1092.

30. McLellan N. *Measuring productivity using the index number approach: an introduction.* Working Paper 04/05. Wellington: New Zealand Treasury; 2004.

31. Grifell-Tatje E, Lovell CAK. The sources of change in Spanish banking. *European Journal of Operational Research* 1997;98(2): 364-380.

32. Fare R, Grosskopf S, Lovell CAK. *Production frontiers.* Cambridge: Cambridge University Press; 1994.

33. Kirikal L, Sorg M, Vensel V. Estonian banking sector performance analysis using Malmquist indexes and DuPoint financial ratio analysis. *International Business and Economic Research Journal* 2004;3(12): 21-36.

34. Republic of Botswana. *National health services situation analysis report.* Gaborone: Ministry of Health; 2005.

35. World Health Organization, Regional Office for Africa. *Hospitals economic efficiency analysis data collection instrument.* Brazzaville: World Health Organization; 2000.

36. English M, Lanata CF, Ngugi I, Smith PC. The district hospital. In: Jamison DT, Breman JG, Measham AR, Alleyne G, Claeson M, Evans DB, Jha P, Mills A, Mugrove P, editors. *Disease Control Priorities in Developing Countries.* 2nd edition. New York: Oxford University Press; 2006. p. 1211-1228.

37. Coelli T: *Guide to DEAP, Version 2.1: a data envelopment analysis [computer] program,* Centre for Efficiency and Productivity Analysis (CEPA)

Working Paper 96/08. Department of Econometrics, University of New England, Armidale, NSW Australia; 1996.

38. Pindyck RS, Rubinfeld DL. *Microeconomics.* New Jersey: Prentice Hall; 1995.

39. Varian HR. *Intermediate microeconomics.* New York: W.W. Norton & Co; 2003.

40. World Health Organization. *Milestones in health promotion statements from global conferences.* Geneva: World Health Organization; 2009.

41. World Health Organization. *Primary health care: now more than ever.* Geneva: World Health Organization; 2008.

42. World Health Organization. *Health financing: a strategy for the African Region.* Brazzaville: World Health Organization Regional Office for Africa; 2006.

43. Carrin G, James C, Evans D. *Achieving universal health coverage: developing the health financing system.* Technical briefs for policy makers. Number 1. Geneva: World Health Organization; 2005.

44. Killick T. Policy economics: a textbook for applied economics on developing countries. London: Heinemann; 1981.

45. Renner A, Kirigia JM, Zere AE, Barry SP, Kirigia DG, Kamara C, Muthuri HK. Technical efficiency of peripheral health units in Pujehun district of Sierra Leone: a DEA application. *BMC Health Services Research* 2005; 5:77.

Appendix 16.1   Millennium Development Goals, health, and national health accounts indicators

Indicators	Botswana	African Region
Health-related Millennium Development Goals indicators		
Low birth weight newborns (per cent)	10	14
Children aged <5 years underweight for age (per cent)	10.7	21.3
Under-5 mortality rate (probability of dying by age 5 per 1,000 live births	40	145
Measles immunisation coverage among 1-year-olds (per cent)	90	74
Maternal mortality ratio (per 100,000 live births)	380	900
Births attended by skilled health personnel (per cent)	94	46
Contraceptive prevalence (per cent)	44.4	24.4
Adolescent fertility rate (per 1,000 girls aged 15–19 years)	51	117
Antenatal care coverage (per cent) : at least 1 visit	97	73
Prevalence of HIV among adults aged >=15 years per 100,000 population	22,757	4,735
Antiretroviral therapy coverage among people with advanced HIV infection (per cent)	79	30
Malaria mortality rate per 100,000 population	2	104
Tuberculosis treatment success under DOTS (per cent)	72	75
Access to improved drinking water sources (per cent)	96	59
Access to improved sanitation (per cent)	47	33
Global health indicators		
Life expectancy at birth in years	56	52
Healthy life expectancy (HALE) at birth (years)	49	45
Neonatal mortality rate (per 1,000 live births)	46	40
Infant mortality rate (probability of dying between birth and age 1 per 1,000 live births)	32	88
Adult mortality rate (probability of dying between 15 and 60 years per 1,000 population)	514	401
HIV/AIDS -specific mortality rate (per 100,000 population)	585	198
Malaria -specific mortality rate (per 100,000 population)	2	104
TB among HIV-negative people (per 100,000 population)	37	45
TB among HIV-positive people (per 100,000 population)	156.5	47.6
Age-standardised mortality rates from non-communicable diseases (per 100,000 population)	594	841
Prevalence of tuberculosis (per 100,000 population)	622	475
Incidence of tuberculosis (per 100,000 population per year)	731	363
Prevalence of HIV among adults aged >15 years (per 100,000 population)	22,757	4,735
Health service coverage		
Antenatal care coverage (per cent) - at least 1 visit	97	73
Antenatal care coverage (per cent) - at least 4 visit	97	45
Births attended by skilled health personnel (per cent)	94	46
Births by caesarean section (per cent)	7.7	3.3
Neonates protected at birth against neonatal tetanus (per cent)	78	31
Immunisation coverage among 1-year-olds (per cent) - MDG 4 Measles	90	74

.../cont.

Appendix 16.1 (cont.)

Indicators	Botswana	African Region
Immunisation coverage among 1-year-olds (per cent) - MDG 4 DPT3	97	74
Immunisation coverage among 1-year-olds (per cent) - MDG 4 HepB3	85	69
Antiretroviral therapy coverage (per cent) - Pregnant women (PMTCT)	95	34
Antiretroviral therapy coverage (per cent) - People with advanced HIV infection	79	30
Tuberculosis detection rate under DOTS (per cent)	57	47
Tuberculosis treatment success under DOTS (per cent)	72	75
Health workforce and infrastructure		
Physicians	715	150,708
Physicians - Density (per 10,000 population)	4	2
Nursing and midwifery personnel	4,753	792,361
Nursing and midwifery personnel (per 10,000 population)	27	11
Dentistry personnel	38	23,964
Dentistry personnel (per 10,000 population)	<1	1
Other health service providers	1,611	257,520
Other health service providers (per 10,000 population)	9	4
Hospital beds (per 10,000 population)	24	10
Health expenditure (2008)		
Total expenditure on health as per cent of gross domestic product	5.6	5.7
General government expenditure on health as per cent of total expenditure on health	74.3	50.5
Private expenditure on health as per cent of total expenditure on health	25.7	49.5
General government expenditure on health as per cent of total government expenditure	11.7	10.1
External resources for health as per cent of total expenditure on health	5.7	20.8
Social security expenditure on health as per cent general government expenditure on health	0.0	3.4
Out-of-pocket expenditure as per cent of private expenditure on health	27.3	73.3
Private prepaid plans as per cent of private expenditure on health	5.2	7.1
Per capita total expenditure on health at average exchange rate (US$)	392.5	101.8
Per capita total expenditure on health (PPP int.$)	779.3	172.1
Per capita government expenditure on health at average exchange rate (US$)	291.5	59.8
Per capita government expenditure on health (PPP int.$)	578.8	99.8

Source: WHO [3].

Appendix 16.2   Hospital technical and scale efficiency during 2006-2008

Hospital	Efficiency 2006				Efficiency 2007				Efficiency 2008			
	CRSTE	VRSTE	Scale	Returns to scale	CRSTE	VRSTE	Scale	Returns to scale	CRSTE	VRSTE	Scale	Returns to scale
Rakops	0.511	0.54	0.946	DRS	0.559	0.615	0.909	IRS	0.552	0.587	0.94	IRS
Masunga	0.277	0.315	0.879	DRS	0.263	0.272	0.964	IRS	0.272	0.278	0.978	IRS
Mmadinare	0.536	0.557	0.962	IRS	0.531	0.54	0.984	IRS	0.473	0.484	0.977	IRS
Bobonong	1	1	1	CRS	1	1	1	CRS	1	1	1	CRS
Palapye	0.834	0.947	0.881	DRS	0.651	0.772	0.844	DRS	0.489	0.633	0.774	DRS
Letlhakane	1	1	1	CRS	1	1	1	CRS	1	1	1	CRS
Sefhare	0.49	0.522	0.939	DRS	0.454	0.485	0.936	IRS	0.444	0.463	0.958	IRS
Thebephatswa	0.352	0.371	0.948	IRS	0.403	0.426	0.946	IRS	0.478	0.514	0.931	IRS
Gweta	0.352	0.37	0.952	DRS	0.257	0.261	0.986	IRS	0.347	0.363	0.955	IRS
Kanye	0.79	1	0.79	DRS	0.973	1	0.973	DRS	0.931	1	0.931	DRS
Orapa	0.467	1	0.467	DRS	0.636	0.991	0.642	DRS	0.619	0.993	0.624	DRS
Maun	0.336	0.463	0.727	DRS	0.354	0.591	0.599	DRS	0.354	0.827	0.428	DRS
Phikwe	0.712	0.93	0.766	DRS	0.7	0.905	0.773	DRS	0.643	1	0.643	DRS
Scottish	0.365	0.506	0.723	DRS	0.513	0.836	0.613	DRS	0.385	0.881	0.437	DRS
Sekgoma	0.394	0.748	0.527	DRS	0.323	0.883	0.366	DRS	0.413	1	0.413	DRS
Athlone	0.409	0.512	0.798	DRS	0.634	0.642	0.988	IRS	0.387	0.59	0.657	DRS
Mahalapye	0.672	0.854	0.788	DRS	0.636	0.965	0.659	DRS	0.525	1	0.525	DRS
Delta	0.447	1	0.447	IRS	0.848	1	0.848	IRS	0.785	1	0.785	IRS
Jwaneng	0.441	0.727	0.606	DRS	0.803	0.809	0.994	IRS	0.622	0.624	0.996	IRS
Bamalete	0.638	0.862	0.74	DRS	1	1	1	CRS	1	1	1	CRS
Deborah	0.416	0.563	0.739	DRS	0.45	0.596	0.755	DRS	0.482	0.791	0.61	DRS
Median	**0.467**	**0.727**	**0.79**		**0.634**	**0.809**	**0.936**		**0.489**	**0.827**	**0.931**	
Mean	**0.467**	**0.704**	**0.792**		**0.618**	**0.742**	**0.847**		**0.581**	**0.763**	**0.789**	
STDEV	**0.215**	**0.246**	**0.169**		**0.245**	**0.248**	**0.179**		**0.231**	**0.249**	**0.216**	

Appendix 16.3   Output (input) increases (reductions) needed to make individual inefficient hospitals efficient during 2006-2008

Hospital	2006				2007			
	Outputs		Inputs		Outputs		Inputs	
	Outpatient visits	Inpatient days	Outpatient visits	Inpatient days	Outpatient visits	Inpatient days	Outpatient visits	Inpatient days
Rakops	16,029	0	25	0	19,373	0	0	0
Masunga	16,807	0	2	0	19,413	0	0	0
Mmadinare	0	4,887	0	24	0	12,872	0	0
Bobonong	0	0	0	0	0	0	0	0
Palapye	10,333	0	90	0	10,419	0	31	0
Letlhakane	0	0	0	0	0	0	0	0
Sefhare	11,509	0	6	0	14,354	0	0	0
Thebephatswa	0	7,370	0	15	0	7,779	0	0
Gweta	12,518	0	0	16	0	2,350	0	0
Kanye	0	0	0	0	0	0	0	0
Orapa	0	0	0	0	0	12,732	54	0
Maun	35,969	0	51	0	4,186	0	165	0
Phikwe	38,844	0	103	0	46,590	0	77	0
Scottish	25,197	0	42	0	49,543	0	127	0
Sekgoma	64,196	0	94	183	55,601	0	160	183
Athlone	28,688	0	0	17	27,187	0	0	43
Mahalapye	33,365	0	174	0	42,660	0	143	0
Delta	0	0	0	0	0	0	0	0
Jwaneng	0	1,073	0	25	0	13,579	0	0
Bamalete	2,728	0	66	0	0	0	0	0
Deborah	29,739	0	25	0	33,009	0	98	0
Total	**325,922**	**13,330**	**678**	**280**	**322,336**	**49,312**	**857**	**226**
Median	**11,509**	**0**	**2**	**0**	**4,186**	**0**	**0**	**0**
Mean	**15,520**	**667**	**32**	**13**	**15,349**	**2,348**	**41**	**11**
STDEV	**176,499**	**7,696**	**48**	**40**	**175,955**	**28,470**	**61**	**41**

…/cont.

Efficiency Analysis of Health Systems in Africa

Appendix 16.3 (cont.)

Hospital	2008			
	Outputs		Inputs	
	Outpatient visits	Inpatient days	Outpatient visits	Inpatient days
Rakops	23,765	0	0	0
Masunga	17,150	0	0	0
Mmadinare	0	14,345	0	0
Bobonong	0	0	0	0
Palapye	745	0	0	0
Letlhakane	0	0	0	0
Sefhare	13,220	0	0	0
Thebephatswa	0	10,955	0	0
Gweta	5,311	0	0	0
Kanye	0	0	0	0
Orapa	0	14,467	60	0
Maun	0	0	90	11
Phikwe	0	0	0	0
Scottish	7,792	0	0	27
Sekgoma	0	0	0	0
Athlone	26,357	0	67	0
Mahalapye	0	0	0	0
Delta	0	0	0	0
Jwaneng	0	9,648	0	0
Bamalete	0	0	0	0
Deborah	23,287	0	47	0
Total	**117,627**	**49,415**	**264**	**39**
Median	**0**	**0**	**0**	**0**
Mean	**5,601**	**2,353**	**13**	**2**
STDEV	**9,223**	**5,059**	**27**	**6**

Appendix 16.4   Total output (input) increases (reductions) needed to make inefficient hospitals efficient

	2006		2007		2008	
	Total actual values	Shortfall/excess	Total actual values	Shortfall/excess	Total actual values	Shortfall/excess
OPD visits	626,350	325,922 (52%)	652,401	322,336 (49%)	648,185	117,627 (18%)
Inpatient days	368,985	13,330 (4%)	350,057	49,312 (14%)	383,597	49,415 (13%)
Clinical staff	2,803	678 (24%)	2,599	857 (33%)	2,956	264 (9%)
Beds	2,047	280 (14%)	2,067	226 (11%)	2,374	39 (2%)

Appendix 16.5   Malmquist index summary of annual means (output-oriented)

Year	Efficiency change [A = (C × D]	Technical change [B]	Pure efficiency change [C]	Scale efficiency change [D = (A/C]]	Malmquist index of total factor productivity change [E = A × B]
2007	1.119	0.86	1.049	1.067	0.963
2008	0.95	1.061	1.035	0.918	1.008
Mean	**1.035**	**0.955**	**1.042**	**0.990**	**0.985**

Appendix 16.6   Malmquist index summary of firm means

Hospital	Efficiency change [A=(C × D)]	Technical change [B]	Pure efficiency change [C]	Scale efficiency change [D=(A/C)]	Malmquist index of total factor productivity change [E=A × B]
Rakops	1.039	1.034	1.042	0.997	1.074
Masunga	0.991	0.95	0.94	1.054	0.942
Mmadinare	0.939	0.816	0.932	1.007	0.766
Bobonong	1	0.997	1	1	0.997
Palapye	0.766	1.198	0.817	0.937	0.918
Letlhakane	1	1.012	1	1	1.012
Sefhare	0.951	0.948	0.942	1.01	0.902
Thebephatswa	1.165	0.818	1.176	0.991	0.953
Gweta	0.992	0.912	0.99	1.002	0.905
Kanye	1.086	0.937	1	1.086	1.018
Orapa	1.152	0.845	0.997	1.156	0.973
Maun	1.026	0.993	1.337	0.768	1.019
Phikwe	0.95	1.071	1.037	0.917	1.018
Scottish	1.026	0.916	1.32	0.778	0.94
Sekgoma	1.024	0.975	1.156	0.885	0.998
Athlone	0.974	0.963	1.073	0.907	0.938
Mahalapye	0.884	1.217	1.082	0.816	1.075
Delta	1.325	0.816	1	1.325	1.082
Jwaneng	1.188	0.816	0.926	1.282	0.969
Bamalete	1.252	0.978	1.077	1.162	1.224
Deborah	1.077	0.97	1.185	0.909	1.045
Mean	**1.031**	**0.955**	**1.042**	**0.99**	**0.985**

Note: All Malmquist index averages are geometric means

-17-

Technical Efficiency, Efficiency Change, Technical Progress, and Productivity Growth Among National Health Systems in African Continent*

Joses Muthuri Kirigia; Eyob Zere Asbu;
William Greene; Ali Emrouznejad

ABSTRACT

In May 2006, the Ministers of Health of all the countries in the African continent, at a special session of the African Union, undertook to institutionalise efficiency monitoring within their respective national health information management systems. The specific objectives of this study were to assess the technical efficiency of National Health Systems (NHSs) of African countries for producing male and female life expectancies and to assess changes in health productivity over time with a view to analysing changes in efficiency and changes in technology.

The analysis was based on a five-year panel data (1999-2003) from all the 53 countries of continental Africa. Data envelopment analysis (DEA) – a non-parametric linear programming approach – was employed to assess technical efficiency. The Malmquist total factor productivity (MTFP) was used to analyse efficiency and productivity change over time among the national health systems of the 53 countries. The data consisted of two outputs (male and female life expectancies) and two inputs (per capital total health expenditure and adult literacy).

---

* The original article appeared in *Eastern Africa Social Sciences Research Review* 2007;23(2):19-14. Reproduced with the permission of Organisation for Social Science Research in Eastern and Southern Africa (OSSREA).

The DEA revealed that 49 (92.5%) countries' national health systems were run inefficiently in 1999 and 2000 while 50 (94.3%), 48 (90.6%), and 47 (88.7%) were operated inefficiently in 2001, 2002, and 2003 respectively. Fifty-two countries did not experience any change in scale efficiency, while thirty (56.6%) countries' national health systems had a pure efficiency change (PEFFCH) index of less than one signifying that those countries' NHSs pure efficiency contributed negatively to productivity change.

All the 53 countries' national health systems registered improvements in total factor productivity attributable mainly to technical progress. Over half of the countries' national health systems had a pure efficiency index of less than one signifying that those countries' NHSs pure efficiency contributed negatively to productivity change. African countries may need to critically evaluate the utility of institutionalising of the Malmquist TFP type of analyses to monitor the changes in health systems economic efficiency and productivity over time.

Keywords: African national health systems; per capital total health expenditure, technical efficiency; scale efficiency; Malmquist indices of productivity change; DEA.

INTRODUCTION

A national health system (NHS) has been described as representing all the activities whose primary purposes are to promote, restore, or maintain health (i.e., quantity and health-related quality of life) [1]. It performs the functions of stewardship (oversight); health financing (revenue collection, pooling of resources, sharing of financial risk, and purchasing of health services); creating resources/inputs (including human resources for health) for producing health and providing health services with a view to improving responsiveness to people's non-medical expectations; ensuring fair financial contribution to health systems and ultimately improving health (the three being goals of the health system) [1]. The *World Health Report 2000* ranked the 191 Member States of the World Health Organization (WHO) on the basis of their overall health system goals performance. In this ranking, the national health of a majority of countries on the African continent performed poorly [2].

In August 2005, the fifty-fifth session of the WHO Regional Committee for Africa, consisting of Ministers of Health of 46 Member States, recommended that WHO and the World Bank should support countries to institutionalise mechanisms for monitoring efficiency in the use of health sector resources [3]. Subsequently, in May 2006, the Ministers of Health of the countries in the African continent at a special session of the African Union decided to undertake a number of measures to strengthen the health financing function of their health systems [4] with a view to mobilising more domestic resources for massive expansion in the coverage of health interventions envisaged in the United Nations MDGs [5]. The Health Ministers undertook to institutionalise efficiency monitoring within the national health information management systems. In August 2006, the fifty-sixth session of the WHO Regional Committee for Africa adopted a strategy for health financing; the specific objective of which is to ensure efficiency in the allocation and use of health sector resources [6]. Thus, there is a growing awareness among the African Ministers of Health that as they attempt to mobilise more domestic and external resources, it is important to ensure that available and future health-related sector resources are optimally used to produce health outcomes.

The current study aimed at contributing to establishment of baseline efficiency and productivity growth scores that the African Union can use to monitor changes in the performance of NHSs as countries strive to implement the above-mentioned decision [4]. The study's specific objectives were to: *(a)* assess the technical efficiency of NHSs of African continent countries for producing male and female life expectancies, and *(b)* assess changes in health productivity over time with a view to analysing changes in efficiency and changes in technology.

METHODOLOGY

Concept and Measurement of Technical Efficiency and Productivity of National Health Systems

A national health system is endowed with a limited supply of health-producing resources including human resources, pharmaceutical and non-pharmaceutical supplies, clinical technologies, beds, building space, and ambulances among others. Although people's health needs are unlimited (and thus insatiable), resource scarcity limits a health system's ability to meet all the needs. A fundamental economic problem is how to empower the system to avoid waste, that is be technically efficient.

Technical efficiency means producing maximum health outcomes (measured, for example, in terms of life expectancy at birth) from available resources or minimising the use of available resources to produce a given level of health outcome. The concept and measurement of technical efficiency is illustrated in Figure 17.1 [7,8]. It depicts a single input, per capita total health expenditure (THE) and a single output (life expectancy in years) production technology under constant returns to scale (CRS) and variable returns to scale (VRS) assumptions. Graphically, under the CRS assumption the production frontier (0FC) is a straight line. Contrastingly, the frontier (ABCD) under the VRS assumption is concave.

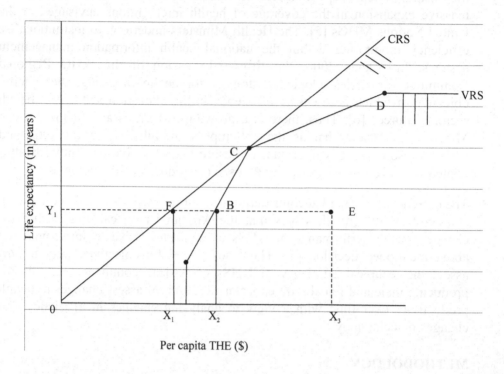

Figure 17.1   Concept and measurement of technical efficiency

We shall use a national health system "E" to demonstrate the estimation of overall technical efficiency and its decomposition into pure technical efficiency and scale efficiency. This NHS uses $0X_3$ units of input (per capita THE) to produce $0Y_1$ units of health outcome (years of life expectancy). Under the CRS technology, the national health system E could have produced the current level of life expectancy ($0Y_1$) with fewer international dollars per capita ($0X_1$). Likewise, under the VRS technology, the same outcome level could have been produced using only $0X_2$ international dollars per capita. The technical efficiency of national health system E under constant returns to scale (TE_{CRS}) is:

$$TE_{CRS} = \frac{0X_1}{0X_3} \qquad (1)$$

On the other hand, the pure technical efficiency of hospital E under variable returns to scale (TE_{VRS}) is:

$$TE_{VRS} = \frac{0X_2}{0X_3} \qquad (2)$$

Technical efficiency takes values between one (or 100%) and zero (or 0%). A technically efficient NHS will have a technical efficiency score of one, while the inefficient ones have a score of less than one. For illustration purpose, let us assume that the pure technical efficiency of E is 70%. This implies that the NHS could have produced the same number of years of life expectancy with approximately 30 per cent fewer international dollars per capita than it is currently employing. Scale efficiency refers to the extent to which an NHS can take advantage of returns to scale by altering its size towards optimal scale (which is defined as the region in which there are constant returns to scale in the relationship between outputs and inputs).

$$\text{Scale efficiency} = \frac{0X_1}{0X_2} = \frac{TE_{CRS}}{TE_{VRS}} \tag{3}$$

The distances X_1X_3 and X_2X_3 represent technical inefficiencies under the CRS and VRS assumptions respectively. Scale inefficiency equals the difference between the two. Scale efficiency takes values between one and zero. Scale efficient national health systems have a score of one whereas the inefficient ones have a score of less than one. For instance, if the scale efficiency score for national health system E is 75%, it implies an inefficiency level of about 25%, which is explained by inappropriate NHS size (inefficiently large or small).

Whilst technical efficiency means producing maximum health outcomes from available resources, productivity is the measure of the physical health system output produced from the use of a given quantity of health system inputs. This may include all health system inputs and all health system outputs (total factor productivity) or a subset of health system inputs and health system outputs (partial productivity). The productivity of national health systems varies as a result of differences in production technology, differences in the technical efficiency of the health system or its component, and the external environment in which production occurs.

The two approaches to the measurement of efficiency are parametric methods that include the estimation of production [9] and cost functions with *a priori* well-defined functional form and construction of index numbers using non-parametric methods including data envelopment analysis (DEA) and Free Disposal Hall (FDH) [10,11]. Data envelopment analysis is the preferred method of efficiency analysis in the non-profit sector [12]. It has the advantage of easily accommodating multiple input, multiple output production and does not make behavioural assumptions (such as profit maximisation) about the NHS (decision-making unit). For these reasons we opted to employ DEA in estimating the technical efficiency and productivity of national health systems in the African continent.

Data Envelopment Analysis

Coelli, Rao, and Battese [12] provide a very good introduction to efficiency and productivity analysis and discuss in an accessible manner the DEA and the Malmquist total factor productivity (TFP) indices among others. Data envelopment analysis generates an efficiency index (E) that is the ratio of the weighted sum of outcomes of a NHS to its weighted sum of inputs [12].

Let us assume that there are n national health systems each using varying amounts of m different health system inputs to produce s different outputs. Specifically, NHS_j $(j = 1,...,n)$ uses amounts $x_i (i = 1,2,...,m)$ of input and produces amounts $y_r (r = 1,2,...,s)$ of output. The relative efficiency (Θ_j) of jth NHS can be evaluated by solving the following DEA-BCC output-oriented model [13]:

$$Max: \Theta` + \varepsilon \sum_r s_r^+ + \varepsilon \sum_i s_i^- \qquad (4)$$

$$subject\ to: \quad \Theta_{y^o} - \sum_{r=1}^{s} y_{rj}\lambda_j + s_r^+ = 0$$

$$x_{i^o} = \sum_{j=1}^{n} x_{ij}\lambda_j + s_i^-$$

$$\sum_{j=1}^{J} \lambda_j = 1$$

$$\lambda_j, s_r^+, s_i^- \geq 0.$$

where: Θ is the efficiency score value; y_r = observed quantity of output r; x_i = observed quantity of input i; s_i^-; s_r^+; and λ_j.

The first constraint indicates that all observed input combinations for j^{th} NHS lie on or below the production frontier. The second constraint signifies that the output levels of inefficient observations are compared to the output levels of a reference DMU that is composed of a convex combination of observed outputs. The third constraint ensures that all values of the production convexity weights are greater than or equal to zero so that the hypothetical reference DMU is within the possibility set. The last constraint allows for variable returns to scale. If the analysis reveals that: *(a)* $\Theta < 1$, then NHS_j is deemed to be inefficient; *(b)* $\Theta = 1$, $s_i^- \neq 0$, and $s_r^+ \neq 0$ then NHS_j is radial efficient; and *(c)* $\Theta = 1$, $s_i^- = 0$, and $s_r^+ = 0$ then NHS_j is BCC efficient or Pareto-Koopmans efficient.

Malmquist Total Factor Productivity Index

We have used the DEA-based Malmquist total factor productivity (MTFP) index [14,15] to measure changes in total output of relative to inputs. The output-oriented MTFP index can be formulated as the geometric mean of productivity indices of two periods $t, t+1$, and subsequently decomposed into various sources of productivity change as follows [8]:

$$MTFP_o^{t+1}\left(x^t, y^t, x^{t+1}, y^{t+1}\right) = \left[\frac{D_o^{t+1}\left(x^{t+1}, y^{t+1}\right)}{D_o^t\left(x^t, y^t\right)}\right] \times$$

$$\left[\frac{D_o^t\left(x^{t+1}, y^{t+1}\right)}{D_o^{t+1}\left(x^{t+1}, y^{t+1}\right)} \times \frac{D_o^t\left(x^t, y^t\right)}{D_o^{t+1}\left(x^t, y^t\right)}\right]^{\frac{1}{2}} \tag{5}$$

$$\text{Efficiency change (EFFCH)} = \left[\frac{D_0^{t+1}(x^{t+1}, y^{t+1})}{D_0^t(x^t, y^t)}\right]$$

$$\text{Technical change (TECH)} = \left[\frac{D_0^t(x^{t+1}, y^{t+1})}{D_0^{t+1}(x^{t+1}, y^{t+1})} \times \frac{D_0^t(x^t, y^t)}{D_0^{t+1}(x^t, y^t)}\right]^{\frac{1}{2}}$$

where $D_o^t\left(D_o^{t+1}\right)$ represents the distance function relative to the CRS frontier at time t ($t+1$); x^t and y^t (x^{t+1} and y^{t+1}) are the input and output vectors at time t ($t+1$). Therefore, the MTFP is a product of efficiency change (EFFCH) and technical change (TECH). In turn EFFCH is a product of pure efficiency change (PECH) and scale change (SECH). The MTFP attains a value greater than, equal to, or less than unity if a firm (NHS) has experienced productivity growth, stagnation, or productivity decline net of the contribution of scale economies between periods t and $t+1$ [16].

Data

Variables

The unit of analysis in this study was a country NHS, that is the decision-making unit (DMU). The country health system DEA model had a total of four variables including two ultimate outputs (or outcomes) and two inputs. The two outputs for each individual country NHS were life expectancy at birth (in years) for males and life expectancy at birth (in years) for females. The input variables included per capita total health expenditure (international dollars) and adult literacy rate as the percentage of people aged 15 years and above who can, with understanding, both read and write a short, simple statement about their everyday life out of the whole population of ages 15 and older [17]. The choice of outputs and input variables was guided by past studies [9,10,11] and availability of data from secondary sources mentioned below. Inclusion of adult literacy as an input acknowledges that levels of life expectancy are not solely affected by health systems [9].

Data sources

The male and female life expectancies data used in this paper were obtained from the tabular annexes of the World Health Reports [2,18-22]. Information on per capita total health expenditures for the years 1999 to 2003 was extracted from the *World Health Report 2006* [23]. The above-mentioned reports contain data for all the 53 countries in the African continent. The adult literacy data were obtained from the United Nations Development Programme Human Development reports [24-28].

Analysis

The technical efficiency scores and the MTFP indices were estimated using the data envelopment analysis programme called DEAP Version 2.1 [29]. Firstly, in order to assess technical efficiency of National Health Systems (NHSs) of African continent countries for producing male and female life expectancies, equation (4) was estimated for each of the five years separately. This provides the technical efficiency trend for each of the NHSs. Secondly, to assess changes in health productivity over time equation (5) was estimated with the combined data set for the five years. The year 1999 was used as the year of comparison. The latter estimation yielded the efficiency change, technical change, pure efficiency change, scale efficiency change, and MFTP scores.

Limitations of the study

The reader should refer to Anand *et al.* [30], Hollingsworth and Wildman [31], and Richardson *et al* [32] for a detailed critique of health system performance evaluations, functional specifications, choice of variables, and quality of data. Thus, in this section we provide an overview of some of the limitations that the reader should be aware about.

Variables

1. The use of male and female life expectancies as NHSs outcome indicators ignores the multi-dimensional health-related quality of life aspect. In addition, not all changes in life expectancy are attributable to existence and functionality of NHSs [31].

2. Adult literacy may be an inadequate proxy for the many non-health systems related factors that influence health outcomes.

3. The per capita total health expenditure input variable says nothing about the available quantity and quality of health system inputs.

Data

1. The vital registration systems of births and deaths in majority of the African countries are weak and as a result many births and deaths that occur outside the healthcare system may not be captured. Therefore, critiques may question the accuracy and reliability of the life expectancy data reported in the World Health reports and which we used in our analysis [30].

2. Many countries in the continent have never undertaken national health accounts. Thus, per capital total health expenditure data for African countries reported in the World Health Report are estimates. We do not know the magnitudes of the measurement errors inherent in the data. Anand *et al.* [30, p.850] questioned the NHA estimates "on the basis that the quality, validity and reliability of the data available in the countries is variable and frequently poor".

3. Due to lack of elaborate population-based surveys for ascertaining the adult literacy levels, it is difficult to know the level of precision of the estimates reported in UNDP human development reports and other sources.

Weaknesses of DEA

1. DEA is non-stochastic. It does not capture random noise (e.g., epidemics, weather, strikes, civil war, etc). Any deviation from the estimated frontier is interpreted as being due to inefficiency [12].

2. DEA is non-statistical in the sense that it is not possible to conduct statistical tests of hypothesis regarding the inefficiency and the structure of the production technology [12].

3. DEA is good at estimating "relative" efficiency of a DMU but it converges very slowly to "absolute" efficiency. In other words, it can tell you how well you are doing compared to your peers but not compared to a "theoretical maximum" [33].

4. Since a standard formulation of DEA creates a separate linear programme for each DMU, large problems can be computationally intensive [33].

5. The study does not capture the time lags that exist between public health investments and the production of health outcomes [30].

RESULTS AND DISCUSSION

Appendix 17.1 presents descriptive statistics (mean, median, standard deviation, maximum value, minimum value) of the health outcomes, the per capita total health expenditure, and adult literacy rate. The average male life expectancy increased marginally from 49 years in 1999 to 50 years in 2003. The average female life expectancy grew from 51 years in 1999 to 53 years in 2003. The per capita total health expenditure increased from 109 international dollars in 1999 to 129 international dollars in 2003. The median adult literacy rate increased from 59% in 1999 to 64% in 2003. As indicated by the standard deviations and the range, there were large variations in both the health outcomes and the two inputs across the countries.

Technical Efficiency

Figure 17.2 portrays the frequency (and percentage) distribution of constant returns to scale technical efficiency scores for the national health systems on the African continent during 1999-2003.

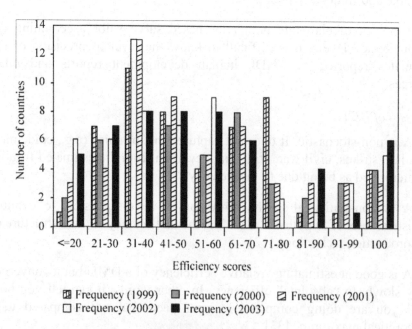

Figure 17.2   Frequency distribution of technical efficiency scores of national health systems in Africa (1999-2003)

Appendix 17.2 presents the individual NHS technical efficiency scores during the five years. As can be seen in the table, out of the 53 countries, only 4 (7.5%) NHSs had a technical efficiency of unity in years 1999 and 2000; 3 (5.7%) in year 2001; 5 (9.4%) in year 2002; and 6 (11.3%) in year 2003. Values of unity imply that the NHS was on the population frontier (or technically efficient) in the associated year. The DEA revealed that the NHSs of 49 (92.5%) countries were run inefficiently in 1999 and 2000; 50 (94.3%), 48 (90.6%), and 47 (88.7%) were operated inefficiently in 2001, 2002 and 2003, respectively. The average CRS technical efficiency scores were 54.6% (STDEV=22.9%) in 1999, 53.5% (STDEV=24.2%) in 2000, 58.8% (STDEV=23.5%) in 2001, 53.1% (STDEV=25.3%) in 2002, and 52.1% (STDEV=26.0%) in 2003. These findings imply that if the NHSs were operating efficiently during the period covered they could, on average, have produced 45.4%, 46.5%, 41.2%, 46.9%, and 47.9% more outputs (male and female life expectancies) respectively using their existing levels of input endowment.

Productivity Growth

In the application of the Malmquist total factor productivity (MTFP) index to analyse the temporal differences in productivity, the year 1999 has been taken as the technology reference. The reader will recall that if the value of the Malmquist index or any of its components is less than one, it denotes regress or deterioration in performance whereas values greater than one denote improvement in the relevant performance.

Appendix 17.3 presents the MTFP index summary of annual geometric means. In the last row (last column), we observe that, on average, the total factor productivity increased by 40.1% [= (1.401-1) × 100] over the 1999-2003 period for the African countries' national health systems. On average, that growth was due to technology change (innovation) rather than improvements in efficiency. Whereas efficiency deteriorated by 0.50%, technical change (innovation) grew by 40.9% per annum. The efficiency change was attributed entirely to the pure efficiency decline of 0.50%; the scale efficiency change was, on average, stagnant. The total factor productivity change was highest in 2000 (MTFP=1.738) and lowest in 2003 (MTFP=1.220).

We now turn to an examination of the magnitude and sources of productivity change within each country's NHS. Appendix 17.4 provides a summary of the average annual values of the MTFP index and its components for each country's NHS. All the 53 national health systems registered improvements in total factor productivity since they had MTFP indices of greater than one. The average MTFP index for all the countries was 1.406 (STDEV=0.111); the median was 1.432; and the range was 0.41. Uganda experienced the least total factor productivity growth of 15.9% and Angola registered the highest growth of 56.9%. Eleven countries (Angola, Botswana, Burundi, Cameroon, Central African Republic, Chad, Cote d'Ivoire, Democratic Republic of Congo, Equatorial Guinea, Gambia, Lesotho) experienced TFP growth of 50% and above.

On the other hand, Angola, Lesotho, and Botswana had the highest TFP growth of 56.9%, 54.4%, and 52.8% respectively. From an analysis of the decomposition of the MTFP, the productivity growth in Botswana and Lesotho was brought about by a combination of technological improvements of 48.9% and 47.5% respectively and improvements in efficiency of 2.6% and 4.7% respectively. On the other hand, Uganda, Tunisia, and Zambia displayed the lowest MTFP growth of 15.9%, 18.7%, and 18.6% respectively. The three countries experienced an efficiency decline of 4.7%, 3.1%, and 1.8% and a technical progress of 21.6%, 22.5%, and 20.8% respectively.

Pure Efficiency Change

The efficiency change component of the MTFP provides a measure of the contribution to productivity change of a change in technical efficiency between years t (1999 in our case) and $t+1$ (years 2000, 2001, 2002, and 2003). Efficiency change is a product of pure efficiency change (PEFFCH) and scale efficiency change (SCH) [8]. The PEFFCH index is greater than, equal to, or less than unity if the relative technical efficiency of a country's NHS (firm) has increased, remained the same, or decreased between time periods t and $t+1$.

The national health systems of twenty (37.7%) countries attained a PEFFCH index value of greater than one implying that their pure efficiency increased and contributed positively to productivity change. Kenya, Somalia and Zimbabwe were the only countries with a pure efficiency score of one (100%) which means their NHS pure efficiency of production remained constant and did not contribute at all to productivity change. The NHSs of thirty (56.6%) countries had a PEFFCH index of less than one signifying that those countries' NHSs production contributed negatively to productivity change. Swaziland had a PEFFCH score of 1.061, which meant that the pure efficiency of its NHS increased by 6.1% per annum; it was the highest in the African continent. The average PEFFCH score was 0.995 (STDEV=0.025) implying that the pure efficiency of production, on average, contributed negatively to efficiency change by 0.5%.

Scale Efficiency Change

The scale efficiency change index attains a value greater than, equal to, or less than unity if a country's national health system's (firm's) scale of production contributes positively, not at all, or negatively to productivity change [16]. Fifty-two (98.1%) countries' national health systems attained a scale index value of one implying that their NHS scale efficiency of production did not contribute at all to productivity change. Zimbabwe was the only country with a scale efficiency score of slightly greater than one implying that her scale of production had a small positive contribution to productivity change.

Technical Change

The second component of the MTFP provides a measure of the contribution to productivity change of whatever technical change (innovative) occurred between 1999 and 2000, 2001, 2002, and 2003. This index attains a value of greater than, equal to, or less than one if technical progress, stagnation, or technical regress had occurred along a ray through a NHS's data between 1999 and 2000, 2001, 2002 and 2003. All the 53 countries' national health systems had technical change index greater than one, which means that they all experienced technical progress. The average technical change score was 1.413 (STDEV=0.102) indicating about 41.3% technical progress. Zimbabwe had the least technical change of 1.206 implying a technical progress of 20.6%. The NHSs of Angola, Cape Verde, DRC, Djibouti, and Gambia registered the highest technical change of 1.495 and above (i.e., a technical progress of 49.5% and above). In terms of distribution, 12 (22.6%) countries experienced a technical growth of between 20% and 30%; 5 (9.4%) countries a technical growth of between 31% and 40%; and 36 (67.9%) countries a technical growth of over 41%.

CONCLUSION

This study assessed the technical efficiency of NHSs of countries on the African continent for producing male and female life expectancies and the changes in health productivity over time with a view to analysing changes in efficiency and changes in technology. The findings indicate that NHSs of 49 (92.5%) countries were run inefficiently in 1999 and 2000; 50 (94.3%) were operated inefficiently in 2001; 48 (90.6%) ran inefficiently in 2002; and 47 (88.7%) operated inefficiently during 2003. All the 53 countries' national health systems registered improvements in total factor productivity attributable mainly to technical progress. Fifty-two countries did not experience any change in scale efficiency. Thirty (56.6%) countries' national health systems had a PEFFCH index of less than one signifying that those countries' NHSs pure efficiency contributed negatively to productivity change.

African countries may need to critically evaluate the utility of institutionalising the Malmquist TFP type of analyses to monitor the changes in health systems economic efficiency and productivity over time. If they decide to institutionalise these kinds of analyses, it would be necessary to strengthen the national and district health management information systems to routinely capture the input, input prices, and output data.

ACKNOWLEDGEMENTS

We are immensely grateful to Jehovah Jireh for [His] multifaceted support at all stages of preparing this manuscript; to Mr. A Kochar for editorial help and the anonymous reviewers of OSSREA for their suggestions and comments.

The manuscript contains the analyses and views of the authors only and does not represent the decisions or stated policies of the institutions they work for.

REFERENCES

1. Murray CJL, Frenk J. A framework for assessing the performance of health systems. *Bulletin of the World Health Organization* 2000;78(6):717-731.

2. World Health Organization. *The world health report 2000 – improving performance of health systems.* Geneva: World Health Organization; 2000.

3. World Health Organization Regional Office for Africa. *Fifty-fifth WHO Regional Committee for Africa final report.* Brazzaville: WHO/AFRO; 2005.

4. African Union. *Universal access to HIV/AIDS, tuberculosis and malaria services by a united Africa by 2010.* Resolution Sp/Assembly/ATM/5(I) Rev. 3 of the Ministers of Health on health financing in Africa. Addis Ababa: African Union; 2006.

5. United Nations. *Millennium Development Declaration. Resolution A/55/L.2.* New York: United Nations; 2000.

6. World Health Organization. *The world health report 2006: Working together for health.* Geneva: World Health Organization; 2006.

7. Zere EA, Addison T, McIntyre D. Hospital efficiency in sub-Saharan Africa: Evidence from South Africa. *South African Journal of Economics* 2000; 69(2):336-358.

8. Fare R, Grosskopf S, Norris M, Zhang Z. Productivity growth, technical progress, and efficiency change in industrialized countries. *The American Economic Review* 1994; 84(1):66-83.

9. Evans DB, Tandon A, Murray CJL, Lauer JA. Comparative efficiency of national health systems: cross national econometric analysis. *British Medical Journal* 2001;323:307-310.

10. Tandon A, Lauer JA, Evans DB, Murray CJL. Health systems efficiency: concepts. In: Murray CJL, Evans DB, editors. *Health systems performance assessment: debates, methods and empiricism.* Geneva: World Health Organization; 2003. p 683-691.

11. Evans DB, Lauer JA, Tandon A, Murray CJL. Determinants of health system performance: second-stage efficiency analysis. In: Murray CJL , Evans DB, editors. *Health systems performance assessment: debates, methods and empiricism.* Geneva: World Health Organization; 2003. p 693-703.

12. Coelli T, Rao DSP, Battese G. *An introduction to efficiency and productivity analysis.* Boston: Kluwer Academic Publishers; 1998.

13. Banker RD, Charness A, Cooper WW. Some models for estimating technical and scale inefficiencies in data envelopment analysis. *Management Science* 1984;30(1):1078-1092.

14. Malmquist S. Index numbers and indifference curves. *Trabajos de Estatistica* 1953; 4(1):209-42.

15. Caves DW, Christensen LR, Diewert WE. The economic theory of index numbers and measurement of input, output and productivity. *Econometrica* 1982;50(6):1393-1414.

16. Grifell-Tatje E, Lovell CAK. The sources of productivity change in Spanish banking. *European Journal of Operational Research* 1997;98(2):364-380.

17. World Bank. GenderStats database of gender statistics. Available at: http://devdata.worldbank.org, accessed 2 May, 2007.

18. World Health Organization. *The world health report 2001: Mental health: new understanding, new hope.* Geneva: World Health Organization; 2001.

19. World Health Organization. *The world health report 2002: Reducing health risks, promoting healthy life.* Geneva: World Health Organization; 2002.

20. World Health Organization. *The world health report 2003: Shaping the future.* Geneva: World Health Organization; 2003.

21. World Health Organization. *The world health report 2004: Changing history.* Geneva: World Health Organization; 2004.

22. World Health Organization. *The world health report 2005: Make every mother and child count.* Geneva: World Health Organization; 2005.

23. World Health Organization. *The world health report 2006: working together for health.* Geneva: World Health Organization; 2006.

24. United Nations Development Programme. *Human development report 2001.* New York: Oxford University Press; 2001.

25. United Nations Development Programme. *Human development report 2002.* New York: Oxford University Press; 2002.

26. United Nations Development Programme. *Human development report 2003.* New York: Oxford University Press; 2003.

27. United Nations Development Programme. *Human development report 2004.* New York: Oxford University Press; 2004.

28. United Nations Development Programme. *Human development report 2005.* New York: Oxford University Press; 2005.

29. Coelli TJ: *A guide to DEAP version 2.1: a data envelopment analysis [computer] program,* Centre for Efficiency and Productivity Analysis (CEPA) Working Paper 96/08. Department of Econometrics, University of New England, Armidale, NSW Australia; 1996.

30. Anand S, Ammar W, Evans T, Hasegawa T, Kissomova-Skarbek K, Langer A, Lucas AO, Makubalo L, Marandi A, Meyer G, Podger A, Smith P, Wibulpolprasert S. Report of the scientific peer review group on health systems performance assessment. In: Murray CJL, Evans DB, editors. *Health*

   systems performance assessment: debates, methods and empiricism. Geneva: World Health Organization; 2003. p 839-913.

31. Hollingsworth B, Wildman J. The efficiency of health production: re-estimating the WHO panel data using parametric and non-parametric approaches to provide additional information. *Health Economics* 2003;12:493-504.

32. Richardson J, Wildman J, Robertson IK. A critique of the World Health Organization's evaluation of health systems performance. *Health Economics* 2003; 12:355-366.

33. Anderson T: Data Envelopment Analysis Home Page http://www.emp.pdx.edu/dea/homedea.html.

34. Charnes A, Cooper WW, Rhodes E. Measuring efficiency of decision-making units. *European Journal of Operational Research* 1978; 2(6):429-444.

35. World Health Organization Regional Office for Africa. 2006. *Health financing: a strategy for the African Region.* Document AFR/RC56/10. Brazzaville: World Health Organization Regional Office for Africa.

Appendix 17.1   Descriptive statistics of health outcome, per capita health expenditure and adult literacy rate by year

Year	Male life expectancy	Female life expectancy	Per capita total health expenditure (in purchasing power parity)	Adult literacy rate
1999				
Mean	49	51	109	59
Median	47	48	55	60
STD	9	10	128	19
Max.	68	74	595	88
Min.	33	35	12	15
2000				
Mean	50	52	110	60
Median	48	50	50	61
STD	9	10	130	19
Max.	69	75	579	89
Min.	37	38	13	16
2001				
Mean	50	52	120	60
Median	48	50	55	63
STD	10	11	139	19
Max.	69	77	626	91
Min.	33	36	10	17
2002				
Mean	50	53	125	60
Median	48	51	55	63
STD	10	11	142	20
Max.	70	77	649	92
Min.	32	36	11	13
2003				
Mean	50	53	129	59
Median	48	50	59	64
STD	10	11	150	20
Max.	71	77	669	92
Min.	33	36	14	13

Appendix 17.2   Distribution of technical efficiency scores of national health systems in Africa: 1999-2003

DMUs	CRSTE (1999)	CRSTE (2000)	CRSTE (2001)	CRSTE (2002)	CRSTE (2003)
Algeria	0.421	0.387	0.401	0.377	0.346
Angola	0.622	0.675	0.437	0.567	0.393
Benin	0.799	0.781	0.731	0.772	0.841
Botswana	0.213	0.215	0.198	0.171	0.140
Burkina Faso	0.789	0.664	0.670	1	1
Burundi	1	1	0.856	0.944	0.953
Cameroon	0.415	0.409	0.407	0.411	0.399
Cape Verde	0.368	0.355	0.367	0.351	0.329
CAR	0.551	0.446	0.47	0.485	0.491
Chad	0.697	0.637	0.606	0.617	0.665
Comoros	0.754	0.886	1	1	1
Congo	0.716	0.833	0.707	0.794	0.831
Côte d'Ivoire	0.425	0.375	0.413	0.461	0.505
DRC	1	1	1	1	1
Djibouti	0.411	0.361	0.409	0.425	0.441
Egypt	0.484	0.453	0.462	0.394	0.371
Equatorial Guinea	0.282	0.288	0.250	0.243	0.216
Eritrea	0.531	0.515	0.530	0.626	0.619
Ethiopia	0.952	0.919	0.931	1	1
Gabon	0.356	0.290	0.325	0.291	0.264
Gambia	0.645	0.581	0.616	0.586	0.529
Ghana	0.362	0.316	0.357	0.372	0.427
Guinea	0.543	0.459	0.501	0.494	0.446
Guinea-Bissau	0.619	0.625	0.661	0.591	0.615
Kenya	0.380	0.378	0.381	0.403	0.406
Lesotho	0.288	0.232	0.226	0.192	0.231
Liberia	0.846	0.929	0.955	0.971	1
Libya	0.338	0.321	0.346	0.287	0.283
Madagascar	0.762	0.924	0.883	0.882	0.870
Malawi	0.399	0.421	0.372	0.463	0.426
Mali	0.728	0.651	0.806	0.938	0.859
Mauritania	0.79	0.793	0.714	0.618	0.521
Mauritius	0.332	0.32	0.337	0.272	0.254
Morocco	0.557	0.521	0.547	0.46	0.429
Mozambique	0.624	0.487	0.584	0.539	0.545
Namibia	0.219	0.194	0.23	0.198	0.187
Niger	1	1	1	1	1
Nigeria	0.481	0.57	0.501	0.507	0.435
Rwanda	0.498	0.491	0.508	0.568	0.556
STP	0.399	0.379	0.346	0.389	0.369
Senegal	0.756	0.667	0.644	0.64	0.635
Seychelles	0.303	0.305	0.321	0.252	0.233
Sierra Leone	0.774	0.716	0.651	0.599	0.664
Somalia	1	1	0.975	0.599	0.653
South Africa	0.229	0.221	0.224	0.184	0.169

.../cont.

Appendix 17.2 (cont.)

DMUs	CRSTE (1999)	CRSTE (2000)	CRSTE (2001)	CRSTE (2002)	CRSTE (2003)
Sudan	0.61	0.649	0.616	0.647	0.594
Swaziland	0.239	0.209	0.197	0.162	0.137
Togo	0.482	0.524	0.478	0.533	0.509
Tunisia	0.394	0.374	0.389	0.303	0.277
Uganda	0.393	0.369	0.361	0.388	0.376
Tanzania	0.637	0.666	0.584	0.637	0.603
Zambia	0.356	0.375	0.332	0.368	0.374
Zimbabwe	0.191	0.191	0.164	0.166	0.181
Mean	**0.546**	**0.535**	**0.528**	**0.531**	**0.521**
Median	**0.498**	**0.487**	**0.478**	**0.494**	**0.446**
STDEV	**0.229**	**0.242**	**0.235**	**0.253**	**0.260**
Max.	**1.000**	**1.000**	**1.000**	**1.000**	**1.000**
Min.	**0.191**	**0.191**	**0.164**	**0.162**	**0.137**

Appendix 17.3   Malmquist index summary of annual means (input oriented)

Year	Efficiency change (A = C × D)	Technical change (B)	Pure efficiency change (C)	Scale efficiency Change (D=A/C)	Malmquist index or total factor productivity change (E = A × B)
2000	1.065	1.632	1.067	0.998	1.738
2001	0.924	1.544	0.922	1.002	1.426
2002	0.988	1.29	0.988	1	1.275
2003	1.006	1.213	1.006	1	1.220
Median	**0.997**	**1.417**	**0.997**	**1**	**1.351**
Mean	**0.995**	**1.409**	**0.995**	**1**	**1.401**

Appendix 17.4   Malmquist index summary of annual means (input-oriented)

Decision-making unit	Efficiency Change (A=C × D)	Technical change (B)	Pure efficiency change (C)	Scale efficiency change (D=A/C)	Malmquist index or total factor productivity change (E=A × B)
Algeria	0.993	1.494	0.993	1	1.484
Angola	1.048	1.497	1.048	1	1.569
Benin	1.001	1.490	1.001	1	1.491
Botswana	1.026	1.489	1.026	1	1.528
Burkina Faso	1.003	1.488	1.003	1	1.492
Burundi	1.005	1.500	1.005	1	1.508
Cameroon	1.025	1.488	1.025	1	1.524
Cape Verde	0.988	1.497	0.988	1	1.48
CAR	1.015	1.488	1.015	1	1.511
Chad	1.020	1.493	1.02	1	1.523
Comoros	0.973	1.494	0.973	1	1.453
Congo	1.005	1.491	1.005	1	1.498
Côte d'Ivoire	1.018	1.489	1.018	1	1.516
DRC	1.008	1.495	1.008	1	1.506
Djibouti	0.951	1.495	0.951	1	1.421
Egypt	0.992	1.491	0.992	1	1.48
Equatorial Guinea	1.017	1.487	1.017	1	1.513
Eritrea	0.938	1.492	0.938	1	1.400
Ethiopia	0.963	1.491	0.963	1	1.435
Gabon	0.994	1.487	0.994	1	1.478
Gambia	1.004	1.495	1.004	1	1.501
Ghana	0.985	1.49	0.985	1	1.468
Guinea	0.984	1.488	0.984	1	1.465
Guinea-Bissau	0.999	1.486	0.999	1	1.484
Kenya	1	1.483	1	1	1.483
Lesotho	1.047	1.475	1.047	1	1.544
Liberia	1.015	1.475	1.015	1	1.497
Libya	0.973	1.472	0.973	1	1.432
Madagascar	0.952	1.458	0.952	1	1.388
Malawi	0.982	1.453	0.982	1	1.426
Mali	0.993	1.442	0.993	1	1.432
Mauritania	1.006	1.433	1.006	1	1.442
Mauritius	0.990	1.425	0.990	1	1.411
Morocco	0.982	1.419	0.982	1	1.394
Mozambique	0.993	1.408	0.993	1	1.398
Namibia	0.953	1.408	0.953	1	1.342
Niger	0.996	1.383	0.996	1	1.378
Nigeria	1.016	1.377	1.016	1	1.399
Rwanda	0.983	1.355	0.983	1	1.333
STP	1.024	1.351	1.024	1	1.384

.../cont.

Appendix 17.4 (cont.)

Decision-making unit	Efficiency change (A = C × D)	Technical change (B)	Pure efficiency change (C)	Scale efficiency change (D=A/C)	Malmquist index or total factor productivity change (E = A × B)
Senegal	1.001	1.328	1.001	1	1.329
Seychelles	0.991	1.297	0.991	1	1.285
Sierra Leone	0.980	1.287	0.980	1	1.261
Somalia	1	1.287	1	1	1.286
South Africa	0.997	1.266	0.997	1	1.262
Sudan	0.965	1.258	0.965	1	1.214
Swaziland	1.061	1.251	1.061	1	1.327
Togo	0.978	1.233	0.978	1	1.206
Tunisia	0.969	1.225	0.969	1	1.187
Uganda	0.953	1.216	0.953	1	1.159
Tanzania	0.989	1.205	0.989	1	1.192
Zambia	0.982	1.208	0.982	1	1.186
Zimbabwe	1.002	1.206	1	1.002	1.207
Mean	**0.995**	**1.413**	**0.995**	**1.000**	**1.406**
Median	**0.994**	**1.475**	**0.994**	**1**	**1.432**
STD	**0.025**	**0.102**	**0.025**	**0.000**	**0.111**
Max.	**1.061**	**1.500**	**1.061**	**1.002**	**1.569**
Min.	**0.938**	**1.205**	**0.938**	**1**	**1.159**

Note: Note that all Malmquist index averages are geometric means.

Part III

Case Studies for Developing Skills in Economic Efficiency Analysis

Learning Objectives

By the end of Part 3 you should have developed skills for:

1. Measuring and interpreting technical efficiency scores of health system decision-making units.

2. Measuring and interpreting total cost efficiency or economic efficiency scores of health system decision-making units.

3. Measuring and interpreting the Malmquist total factor productivity indices of health system decision-making units.

-18-

Technical Efficiency Analysis: *A Case Study of Muthuleni Health Centres*

Joses M. Kirigia

BACKGROUND

The Government of Muthuleni, through the Ministry of Health, finances 85 per cent of the annual total health expenditure of M$300 million and provides 75 per cent of the country's health services. The fixed public health facilities (i.e., hospitals, health centres, and dispensaries) consume 90 per cent of the recurrent yearly health budget. Competing demands for exchequer funds from the various social sectors such as education, water, housing, and sanitation and pressure from the World Bank and the International Monetary Fund (IMF) have led to implementation of many healthcare reforms in Muthuleni State. Some of the reforms concern out-of-pocket payments, service contracting, and decentralisation. Unfortunately, implementation of the reforms was not preceded by gathering of baseline data against which to monitor and evaluate their effect nor was it followed by economic analyses of how efficiently the resource endowment was used to realise the goals of equitable and sustainable improvement of access to quality health service and, ultimately, the citizens' health needs.

Although fixed health facilities consume a substantive portion of the national budget, no study has been conducted to assess their efficiency. Due to the negative effects of out-of-pocket payments on access to and equity of health services, the Muthuleni government is considering the termination of some of the reforms and instead explore whether the current resource endowment could be stretched to cater for the healthcare needs of more citizens. For this reason, Professor Lenity Muthongi, Minister for Health, decided to constitute a team of experts to analyse the efficiency of the 32 health centres in Muthuleni. The team consisted of Professor Josphat Aburi, a seasoned health economist;

Professor Phineas Nkanata, the Director of Medical Services; Dr Rose-Nabi Mwaana, a provincial medical officer of health, and Dr Gakii Athamba, a district medical officer.

The Minister for Health, who is also a leading African public health and health economics specialist, formulated the specific questions that the efficiency team needed to address as follows:

1. What are the constant, variable, and scale technical efficiency scores for each of the 32 primary health centres?

2. What input or output levels are needed to turn around inefficient health centres to become efficient in delivering health services?

3. What course of action should healthcare policy makers and managers take to improve efficiency of the inefficient health centres?

INPUT AND OUTPUT DATA

Inputs

After reviewing literature on the economics of health centres, the team concluded that health centres have mainly three categories of inputs: labour, supplies (including pharmaceutical and non-pharmaceutical provisions), and capital goods (such as equipment, vehicles, and building space). Interactive interviews with technical people at the Ministry of Health headquarters and in a sample of health centres indicated that it would be very difficult to obtain information on physical quantities of pharmaceutical and non-pharmaceutical supplies or capital items. However, information was available on personnel, beds, and aggregated non-wage recurrent expenditure. The study team discussed this matter with the Minister for Health and agreed that the team would gather data on the following inputs:

1. Input 1: Number of clinical officers, nurses, community health workers, laboratory technicians, and public health technicians

2. Input 2: Number of administrative and support staff

3. Input 3: Number of beds

4. Input 4: Non-wage recurrent expenditure in Muthuleni dollars (Appendix 18.1).

Proxy Outputs

In order to identify the key outputs of the health centres, the study team reviewed both internationally published and grey literature on efficiency of health centres and the health service records at three health centres and held interactive discussions with the staff in charge of the three health centres. In close consultation with the Minister for Health, the team concluded that outputs of health centres could be grouped into four main types as follows:

1. Output 1: Number of visits for diarrhoea, malaria, sexually transmitted infections, urinary tract infections, intestinal worms, and respiratory diseases plus other general curative outpatient conditions

2. Output 2: Antenatal and postnatal care visits

3. Output 3: Immunisation visits

4. Output 4: Family planning attendances (Appendix 18.1)

CONSENSUS BUILDING MEETING WITH STAKEHOLDERS

The study team held a meeting with the Minister for Health; permanent secretaries of the ministries of health, economic planning, and finance; chairperson of Muthuleni Medical Association; chairperson of Muthuleni Nursing and Allied Professionals Association; a representative of the civil societies in Muthuleni; a representative of the faiths-based Health Services Association; a representative of the private sector Health Services Association; a World Health Organization country representative; social sector focal persons from the World Bank and the IMF country offices; and sectoral officers from bilateral donors represented in the country.

The team took the opportunity to define the concepts of efficiency, to build consensus on the inputs and outputs of the health centres that they were going to assess, and to agree on the research proposal and the questionnaire. All the stakeholders were very supportive of the study. The donors represented at the meeting made financial commitments for the study in addition to committing themselves to support the Government of Muthuleni in implementing the recommendations emanating from the study.

After the meeting, the team revised the research proposal and data collection instruments and submitted them to the National Scientific and Ethical Review Committee (SERC). After about a week the team received clearance from SERC. The team then immediately submitted to the Office of the President the research proposal, the clearance letter from SERC, a supporting letter from the Minister of Health emphasising the importance of the study to government efforts to monitor and improve efficiency in the allocation and use of the scarce resources, and duly completed research permit application forms. The team was granted the research permit from the Office of the President within a week.

SAMPLING AND DATA COLLECTION

The Minister for Health made it very clear to the study team that she wanted technical efficiency scores of every individual unit in the entire population of health centres. Thus, there was no need to sample the health centres. Discussions with the Director of Health Management Information Systems (HMIS) at the Ministry of Health revealed that the data available at the HMIS were unreliable. Thus, it became necessary for the team to gather data from the individual health centres. The team then took the following steps:

1. Pilot-testing of the questionnaire in three health centres and revising it accordingly,

2. Recruiting eight fresh graduates of Muthuleni National University as research assistants,

3. Holding intensive training for research assistants on research ethics, the questionnaire, possible sources of data, and the relevant people to interview at the individual health centres.

The four-member study team divided the health centres among themselves. Each principal investigator took two research assistants to the field to collect data. Owing to inaccessibility of some of the health centres, it took the study team two weeks to collect data from all the health facilities.

DATA ENTRY AND ANALYSIS PROCEDURE

Analysis using EMS software

The study team had the options of parametric econometric production frontier estimation methods and non-parametric mathematical programming methods such as data envelopment analysis. Since econometric approaches usually provide an average picture, Professor Aburi advised the team that these approaches could not answer the questions the study was meant to address. He instead recommended data envelopment analysis (DEA) because it has the ability to handle multiple inputs and outputs and would yield the information required by the Minister.

The team decided to use the free DEA software called EMS (Efficiency Measurement Systems) developed by Dr. Helger Scheel of Dortmund University in Germany. The strength of the software lies in the ability to handle multiple inputs and outputs. The EMS is a user-friendly, Windows-based software, and can be downloaded from the Internet. The study team followed the steps provided below in formatting the data to make it suitable for EMS.

1. Enter the data in Appendix 18.1 in an Excel spreadsheet by assigning the data to columns as follows:

a)   Column 1: Names of health centres

b)   Column 2: Input1{I} = Number of clinical officers, nurses, and other technical staff

c)   Column 3: Input2{I} = Number of administrative and support staff

d)   Column 4: Input3{I} = Number of beds per health centre

e)   Column 5: Input4{I} = Non-wage recurrent expenditure

f)   Column 6: Output1{O} = Number of curative visits

g)   Column 7: Output2{O} = Antenatal care visits

h)   Column 8: Output3{O} = Number of immunisation visits

i)   Column 9: Output4{O} = Number of family planning attendances

2.   Choose **Start**, **Program**, and **EMS**. This will open a window containing five items (File, Edit, DEA, Window, and Help) at the top right corner.

3.   Select **File** and then **Load Data**. You will be prompted to type Filename, e.g. C:\HEC\WHO8.XLS and to indicate file type e.g., Excel 5.0 (*.xls) or Text (*.txt). Lastly, at the EMS menu, select **Open**. If the data retrieval process has been successful, Input Output Data C:\HEC\WHO8.XLS will appear at the bottom left corner of the window.

4.   Select **DEA** and then choose **Run Model**. This will lead you to a window titled E Run Model Window. At the menu, select **Model**. The programme will take you to a window containing the attributes of structure with the options convex and non-convex models; returns to scale with the options Constant, Variable, Non-increasing, and Non-decreasing; distance with the choices of Radial or Additive; and orientation with Input and Output as the options. Once you have made your choices, select the **Start** icon for the model to run. In a few seconds EMS will produce a sheet containing the results, which will include:

a)   The DMU (health centre) name in column 1

b)   Efficiency score in column 2

c)   Input1{I} in column 3

d)   Input2{I} in column 4

e)   Input3{I} in column 5

f)   Input4{I} in column 6

g)   Output1{O} in column 7

h)   Output2{O} in column 8

    i)   Output3{O} in column 9

    j)   Output4{O} in column 10

    k)   Benchmarks in column 11

    l)   Slacks per input in columns 12 to 15

    m) Slacks per output in columns 16 to 19

5.   To obtain the total input reductions or output increases required to make inefficient health centres efficient, you should add the slacks across all the DMUs. If you are using the Excel software, simply go to the bottom of the column containing the slacks for a specific input and click on the summation sign (Σ). Note that some cells will be empty, so after clicking on Σ in the menu you will need to manually specify the range (e.g., =sum(P2:P56).

6.   Remember that scale efficiency score = CRS score $\div$ VRS score. Thus, to obtain scale efficiency scores you will need to run the EMS model twice (i.e., once using CRS and once using VRS model specifications).

7.   Summarise the VRS technical efficiency scores in Table 18.1.

8.   Summarise the scale efficiency scores in Table 18.2.

9.   Provide a summary of excess inputs and output deficits in Table 18.3.

10.   Next answer these two questions:

    a)   What course of action should the Minister for Health take to reduce the level of inefficiency in the use of various cadres of personnel, non-wage expenditures, and beds?

    b)   Would it be advisable for the Minister to work to increase outputs among the inefficient facilities? Provide justification for your answer.

Table 18.1 Summary of the health centres' technical efficiency scores

Technical efficiency score (%)	Frequency distribution (i.e., number of health centres per group)	Percentage distribution (%)
1–10		
1–20		
21–30		
31–40		
41–50		
51–60		
61–70		
71–80		
81–90		
91–99		
100		

Table 18.2 Summary of health centres' efficiency scores

Scale efficiency score (%)	Frequency distribution (i.e., number of health centres per group)	Percentage distribution (%)
1–10		
11–20		
21–30		
31–40		
41–50		
51–60		
61–70		
71–80		
81–90		
91–99		
100		

Table 18.3 Summary of excess inputs and output deficits

Variable	Excess inputs	Output deficits
Input 1		
Input 2		
Input 3		
Input 4		
Output 1		
Output 2		
Output 3		
Output 4		

Analysis using DEAP Version 2.1 software

The study team could also have used the free DEAP software developed by Professor Tim Coelli of the University of New Queensland, Australia. Assuming that the team chose to use DEAP, they would have followed the following steps:

1. Download the DEAP Version 2.1 software from http://www.uq.edu/economics/cepa/ deap.htm into a folder in your computer.

2. Enter data in Appendix 18.1 on Excel spreadsheet as follows:

    a) Column 1: Names of health centres

    b) Column 2: Output1{O} = Number of curative visits

    c) Column 3: Output2{O} = Antenatal care visits

    d) Column 4: Output3{O} = Number of immunisation visits

    e) Column 5: Output4{O} = Number of family planning attendances

    f) Column 6: Input1{I} = Number of clinical officers, nurses and other technical staff

    g) Column 7: Input2{I} = Number of administrative and support staff

    h) Column 8: Input3{I} = Number of beds per health centre

    i) Column 9: Input4{I} = Non-wage recurrent expenditure

    Note that unlike EMS, for DEAP you should first list all outputs and then inputs.

3. Using the computer mouse, copy only the data values of outputs and inputs without the names of health centres' outputs or inputs.

4. Choose **Start, Program, Accessories,** and then **Notepad** to open this software.

5. While in Notepad, choose **File** then **Open**. Browse for the folder in which you saved the DEAP software. Click on, for example, Eg1.dta file and open it. Delete the file contents, paste your data, and choose **Save**. The data once pasted on Notepad will appear like the contents of Appendix 18.2.

6. Choose **File** then **New**. Locate the DEAP instruction file called EG1.ins and open it. The contents of this file will appear as in Appendix 18.3. Modify the instruction file to reflect the data file name = eg1.dta; output file name = eg1.out; number of firms = 32; number of time periods = 1; number of outputs = 4; number of inputs = 4; model orientation = 0 (input oriented) or 1 (output oriented); type of model: 0 = CRS and 1 =

VRS; and type of model for cost efficiency. For technical efficiency estimation, the study team could have used 0 = DEA (MULTI-STAGE), 3 = DEA (1-STAGE) or 4 = DEA (2-STAGE). The DEA manual that comes with the software has more information.

7. Close Notepad and go to the folder where you saved the DEAP software. Locate and select the DEAP.EXE file.

8. The DEAP program will prompt you to enter the instruction filename. At the prompt, type EG1.INS. Within a few seconds the estimations will be processed and the output sent to your output file EG1.OUT.

9. Choose the EG1.OUT file and you will be prompted to indicate the software in which it should be opened. If you select, for example, Excel, the listing of your output will contain an efficiency summary (of firm efficiency, constant returns to scale technical efficiency, variable returns to scale technical efficiency, and scale efficiency); summaries of output slacks, input slacks, peers, peer weights, peer count, output targets, and input targets; and firm by firm results as shown in Appendix 18.4. Note that the figures in this case have been rearranged for clarity.

10. You can then answer questions (7) to (10) in the previous subsection under EMS software.

Appendix 18.1   Health centres' inputs and outputs in a hypothetical country called Muthuleni

Health centre	Curative visits	Antenatal care visits	Immunisation visits	Family planning attendances	Clinical officers + nurses + other technical staff	Administrative staff	Beds	Non-wage recurrent expenditure
Athi-River	8,744	1,333	6,271	858	8	8	5	667,867
Bissel	9,582	427	3,440	171	3	2	14	667,608
Enkorika	1,912	36	270	165	2	1	7	263,010
Githunguri	15,899	2,050	6,991	374	16	7	2	1,001,197
Isinya	4,564	260	978	289	17	11	24	607,150
Karuri	12,589	2,102	15,986	9,796	34	12	8	570,996
Kasigau	6,077	1,106	5,274	890	5	5	12	559,703
Kaviani	7,073	2,221	8,914	1,503	5	5	3	431,668
Kigumo	29,215	3,789	7,633	2,966	17	10	11	1,602,878
Kihara	21,070	1,287	2,371	940	13	8	6	588,704
Kitengela	16,690	2,420	762	1,327	21	9	10	1,718,539
Lari	27,784	3,105	6,253	1,559	14	7	6	967,426
Limuru	19,437	2,158	5,371	1,631	14	6	17	690,365
Lusigeti	10,516	1,362	3,084	1,609	8	5	7	715,336
Masii	8,726	1,848	5,716	2,578	10	5	5	590,359
Mbale	4,864	441	1,059	394	3	5	10	331,572
Mitaboni	7,249	1,324	6,151	1,591	3	5	3	495,147
Mpinzinyi	3,444	321	698	641	3	0	2	399,402
Muthetheni	5,090	750	6,288	19	2	3	5	477,953
Mwala	5,322	2,040	6,343	2,081	7	6	5	514,028
Mwatate	9,120	1,807	4,539	2,045	7	1	0	311,156
Namanga	8,532	447	3,276	1,156	9	5	27	782,663
Ndeiya	7,892	1,287	1,999	940	11	5	18	578,467
Ngewa	16,999	1,192	5,773	1,648	13	6	8	659,139
Ngong	5,508	698	548	586	17	7	20	762,693

.../cont.

Appendix 18.1 (cont.)

Health centre	Curative visits	Antenatal care visits	Immunisation visits	Family planning attendances	Clinical officers + nurses + other technical staff	Administrative staff	Beds	Non-wage recurrent expenditure
Nyanche	2,699	257	2,002	435	3	7	10	289,656
O-Rongai	5,271	1,337	3,798	1,059	14	5	11	728,622
Sagala	8,044	537	2,081	1,351	4	6	16	615,758
Simba	7,265	428	2,387	819	6	4	24	707,426
Thinu	6,634	700	3,710	2,447	4	4	4	377,819
Wangige	6,571	1,172	7,879	1,954	19	5	8	1,477,471
Wundanyi	10,506	2,477	4,414	2,810	11	6	35	336,784

Note: For DEAP, the output variables are listed first then the inputs.

Copy only the data, without the names of the health centres or the variables for pasting on Notepad.

Appendix 18.2   Listing of the data file EG4.DTA

8744	1333	6271	858	8	8	5	667867
9582	427	3440	171	3	2	14	667608
1912	36	270	165	2	1	7	263010
15899	2050	6991	374	16	7	2	1001197
4564	260	978	289	17	11	24	607150
12589	2102	15986	9796	34	12	8	570996
6077	1106	5274	890	5	5	12	559703
7073	2221	8914	1503	5	5	3	431668
29215	3789	7633	2966	17	10	11	1602878
21070	1287	2371	940	13	8	6	588704
16690	2420	762	1327	21	9	10	1718539
27784	3105	6253	1559	14	7	6	967426
19437	2158	5371	1631	14	6	17	690365
10516	1362	3084	1609	8	5	7	715336
8726	1848	5716	2578	10	5	5	590359
4864	441	1059	394	3	5	10	331572
7249	1324	6151	1591	3	5	3	495147
3444	321	698	641	3	0	2	399402
5090	750	6288	19	2	3	5	477953
5322	2040	6343	2081	7	6	5	514028
9120	1807	4539	2045	7	1	0	311156
8532	447	3276	1156	9	5	27	782663
7892	1287	1999	940	11	5	18	578467
16999	1192	5773	1648	13	6	8	659139
5508	698	548	586	17	7	20	762693
2699	257	2002	435	3	7	10	289656
5271	1337	3798	1059	14	5	11	728622
8044	537	2081	1351	4	6	16	615758
7265	428	2387	819	6	4	24	707426
6634	700	3710	2447	4	4	4	377819
6571	1172	7879	1954	19	5	8	1477471
10506	2477	4414	2810	11	6	35	336784

Appendix 18.3   Listing of the instruction file EG4.ins

Eg1.dta	DATA FILE NAME
Eg1.out	OUTPUT FILE NAME
32	NUMBER OF FIRMS
1	NUMBER OF TIME PERIODS
4	NUMBER OF OUTPUTS
4	NUMBER OF INPUTS
1	0=INPUT AND 1=OUTPUT ORIENTATED
1	0=CRS AND 1=VRS
0	0=DEA (MULTI-STAGE), 1=COST-DEA, 2=MALMQUIST-DEA, 3=DEA (1-STAGE), 4=DEA (2-STAGE)

Appendix 18.4   Listing of the output file EG4.OUT

Results from DEAP Version 2.1
Instruction file = Eg4.ins
Data file = eg4.dta
Output orientated DEA
Scale assumption: VRS
Slacks calculated using multi-stage method

Efficiency summary

Firm	CRSTE	VRSTE	Scale	
1	0.638	0.724	0.881	drs
2	1.000	1.000	1.000	-
3	0.423	1.000	0.423	irs
4	0.669	1.000	0.669	drs
5	0.220	0.224	0.982	drs
6	1.000	1.000	1.000	-
7	0.657	0.688	0.955	drs
8	1.000	1.000	1.000	-
9	0.876	1.000	0.876	drs
10	1.000	1.000	1.000	-
11	0.455	0.678	0.671	drs
12	1.000	1.000	1.000	-
13	0.894	0.949	0.943	drs
14	0.698	0.743	0.941	drs
15	0.715	0.892	0.802	drs
16	0.721	1.000	0.721	irs
17	1.000	1.000	1.000	-
18	1.000	1.000	1.000	-
19	1.000	1.000	1.000	-
20	0.859	0.965	0.889	drs
21	1.000	1.000	1.000	-
22	0.501	0.553	0.906	drs
23	0.472	0.508	0.930	drs
24	0.857	0.907	0.945	drs
25	0.223	0.250	0.894	drs
26	0.494	1.000	0.494	irs
27	0.324	0.534	0.607	drs
28	0.831	0.875	0.949	drs
29	0.552	0.574	0.963	drs
30	1.000	1.000	1.000	-
31	0.477	0.888	0.537	drs
32	1.000	1.000	1.000	-
Mean	0.736	0.842	0.874	

Summary of output slacks

Firm	1*	2*	3*	4*
1	0.000	698.505	0.000	705.130
2	0.000	0.000	0.000	0.000
3	0.000	0.000	0.000	0.000
4	0.000	0.000	0.000	0.000
5	0.000	334.442	0.000	839.910
6	0.000	0.000	0.000	0.000
7	0.000	312.165	0.000	102.020
8	0.000	0.000	0.000	0.000
9	0.000	0.000	0.000	0.000
10	0.000	0.000	0.000	0.000
11	2,369.453	0.000	6165.500	906.738
12	0.000	0.000	0.000	0.000
13	0.000	42.159	0.000	402.339
14	0.000	0.000	1,019.211	0.000
15	0.000	0.000	1,670.136	0.000
16	0.000	0.000	0.000	0.000
17	0.000	0.000	0.000	0.000
18	0.000	0.000	0.000	0.000
19	0.000	0.000	0.000	0.000
20	1,924.764	0.000	2,507.180	0.000
21	0.000	0.000	0.000	0.000
22	0.000	1,468.575	0.000	0.000
23	1,317.143	0.000	1,287.545	239.787
24	0.000	1,135.941	0.000	676.357
25	0.000	0.000	4009.884	0.000
26	0.000	0.000	0.000	0.000
27	3,818.655	0.000	0.000	93.950
28	0.000	844.192	3697.573	0.000
29	0.000	425.337	57.709	0.000
30	0.000	0.000	0.000	0.000
31	361.514	838.001	0.000	0.000
32	0.000	0.000	0.000	0.000
Mean	305.985	190.604	637.961	123.945

Note:
CRSTE = technical efficiency from CRSDEA
VRSTE = technical efficiency from VRSDEA
Scale = scale efficiency=CRSTE/VRSTE
Note also that all subsequent tables refer to VRS results

*Output

Summary of input slacks						Summary of peers					
Firm	1*	2*	3*	4*		Firm	Peers				
1	0.000	1.909	0.357	0.000		1	12	9	6	8	
2	0.000	0.000	0.000	0.000		2	2				
3	0.000	0.000	0.000	0.000		3	3				
4	0.000	0.000	0.000	0.000		4	4				
5	1.210	2.534	17.739	0.000		5	10	6	12		
6	0.000	0.000	0.000	0.000		6	6				
7	0.000	0.000	8.542	57,243.476		7	17	8	19	12	
8	0.000	0.000	0.000	0.000		8	8				
9	0.000	0.000	0.000	0.000		9	9				
10	0.000	0.000	0.000	0.000		10	10				
11	5.111	0.000	0.222	259,185.667		11	9	21			
12	0.000	0.000	0.000	0.000		12	12				
13	0.648	0.000	12.417	0.000		13	21	12	10	6	
14	0.000	0.000	2.487	58,469.511		14	17	9	30	12	21
15	0.000	0.000	1.618	102,854.791		15	30	21	8	6	9
16	0.000	0.000	0.000	0.000		16	16				
17	0.000	0.000	0.000	0.000		17	17				
18	0.000	0.000	0.000	0.000		18	18				
19	0.000	0.000	0.000	0.000		19	1				
20	0.000	0.567	1.578	75,961.307		20	8	30	6		
21	0.000	0.000	0.000	0.000		21	21				
22	0.000	0.000	22.790	34,664.105		22	17	9	30	21	12
23	0.000	0.000	4.440	0.000		23	32	21	12	8	
24	0.000	0.927	4.224	0.000		24	12	6	21	10	
25	2.681	0.000	6.878	0.000		25	32	12	10	621	
26	0.000	0.000	0.000	0.000		26	26				
27	5.120	0.000	6.863	23,845.066		27	9	8	21		
28	0.000	0.913	12.381	72,243.545		28	2	12	17		
29	0.000	0.000	15.983	87,508.795		29	30	17	12	2	
30	0.000	0.000	0.000	0.000		30	30				
31	11.550	0.000	5.019	1,051,198.822		31	21	8	6		
32	0.000	0.000	0.000	0.000		32	32				
Mean	0.822	0.214	3.861	56,974.221							

*Input

Firm	Peer weights				
1	0.047	0.178	0.015	0.759	
2	1.000				
3	1.000				
4	1.000				
5	0.815	0.130	0.055		
6	1.000				
7	0.275	0.542	0.092	0.092	
8	1.000				
9	1.000				
10	1.000				
11	0.889	0.111			
12	1.000				
13	0.259	0.462	0.211	0.069	
14	0.131	0.132	0.380	0.192	0.166
15	0.077	0.287	0.442	0.128	0.065
16	1.000				
17	1.000				
18	1.000				
19	1.000				
20	0.863	0.065	0.071		
21	1.000				
22	0.286	0.243	0.010	0.354	0.107
23	0.319	0.276	0.393	0.012	
24	0.484	0.092	0.401	0.023	
25	0.245	0.637	0.041	0.060	0.016
26	1.000				
27	0.268	0.398	0.335		
28	0.032	0.091	0.878		
29	0.407	0.002	0.236	0.355	
30	1.000				
31	0.132	0.793	0.075		
32	1.000				

Summary of peer weights
(in same order as summary of peers above)

Peer count summary
(i.e., no. times each firm is a peer for another)

Firm	Peer count
1	0
2	2
3	0
4	0
5	0
6	8
7	0
8	7
9	6
10	4
11	0
12	11
13	0
14	0
15	0
16	0
17	5
18	0
19	1
20	0
21	10
22	0
23	0
24	0
25	0
26	0
27	0
28	0
29	0
30	5
31	0
32	2

Summary of output targets

Firm	1	2	3	4
1	12,083.067	2,540.538	8,665.704	1,890.774
2	9,582.000	427.000	3,440.000	171.000
3	1,912.000	36.000	270.000	165.000
4	15,899.000	2,050.000	6,991.000	374.000
5	20,333.222	1,492.776	4,357.119	2,127.443
6	12,589.000	2,102.000	15,986.000	9,796.000
7	8,837.656	1,920.598	7,669.870	1,396.329
8	7,073.000	2,221.000	8,914.000	1,503.000
9	29,215.000	3,789.000	7,633.000	2,966.000
10	21,070.000	1,287.000	2,371.000	940.000
11	26,982.222	3,568.778	7,289.222	2,863.667
12	27,784.000	3,105.000	6,253.000	1,559.000
13	20,488.641	2,316.918	5,661.599	2,121.584
14	14,161.324	1,834.131	5,172.266	2,166.753
15	9,783.656	2,071.991	8,078.958	2,890.473
16	4,864.000	441.000	1,059.000	394.000
17	7,249.000	1,324.000	6,151.000	1,591.000
18	3,444.000	321.000	698.000	641.000
19	5,090.000	750.000	6,288.000	19.000
20	7,437.129	2,112.970	9,077.066	2,155.436
21	9,120.000	1,807.000	4,539.000	2,045.000
22	15,431.155	2,277.028	5,925.043	2,090.766
23	16,864.769	2,535.453	5,225.673	2,091.633
24	18,750.270	2,450.744	6,367.746	2,494.137
25	22,051.878	2,794.519	6,203.861	2,346.115
26	2,699.000	257.000	2,002.000	435.000
27	13,683.027	2,502.118	7,107.738	2,075.807
28	9,189.314	1,457.651	6,074.869	1,543.357
29	12,667.166	1,171.593	4,219.653	1,427.998
30	6,634.000	700.000	3,710.000	2,447.000
31	7,758.957	2,157.405	8,869.951	2,199.757
32	10,506.000	2,477.000	4,414.000	2,810.000

Summary of input targets

Firm	1	2	3	4
1	8.000	6.091	4.643	667,867.000
2	3.000	2.000	14.000	667,608.000
3	2.000	1.000	7.000	263,010.000
4	16.000	7.000	2.000	1,001,197.000
5	15.790	8.466	6.261	607,150.000
6	34.000	12.000	8.000	570,996.000
7	5.000	5.000	3.458	502,459.524
8	5.000	5.000	3.000	431,668.000
9	17.000	10.000	11.000	1602,878.000
10	13.000	8.000	6.000	588,704.000
11	15.889	9.000	9.778	1459,353.333
12	14.000	7.000	6.000	967,426.000
13	13.352	6.000	4.583	690,365.000
14	8.000	5.000	4.513	656,866.489
15	10.000	5.000	3.382	487,504.209
16	3.000	5.000	10.000	331,572.000
17	3.000	5.000	3.000	495,147.000
18	3.000	0.000	2.000	399,402.000
19	2.000	3.000	5.000	477,953.000
20	7.000	5.433	3.422	438,066.693
21	7.000	1.000	0.000	311,156.000
22	9.000	5.000	4.210	747,998.895
23	11.000	5.000	13.560	578,467.000
24	13.000	5.073	3.776	659,139.000
25	14.319	7.000	13.122	762,693.000
26	3.000	7.000	10.000	289,656.000
27	8.880	5.000	4.137	704,776.934
28	4.000	5.087	3.619	543,514.455
29	6.000	4.000	8.017	619,917.205
30	4.000	4.000	4.000	377,819.000
31	7.450	5.000	2.981	426,272.178
32	11.000	6.000	35.000	336,784.000

FIRM BY FIRM RESULTS

Results for firm: 1

Technical efficiency = 0.724
Scale efficiency = 0.881 (drs)

Projection summary

Variable	Original value	Radial movement	Slack movement	Projected value
output 1	8,744.000	3,339.067	0.000	12,083.067
output 2	1,333.000	509.032	698.505	2,540.538
output 3	6,271.000	2,394.704	0.000	8,665.704
output 4	858.000	327.644	705.130	1,890.774
input 1	8.000	0.000	0.000	8.000
input 2	8.000	0.000	-1.909	6.091
input 3	5.000	0.000	-0.357	4.643
input 4	667,867.000	0.000	0.000	667,867.000

Listing of peers

Peer	Lambda weight
12	0.047
9	0.178
6	0.015
8	0.759

Results for firm: 2

Technical efficiency = 1.000
Scale efficiency = 1.000 (crs)

Projection summary

Variable	Original value	Radial movement	Slack movement	Projected value
output 1	9,582.000	0.000	0.000	9,582.000
output 2	427.000	0.000	0.000	427.000
output 3	3,440.000	0.000	0.000	3,440.000
output 4	171.000	0.000	0.000	171.000
input 1	3.000	0.000	0.000	3.000
input 2	2.000	0.000	0.000	2.000
input 3	14.000	0.000	0.000	14.000
input 4	667,608.000	0.000	0.000	667,608.000

Listing of peers

Peer	Lambda weight
2	1.000

Results for firm: 3

Technical efficiency = 1.000
Scale efficiency = 0.423 (irs)

Projection summary

Variable	Original value	Radial movement	Slack movement	Projected value
output 1	1,912.000	0.000	0.000	1,912.000
output 2	36.000	0.000	0.000	36.000
output 3	270.000	0.000	0.000	270.000
output 4	1,65.000	0.000	0.000	165.000
input 1	2.000	0.000	0.000	2.000
input 2	1.000	0.000	0.000	1.000
input 3	7.000	0.000	0.000	7.000
input 4	263,010.000	0.000	0.000	263,010.000

Listing of peers

Peer	Lambda weight
3	1.000

Results for firm: 4

Technical efficiency = 1.000
Scale efficiency = 0.669 (drs)

Projection summary

Variable	Original value	Radial movement	Slack movement	Projected value
output 1	15,899.000	0.000	0.000	15,899.000
output 2	2,050.000	0.000	0.000	2,050.000
output 3	6,991.000	0.000	0.000	6,991.000
output 4	374.000	0.000	0.000	374.000
input 1	16.000	0.000	0.000	16.000
input 2	7.000	0.000	0.000	7.000
input 3	2.000	0.000	0.000	2.000
input 4	1,001,197.000	0.000	0.000	1,001,197.000

Listing of peers

Peer	Lambda weight
4	1.000

Results for firm: 5

Technical efficiency = 0.224
Scale efficiency = 0.982 (drs)

Projection summary

Variable	Original value	Radial movement	Slack movement	Projected value
output 1	4,564.000	157,69.222	0.000	20,333.222
output 2	260.000	898.334	334.442	1,492.776
output 3	978.000	3,379.119	0.000	4,357.119
output 4	289.000	998.533	839.910	2,127.443
input 1	17.000	0.000	-1.210	15.790
input 2	11.000	0.000	-2.534	8.466
input 3	24.000	0.000	-17.739	6.261
input 4	607,150.000	0.000	0.000	607,150.000

Listing of peers

Peer	Lambda weight
10	0.815
6	0.130
12	0.055

Results for firm: 6

Technical efficiency = 1.000
Scale efficiency = 1.000 (crs)

Projection summary

Variable	Original value	Radial movement	Slack movement	Projected value
output 1	12,589.000	0.000	0.000	12,589.000
output 2	2,102.000	0.000	0.000	2,102.000
output 3	15,986.000	0.000	0.000	15,986.000
output 4	9,796.000	0.000	0.000	9,796.000
input 1	34.000	0.000	0.000	34.000
input 2	12.000	0.000	0.000	12.000
input 3	8.000	0.000	0.000	8.000
input 4	570,996.000	0.000	0.000	570,996.000

Listing of peers

Peer	Lambda weight
6	1.000

Results for firm: 7

Technical efficiency = 0.688
Scale efficiency = 0.955 (drs)

Projection summary

Variable	Original value	Radial movement	Slack movement	Projected value
output 1	6,077.000	2,760.656	0.000	8,837.656
output 2	1,106.000	502.433	312.165	1,920.598
output 3	5,274.000	2,395.870	0.000	7,669.870
output 4	890.000	404.309	102.020	1,396.329
input 1	5.000	0.000	0.000	5.000
input 2	5.000	0.000	0.000	5.000
input 3	12.000	0.000	-8.542	3.458
input 4	559,703.000	0.000	-57,243.476	502,459.524

Listing of peers

Peer	Lambda weight
17	0.275
8	0.542
19	0.092
12	0.092

Results for firm: 8

Technical efficiency = 1.000
Scale efficiency = 1.000 (crs)

Projection summary

Variable	Original value	Radial movement	Slack movement	Projected value
output 1	7,073.000	0.000	0.000	7,073.000
output 2	2,221.000	0.000	0.000	2,221.000
output 3	8,914.000	0.000	0.000	8,914.000
output 4	1,503.000	0.000	0.000	1,503.000
input 1	5.000	0.000	0.000	5.000
input 2	5.000	0.000	0.000	5.000
input 3	3.000	0.000	0.000	3.000
input 4	431,668.000	0.000	0.000	431,668.000

Listing of peers

Peer	Lambda weight
8	1.000

Results for firm: 9

Technical efficiency = 1.000
Scale efficiency = 0.876 (drs)

Projection summary

Variable	Original value	Radial movement	Slack movement	Projected value
output 1	29,215.000	0.000	0.000	29,215.000
output 2	3,789.000	0.000	0.000	3,789.000
output 3	7,633.000	0.000	0.000	7,633.000
output 4	2,966.000	0.000	0.000	2,966.000
input 1	17.000	0.000	0.000	17.000
input 2	10.000	0.000	0.000	10.000
input 3	11.000	0.000	0.000	11.000
input 4	1,602,878.000	0.000	0.000	1,602,878.000

Listing of peers

Peer	Lambda weight
9	1.000

Results for firm: 10

Technical efficiency = 1.000
Scale efficiency = 1.000 (crs)

Projection summary

Variable	Original value	Radial movement	Slack movement	Projected value
output 1	21,070.000	0.000	0.000	21,070.000
output 2	1,287.000	0.000	0.000	1,287.000
output 3	2,371.000	0.000	0.000	2,371.000
output 4	940.000	0.000	0.000	940.000
input 1	13.000	0.000	0.000	13.000
input 2	8.000	0.000	0.000	8.000
input 3	6.000	0.000	0.000	6.000
input 4	588,704.000	0.000	0.000	588,704.000

Listing of peers

Peer	Lambda weight
10	1.000

Results for firm: 11

Technical efficiency = 0.678
Scale efficiency = 0.671 (drs)

Projection summary

Variable	Original value	Radial movement	Slack movement	Projected value
output 1	16,690.000	7,922.769	2,369.453	26,982.222
output 2	2,420.000	1,148.778	0.000	3,568.778
output 3	762.000	361.723	6,165.500	7,289.222
output 4	1,327.000	629.929	906.738	2,863.667
input 1	21.000	0.000	-5.111	15.889
input 2	9.000	0.000	0.000	9.000
input 3	10.000	0.000	-0.222	9.778
input 4	1,718,539.000	0.000	-259,185.667	1,459,353.333

Listing of peers

Peer	Lambda weight
9	0.889
21	0.111

Results for firm: 12

Technical efficiency = 1.000
Scale efficiency = 1.000 (crs)

Projection summary

Variable	Original value	Radial movement	Slack movement	Projected value
output 1	27,784.000	0.000	0.000	27,784.000
output 2	3,105.000	0.000	0.000	3,105.000
output 3	6,253.000	0.000	0.000	6,253.000
output 4	1,559.000	0.000	0.000	1,559.000
input 1	14.000	0.000	0.000	14.000
input 2	7.000	0.000	0.000	7.000
input 3	6.000	0.000	0.000	6.000
input 4	967,426.000	0.000	0.000	967,426.000

Listing of peers

Peer	Lambda weight
12	1.000

Results for firm: 13

Technical efficiency = 0.949
Scale efficiency = 0.943 (drs)

Projection summary

Variable	Original value	Radial movement	Slack movement	Projected value
output 1	19,437.000	1,051.641	0.000	20,488.641
output 2	2,158.000	116.759	42.159	2,316.918
output 3	5,371.000	290.599	0.000	5,661.599
output 4	1,631.000	88.245	402.339	2,121.584
input 1	14.000	0.000	-0.648	13.352
input 2	6.000	0.000	0.000	6.000
input 3	17.000	0.000	-12.417	4.583
input 4	690,365.000	0.000	0.000	690,365.000

Listing of peers

Peer	Lambda weight
21	0.259
12	0.462
10	0.211
6	0.069

Results for firm: 14

Technical efficiency = 0.743
Scale efficiency = 0.941 (drs)

Projection summary

Variable	Original value	Radial movement	Slack movement	Projected value
output 1	105,16.000	3,645.324	0.000	14,161.324
output 2	1,362.000	472.131	0.000	1,834.131
output 3	3,084.000	1,069.055	1,019.211	5,172.266
output 4	1,609.000	557.753	0.000	2,166.753
input 1	8.000	0.000	0.000	8.000
input 2	5.000	0.000	0.000	5.000
input 3	7.000	0.000	-2.487	4.513
input 4	715,336.000	0.000	-58,469.511	656,866.489

Listing of peers

Peer	Lambda weight
17	0.131
9	0.132
30	0.380
12	0.192
21	0.166

Results for firm: 15

Technical efficiency = 0.892
Scale efficiency = 0.802 (drs)

Projection summary

Variable	Original value	Radial movement	Slack movement	Projected value
output 1	8,726.000	1,057.656	0.000	9,783.656
output 2	1,848.000	223.991	0.000	2,071.991
output 3	5,716.000	692.822	1,670.136	8,078.958
output 4	2,578.000	312.473	0.000	2,890.473
input 1	10.000	0.000	0.000	10.000
input 2	5.000	0.000	0.000	5.000
input 3	5.000	0.000	-1.618	3.382
input 4	590,359.000	0.000	-102,854.791	487,504.209

Listing of peers

Peer	Lambda weight
30	0.077
21	0.287
8	0.442
6	0.128
9	0.065

Results for firm: 16

Technical efficiency = 1.000
Scale efficiency = 0.721 (irs)

Projection summary

Variable	Original value	Radial movement	Slack movement	Projected value
output 1	4,864.000	0.000	0.000	4,864.000
output 2	441.000	0.000	0.000	441.000
output 3	1,059.000	0.000	0.000	1,059.000
output 4	394.000	0.000	0.000	394.000
input 1	3.000	0.000	0.000	3.000
input 2	5.000	0.000	0.000	5.000
input 3	10.000	0.000	0.000	10.000
input 4	331,572.000	0.000	0.000	331,572.000

Listing of peers

Peer	Lambda weight
16	1.000

Results for firm: 17

Technical efficiency = 1.000
Scale efficiency = 1.000 (crs)

Projection summary

Variable	Original value	Radial movement	Slack movement	Projected value
output 1	7,249.000	0.000	0.000	7,249.000
output 2	1,324.000	0.000	0.000	1,324.000
output 3	6,151.000	0.000	0.000	6,151.000
output 4	1,591.000	0.000	0.000	1,591.000
input 1	3.000	0.000	0.000	3.000
input 2	5.000	0.000	0.000	5.000
input 3	3.000	0.000	0.000	3.000
input 4	495,147.000	0.000	0.000	495,147.000

Listing of peers

Peer	Lambda weight
17	1.000

Results for firm: 18

Technical efficiency = 1.000
Scale efficiency = 1.000 (crs)

Projection summary

Variable	Original value	Radial movement	Slack movement	Projected value
output 1	3,444.000	0.000	0.000	3,444.000
output 2	321.000	0.000	0.000	321.000
output 3	698.000	0.000	0.000	698.000
output 4	641.000	0.000	0.000	641.000
input 1	3.000	0.000	0.000	3.000
input 2	0.000	0.000	0.000	0.000
input 3	2.000	0.000	0.000	2.000
input 4	399,402.000	0.000	0.000	399,402.000

Listing of peers

Peer	Lambda weight
18	1.000

Results for firm: 19

Technical efficiency = 1.000
Scale efficiency = 1.000 (crs)

Projection summary

Variable	Original value	Radial movement	Slack movement	Projected value
output 1	5,090.000	0.000	0.000	5,090.000
output 2	750.000	0.000	0.000	750.000
output 3	6,288.000	0.000	0.000	6,288.000
output 4	19.000	0.000	0.000	19.000
input 1	2.000	0.000	0.000	2.000
input 2	3.000	0.000	0.000	3.000
input 3	5.000	0.000	0.000	5.000
input 4	477,953.000	0.000	0.000	477,953.000

Listing of peers

Peer	Lambda weight
19	1.000

Results for firm: 20

Technical efficiency = 0.965
Scale efficiency = 0.889 (drs)

Projection summary

Variable	Original value	Radial movement	Slack movement	Projected value
output 1	5,322.000	190.366	1,924.764	7,437.129
output 2	2,040.000	72.970	0.000	2,112.970
output 3	6,343.000	226.886	2,507.180	9,077.066
output 4	2,081.000	74.436	0.000	2,155.436
input 1	7.000	0.000	0.000	7.000
input 2	6.000	0.000	-0.567	5.433
input 3	5.000	0.000	-1.578	3.422
input 4	514,028.000	0.000	-75,961.307	438,066.693

Listing of peers

Peer	Lambda weight
8	0.863
30	0.065
6	0.071

Results for firm: 21

Technical efficiency = 1.000
Scale efficiency = 1.000 (crs)

Projection summary

Variable	Original value	Radial movement	Slack movement	Projected value
output 1	9,120.000	0.000	0.000	9,120.000
output 2	1,807.000	0.000	0.000	1,807.000
output 3	4,539.000	0.000	0.000	4,539.000
output 4	2,045.000	0.000	0.000	2,045.000
input 1	7.000	0.000	0.000	7.000
input 2	1.000	0.000	0.000	1.000
input 3	0.000	0.000	0.000	0.000
input 4	311,156.000	0.000	0.000	311,156.000

Listing of peers

Peer	Lambda weight
21	1.000

Results for firm: 22

Technical efficiency = 0.553
Scale efficiency = 0.906 (drs)

Projection summary

Variable	Original value	Radial movement	Slack movement	Projected value
output 1	8,532.000	6,899.155	0.000	15,431.155
output 2	447.000	361.454	1,468.575	2,277.028
output 3	3,276.000	2,649.043	0.000	5,925.043
output 4	1,156.000	934.766	0.000	2,090.766
input 1	9.000	0.000	0.000	9.000
input 2	5.000	0.000	0.000	5.000
input 3	27.000	0.000	-22.790	4.210
input 4	782,663.000	0.000	-34,664.105	747,998.895

Listing of peers

Peer	Lambda weight
17	0.286
9	0.243
30	0.010
21	0.354
12	0.107

Results for firm: 23

Technical efficiency = 0.508
Scale efficiency = 0.930 (drs)

Projection summary

Variable	Original value	Radial movement	Slack movement	Projected value
output 1	7,892.000	7,655.626	1,317.143	16,864.769
output 2	1,287.000	1,248.453	0.000	2,535.453
output 3	1,999.000	1,939.128	1,287.545	5,225.673
output 4	940.000	911.846	239.787	2,091.633
input 1	11.000	0.000	0.000	11.000
input 2	5.000	0.000	0.000	5.000
input 3	18.000	0.000	-4.440	13.560
input 4	578,467.000	0.000	0.000	578,467.000

Listing of peers

Peer	Lambda weight
32	0.319
21	0.276
12	0.393
8	0.012

Results for firm: 24

Technical efficiency = 0.907
Scale efficiency = 0.945 (drs)

Projection summary

Variable	Original value	Radial movement	Slack movement	Projected value
output 1	16,999.000	1751.270	0.000	18750.270
output 2	1,192.000	122.802	1135.941	2450.744
output 3	5,773.000	594.746	0.000	6367.746
output 4	1,648.000	169.780	676.357	2494.137
input 1	13.000	0.000	0.000	13.000
input 2	6.000	0.000	-0.927	5.073
input 3	8.000	0.000	-4.224	3.776
input 4	659,139.000	0.000	0.000	659139.000

Listing of peers

Peer	Lambda weight
12	0.484
6	0.092
21	0.401
10	0.023

Results for firm: 25

Technical efficiency = 0.250
Scale efficiency = 0.894 (drs)

Projection summary

Variable	Original value	Radial movement	Slack movement	Projected value
output 1	5,508.000	16,543.878	0.000	22,051.878
output 2	698.000	2,096.519	0.000	2,794.519
output 3	548.000	1,645.978	4,009.884	6,203.861
output 4	586.000	1,760.115	0.000	2,346.115
input 1	17.000	0.000	-2.681	14.319
input 2	7.000	0.000	0.000	7.000
input 3	20.000	0.000	-6.878	13.122
input 4	762,693.000	0.000	0.000	762,693.000

Listing of peers

Peer	Lambda weight
32	0.245
12	0.637
10	0.041
6	0.060
21	0.016

Results for firm: 26

Technical efficiency = 1.000
Scale efficiency = 0.494 (irs)

Projection summary

Variable	Original value	Radial movement	Slack movement	Projected value
output 1	2,699.000	0.000	0.000	2,699.000
output 2	257.000	0.000	0.000	257.000
output 3	2,002.000	0.000	0.000	2,002.000
output 4	435.000	0.000	0.000	435.000
input 1	3.000	0.000	0.000	3.000
input 2	7.000	0.000	0.000	7.000
input 3	10.000	0.000	0.000	10.000
input 4	289,656.000	0.000	0.000	289,656.000

Listing of peers

Peer	Lambda weight
26	1.000

Results for firm: 27

Technical efficiency = 0.534
Scale efficiency = 0.607 (drs)

Projection summary

Variable	Original value	Radial movement	Slack movement	Projected value
output 1	5,271.000	4,593.372	3,818.655	13,683.027
output 2	1,337.000	1,165.118	0.000	2,502.118
output 3	3,798.000	3,309.738	0.000	7,107.738
output 4	1,059.000	922.857	93.950	2,075.807
input 1	14.000	0.000	-5.120	8.880
input 2	5.000	0.000	0.000	5.000
input 3	11.000	0.000	-6.863	4.137
input 4	728,622.000	0.000	-23,845.066	704,776.934

Listing of peers

Peer	Lambda weight
9	0.268
8	0.398
21	0.335

Results for firm: 28

Technical efficiency = 0.875
Scale efficiency = 0.949 (drs)

Projection summary

Variable	Original value	Radial movement	Slack movement	Projected value
output 1	8,044.000	1,145.314	0.000	9,189.314
output 2	537.000	76.459	844.192	1,457.651
output 3	2,081.000	296.295	3,697.573	6,074.869
output 4	1,351.000	192.357	0.000	1,543.357
input 1	4.000	0.000	0.000	4.000
input 2	6.000	0.000	-0.913	5.087
input 3	16.000	0.000	-12.381	3.619
input 4	615,758.000	0.000	-72,243.545	543,514.455

Listing of peers

Peer	Lambda weight
2	0.032
12	0.091
17	0.878

Results for firm: 29

Technical efficiency = 0.574
Scale efficiency = 0.963 (drs)

Projection summary

Variable	Original value	Radial movement	Slack movement	Projected value
output 1	7,265.000	5,402.166	0.000	12,667.166
output 2	428.000	318.256	425.337	1,171.593
output 3	2,387.000	1,774.944	57.709	4,219.653
output 4	819.000	608.998	0.000	1,427.998
input 1	6.000	0.000	0.000	6.000
input 2	4.000	0.000	0.000	4.000
input 3	24.000	0.000	-15.983	8.017
input 4	707,426.000	0.000	-87,508.795	619,917.205

Listing of peers

Peer	Lambda weight
30	0.407
17	0.002
12	0.236
2	0.355

Results for firm: 30

Technical efficiency = 1.000
Scale efficiency = 1.000 (crs)

Projection summary

Variable	Original value	Radial movement	Slack movement	Projected value
output 1	6,634.000	0.000	0.000	6,634.000
output 2	700.000	0.000	0.000	700.000
output 3	3,710.000	0.000	0.000	3,710.000
output 4	2,447.000	0.000	0.000	2,447.000
input 1	4.000	0.000	0.000	4.000
input 2	4.000	0.000	0.000	4.000
input 3	4.000	0.000	0.000	4.000
input 4	377,819.000	0.000	0.000	377,819.000

Listing of peers

Peer	Lambda weight
30	1.000

Results for firm: 31

Technical efficiency = 0.888
Scale efficiency = 0.537 (drs)

Projection summary

Variable	Original value	Radial movement	Slack movement	Projected value
output 1	6,571.000	826.442	361.514	7,758.957
output 2	1,172.000	147.404	838.001	2,157.405
output 3	7,879.000	990.951	0.000	8,869.951
output 4	1,954.000	245.757	0.000	2,199.757
input 1	19.000	0.000	-11.550	7.450
input 2	5.000	0.000	0.000	5.000
input 3	8.000	0.000	-5.019	2.981
input 4	147,7471.000	0.000	-1051,198.822	426,272.178

Listing of peers

Peer	Lambda weight
21	0.132
8	0.793
6	0.075

Results for firm: 32

Technical efficiency = 1.000
Scale efficiency = 1.000 (crs)

Projection summary

Variable	Original value	Radial movement	Slack movement	Projected value
output 1	10,506.000	0.000	0.000	10,506.000
output 2	2,477.000	0.000	0.000	2,477.000
output 3	4,414.000	0.000	0.000	4,414.000
output 4	2,810.000	0.000	0.000	2,810.000
input 1	11.000	0.000	0.000	11.000
input 2	6.000	0.000	0.000	6.000
input 3	35.000	0.000	0.000	35.000
input 4	336,784.000	0.000	0.000	336,784.000

Listing of peers

Peer	Lambda weight
32	1.000

-19-

Measurement of Total Cost Efficiency or Economic Efficiency: *A Case Study of Health Centres in the Democratic Republic of Njuri–Ncheke*

Joses M. Kirigia and Eyob Zere Asbu

BACKGROUND

Njuri-Ncheke is a landlocked, low income, and highly indebted country located in southern Afromiola and has a population of 4 million. The country's economy is largely based on petroleum and timber. The last traditional ruler of Njuri-Ncheke gave 200 years' leasehold to two multinational companies from the former colonial master to exploit petroleum and timber. The meagre annual payment largely goes to the family accounts of the current president, who served previously as a military dictator for 20 years. About 80 per cent of Njuri-Ncheke's population lives below the international poverty line of US$1 per day. The adult illiteracy rate in the country is 50 per cent. Sixty per cent and 40 per cent of the population lack access to safe drinking water and adequate sanitation facilities respectively. Njuri-Ncheke has about 300 doctors, 600 clinical officers, and 2000 nurses working in 100 hospitals and 300 health centres.

The vision of the Njuri-Ncheke government is to provide all citizens with equitable access to cost-effective and high quality health services. Since 1992, the government has embarked on implementation of health sector reforms aimed at facilitating the realisation of this vision. The reforms have ranged from introduction of user fees for public health services to launching of community health financing and decentralisation of planning, management, and decision-making for health services to the health district. The control of financial and human resources was retained at the Ministry of Health headquarters. In spite of the sectoral reforms, approximately 50 per cent of the country's population lack access to essential medicines, 68 per cent of infants do not use oral rehydration, 80 per cent of the eligible population does not use contraceptives, and 60 per cent of births occur without assistance of skilled health attendants.

Njuri-Ncheke's health indicators are generally very poor. The average life expectancy at birth is 35 years and the disability-adjusted life expectancy (DALE) is 26 years. The maternal mortality ratio (MMR) is 1,500 per 100,000 live births, the under-five mortality rate is 300 per 1,000 live births, 30 per cent of children under five years of age are underweight, and infant mortality rate is 200 deaths per 1,000 live births. The probability, at birth, of surviving to age 40 was 50 per cent in 2005. These dismal health indicators have largely been attributed to widespread poverty, which has been exacerbated by the growing incidence of HIV. Faced with such widespread poverty, the only sustainable option the country has of providing effective coverage of health services is efficient use of resources at all levels of the national health system.

An assessment of the *World Health Report 2000* [1] of the performance of national health systems of 191 WHO Member States ranked Njuri-Ncheke at number 190. Although Njuri-Ncheke's per capita total health spending was 150 international dollars per year (the fifth highest in Afromiola), the country's performance was worse than that of countries spending less than 34 international dollars per capita per year. The WHO rankings triggered a public outcry and led to the dismissal of the then Minister for Health.

The President of Njuri-Ncheke appointed Professor Koomenjwe, an internationally acclaimed Professor of Public Health and Health Economics, as the Minister for Health. The main terms of reference for the new Health Minister were to improve the performance of Njuri-Ncheke's health system. Professor Koomenjwe constituted the Council for Assessment and Enhancement of Health Systems Performance (CAEHSP). The CAEHSP comprised the Minister; one each of Ph.D-level university academic specialists in public health, health systems organisation and management, efficiency and productivity analysis, and health economics. The Council members also consisted of the directors from the Ministry of Health dealing with health policy and planning, public health and medical services, and primary health care and community-based health services; the director of efficiency monitoring and evaluation from the Ministry of Economic Planning and Finance, and the director of the national bureau of statistics. The others were a representative each of the faiths-based health services organisations, the Private Sector Health Services, and the civil society; chairs of the national Medical Association, the Nursing and Allied Professions Association, and the Sector-Wide Approach Group; one provincial medical officer of health; and one district medical officer of health. The entire CAEHSP held a meeting with the President, who emphasised the importance the country attached to the work that the Council was about to embark on.

From his research, Professor Koomenjwe knew that tertiary, provincial, and district hospitals alone consumed approximately 85 per cent of the country's recurrent and capital budgets of the total health sector budget of N$200 million per year. About 10 per cent of these funds went into the health system's administration, especially at the headquarters, and only 5 per cent was spent on the much-talked-about cost-effective primary health care health centres, dispensaries, health posts, and public health outreach activities. Thus, from the outset the Minister decided that the first priority for CAEHSP was to measure the performance of hospitals and develop an action plan for improving their performance. The specific terms of reference for CAEHSP were to estimate the degree of technical, allocative, and cost efficiency of all public and private for-profit and not-for-profit hospitals and to identify the relative inefficiencies in the use of various inputs among individual hospitals.

CONCEPTUAL FRAMEWORK

The Health Minister, as the chair of CAEHSP, allocated to the university academics the following tasks:

1. To review and document published national and international literature on hospital performance assessment and measurement;

2. To identify and critically review how hospital inputs and outputs were treated in published studies with a view to recommending the appropriate inputs and outputs for the Njuri-Ncheke study;

3. To critically review international methods for measuring hospital efficiency with a view to recommending the most appropriate approach for Njuri-Ncheke;

4. To critically review the performance measurement software in the market and to make recommendations for Njuri-Ncheke.

Hospital Inputs and Outputs

A rigorous review of published studies revealed the inputs, process, and outputs contained in Figure 19.1 as the most common in hospital studies. Those inputs and outputs were discussed at a CAEHSP meeting and deemed appropriate for use in the Njuri-Ncheke study.

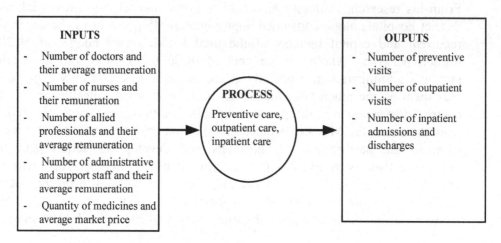

Figure 19.1   Production process for a hospital

Methods for Measuring Hospital Efficiency

A critical review of methods used internationally for measuring hospital efficiency found econometric modelling and data envelopment analysis (DEA) as the common tools. The literature revealed that using econometrics would entail the strong presumptions that hospitals produce only one output and that their objective function is to maximise profits. The four academics also realised that DEA deals very well with multiple input, multiple output production scenarios typical of hospitals; does not require *a priori* function specification; and yields efficiency scores for individual hospitals and input and output targets. The four professors apprised the CAEHSP of the strengths and weaknesses of parametric and non-parametric approaches. In the ensuing discussions, all members of CAEHSP agreed that the most appropriate method for Njuri-Ncheke would be the DEA approach.

Choice of Software

Dr Kauro-Beechau, a professor of efficiency and productivity analysis, informed CAEHSP that commercial and non-commercial DEA software were available in the market. The Minister for Health indicated that there was no need to spend the scarce resources on commercial software when free software was available. The Minister requested Professor Kauro-Beechau to apprise CAEHSP on the strengths and weaknesses of the non-commercial DEA software. Professor Kauro-Beechau informed the Council of the two DEA software available on the Internet for free downloading: DEAP Version 2.1 [2] and EMS (Efficiency Measurement Systems) [3]. He explained that DEAP was used to estimate technical, allocative, and cost efficiencies while EMS could be used only for technical efficiency analysis. The Council decided that DEAP would be used to adequately address the terms of reference.

Data Collection

The four academics informed the Minister for Health of the WHO hospital efficiency data gathering instruments and their availability from the organisation's country office. The Minister immediately contacted Professor Tumbo Kubwa, the WHO Country Representative, and requested for the instruments. An electronic copy of the instruments was delivered to the Minister within one day. The Minister then convened a CAEHSP meeting to review and adapt the instruments for Njuri-Ncheke.

The task of pilot-testing the adapted data collection instruments was given to the provincial medical officer of health, the district medical officer of health, and the representatives of the faiths-based health services and the private sector association. They were each requested to pilot-test the instruments in one hospital and to note the amendments needed. After a week the Minister convened another meeting to discuss the outcomes of the pilot test and to finalise changes to the data collection instruments.

The four academics were also tasked with identifying, for recruitment, 12 research assistants with a minimum of a master's degree qualification in public health or health economics. The Minister instructed the Director of Human Resource Management to recruit the 12 research assistants for three months. The academics then held an intensive training seminar for the research assistants focussing on the objectives of the study, treatment of hospital inputs and outputs, overview of DEA, data collection instruments, data sources in hospitals, persons to interview at the hospitals, transport and logistics, research ethics, duration of the fieldwork, and the work plan among others.

The CAEHSP agreed that data would be collected from all the 100 hospitals in the country and there would be four fieldwork teams each overseen by an academic. Thus, each academic was allocated three research assistants to cover 25 hospitals. The data collection activity took one month, computer data entry and cleaning another month, and data analysis and report writing the third month.

Data Analysis Using DEAP Version 2.1

DEAP Version 2.1 software and its manual, developed by Professor Tim Coelli [2], were closely followed by CAEHSP. For the purpose of this case study, let us trace the steps that CAEHSP followed:

1. Download the DEAP Version 2.1 software from http://www.uq.edu/ economics/cepa/deap.htm into a folder on a computer [2].

2. The data for each hospital should occupy a row. Since this case study aims to estimate cost (or economic) efficiency, there should be a column for each output, each input, and each input price with all outputs listed first, then all the quantities of inputs, and finally all input prices listed from left to right. Given that the case study involves 100 hospitals and observations on three outputs, seven inputs, and seven average input prices there should be 17 columns of data listed in the following order: y1, y2, y3, x1, x2, x3, x4, x5, x6, x7, w1, w2, w3, w4, w5, w6, w7 (a description of the data for each column is provided below). Enter the data in Appendix 19.1 on an Excel spreadsheet.

    Column 1: Names of hospitals
    Outputs
    Column 2: Output1 (y1) = Number of preventive care visits
    Column 3: Output2 (y2) = Number of outpatient care visits
    Column 4: Output3 (y3) = Number of inpatient discharges
    Input quantities
    Column 5: Input1 (x1) = Number of doctors and clinical officers
    Column 6: Input2 (x2) = Number of nurses
    Column 7: Input3 (x3) = Number of allied professionals
    Column 8: Input4 (x4) = Number of administrative and support staff
    Column 9: Input5 (x5) = Quantity of medicines
    Column 10: Input6 (x6) = Quantity of non-medical supplies
    Column 11: Input7 (x7) = Number of beds per hospital
    Input average prices
    Column 12: w1 = Average annual remuneration for input x1 (per doctor or clinical officer)
    Column 13: w2 = Average annual remuneration for input x2 (per nurse)
    Column 14: w3 = Average annual remuneration for input x3 (per allied professional)
    Column 15: w4 = Average annual remuneration for input x4 (per administrative and support staff)
    Column 16: w5 = Average price for input x5 (per basket of medicines)
    Column 17: w6 = Average price for input x6 (per basket of non-medical supplies)
    Column 18: w7 = Average price for input x7 (per new bed)

3. Using the computer mouse, copy only the data values of outputs, inputs, and input prices without the names of hospitals, outputs, or inputs.

4. Choose **Start**, **Program**, **Accessories**, and then **Notepad** to open this software.

5. In Notepad, choose **File** and then **Open**. Browse your computer to locate the folder where you saved the DEAP software. Select, for example, eg4.dta file and open it. Delete the contents, paste your data and choose **Save**. The data, once pasted on Notepad, will appear as indicated in Appendix 19.2.

6. Choose **File** and then **New**. Locate the DEAP instruction file called EG4.ins and open it. The contents of this file will appear as in Appendix 19.3. Modify the instruction file to reflect the data file name, eg1.dta; output file name (eg4.out), number of firms (100), number of time

periods (1), number of outputs (3), number of inputs (7), model orientation (0 for input oriented or 1 for output oriented), type of model (0 for CRS and 1 for VRS), and type of model (4 for cost efficiency). For more information, read the DEA manual that comes with the software.

7. Close Notepad and go to the folder where you saved the DEAP software. Locate the DEAP.EXE file and double click on it.

8. The DEAP programme will prompt you to type in the instruction filename. At the prompt type EG4.INS. Within a few seconds the estimations will be completed and the output sent to your output file EG4.OUT.

9. Choose EG4.OUT and you will be prompted to indicate the software in which the file should be opened. If you select, for example, Excel, your output will look like Appendix 19.4. It will contain summaries of efficiency (for firm efficiency, constant returns to scale technical efficiency, variable returns to scale technical efficiency and scale efficiency), output and input slacks, peers and peer weights, count, and output and input target as well as and firm by firm results.

10. Answer questions 1-10 in the next exercise.

Exercise

1. Estimate the mean and standard deviation of the quantities of outputs and inputs and of input prices. Provide the answers in Table 19.1 and discuss the results.

2. Estimate the technical, allocative, and cost efficiency scores for each hospital. Summarise the results in Table 19.2 and discuss them.

3. Estimate the mean and standard deviation of all the hospitals' technical, allocative, and cost efficiency scores. Summarise these scores in Table 19.3 and discuss the results.

4. Estimate the frequency distribution of the hospitals' efficiency scores by ownership and tabulate the information in Table 19.4. Discuss the results.

5. Estimate the output increases needed to make individual inefficient hospitals efficient. Tabulate the information in Table 19.5 and discuss the results.

6. Estimate the input reductions needed to make individual inefficient hospitals efficient and tabulate the information in Table 19.6. Discuss the results.

7. What course of action should the Minister for Health take to reduce the level of technical, allocative, and cost inefficiency in the use of various inputs in public hospitals?

8. What course of action should the private-for-profit and private-not-for-profit hospital owners take to enhance technical, allocative, and cost efficiency of their hospitals?

9. Would it be advisable for the Minister for Health to try to increase outputs of inefficient facilities? If yes, explain the alternative strategies that could be used to increase outputs. If not, justify your answer.

10. Discuss the weaknesses inherent in this study (e.g., in relation to the choice of inputs and outputs, method of efficiency measurement, etc).

Table 19.1 Descriptive statistics for inputs and outputs

Variable	Privately owned hospitals		Government owned hospitals	
	Mean	Standard deviation	Mean	Standard deviation
Outputs				
y1 = Number of preventive care visits				
y2 = Number of outpatient care visits				
y3 = Number of inpatient discharges				
Inputs				
(x1) = Number of doctors and clinical officers				
(x2) = Number of nurses				
(x3) = Number of allied professionals				
(x4) = Number of admin and support staff				
(x5) = Quantity of medicines				
(x6) = Quantity of non-medical supplies				
(x7) = Number of beds per hospital				
Input prices				
(w1) = Doctors and clinical officers' average monthly remuneration				
(w2) = Nurses' average monthly remuneration				
(w3) = Allied professionals' average monthly remuneration				
(w4) = Administrative and support staff's average monthly remuneration				
(w5) = Average price of medicines				
(w6) = Average price non-medical supplies				
(w7) = Price of a single bed				

Table 19.2 Efficiency scores for individual hospitals

Name of hospitals	Technical efficiency	Allocative efficiency	Cost efficiency

Table 19.3 Descriptive statistics for efficiency scores

Type of efficiency	Privately owned hospitals		Government hospitals	
	Mean	Standard deviation	Mean	Standard deviation
Technical				
Allocative				
Cost				

Table 19.4 Frequency distribution of hospitals' efficiency by ownership

Range	Privately owned hospitals (%)			Government hospitals (%)		
	Technical efficiency	Allocative efficiency	Cost efficiency	Technical efficiency	Allocative efficiency	Cost efficiency
1						
0.90–0.99						
0.80–0.89						
0.70–0.79						
0.60–0.69						
0.50–0.59						
0.40–0.49						
0.30–0.39						
0.20–0.29						
0.10–0.19						
Total						

Table 19.5 Output increases needed to make individual inefficient hospitals efficient

Name of hospital	Outputs		
	Preventive visits	Outpatient curative visits	Inpatient discharges
1.			
2.			
3.			
4.			
.			
.			
n.			

Table 19.6 Input reductions (or increases) needed to make individual inefficient hospitals efficient

Name of hospital	Inputs						
	Doctors and clinical officers	Nurses	Allied professionals	Administrative and support staff	Medicines	Non-medical supplies	Beds
1.							
2.							
3.							
4.							
.							
.							
n.							

REFERENCES

World Health Organization. *The world health report 2000: improving health systems performance*. Geneva: World Health Organization; 2000.

Coelli TJ. *A guide to DEAP version 2.1: a data envelopment analysis [computer] program* , Centre for Efficiency and Productivity Analysis (CEPA) Working Paper 96/08, Department of Econometrics, University of New England, Armidale, NSW Australia; 1996.

Scheel H. *EMS (Efficiency Measurement System)*. Dortmund: University of Dortmund; 1999.

Emrouznejad A. Ali Emrouznejad's Data Envelopment Analysis Homepage 1995-2003, www.DEAzone.com.

Appendix 19.1 Health service outputs and inputs of private and public hospitals in Njuri-Ncheke

Hospital name	Ownership	Preventive visits (y1)	Outpatient visits (y2)	Discharges (y3)	Doctors and clinical officers (x1)	Nurses (x2)	Allied personnel (x3)l	Admin (x4)	Medicines (x5)
Njuri-Ncheke private	1	1,239	6,000	32,000	8	19	10	15	918,000
Kiruka-Ntangi private	1	1,239	13,525	32,000	8	19	10	15	682,600
Kiruka-Mbaine private	1	1,239	6,008	32,000	8	19	20	30	682,600
Kiruka-Thamburu private	1	1,239	55,800	32,000	8	19	5	7.5	625,000
Kiruka-Kibabu private	1	1,239	6,480	32,000	8	19	15	22.5	630,000
Kiruka-Kubai private	1	1,239	1,680	32,000	8	19	5	5	690,000
Kiruka-Kaburia private	1	1,239	10,000	32,000	8	19	10	15	683,000
Kiruka-Kiramana private	1	1,239	3,509	32,000	8	19	15	22.5	683,000
Kiruka-Murungi private	1	1,239	3,348	32,000	8	19	20	30	600,000
Kiruka-Kiruja private	1	1,239	4,200	32,000	8	19	10	15	610,000
Kiruka-Guantai private	1	1,239	3,700	32,000	8	19	15	22.5	547,000
Kiruka-Gichunge private	1	1,239	24,000	32,000	8	19	25	37.5	567,000
Kiruka-Miriti private	1	1,239	4,548	32,000	8	19	5	7.5	538,000
Kiruka-Mbarata private	1	1,239	12,600	32,000	8	19	20	30	460,000
Kiruka-Mathiita private	1	1,239	1,480	32,000	8	19	5	7.5	560,000
Kiruka-Rima private	1	1,239	2,241	32,000	8	19	5	7.5	340,000
Kiruka-Michubu private	1	1,239	3,600	32,000	8	19	5	7.5	344,230
Kiruka-Gitangiira private	1	1,239	4,682	32,000	8	19	15	22.5	271,939
Kiruka-Mbaringo private	1	1,239	9,334	32,000	8	19	15	22.5	271,939
Kiruka-Meeme private	1	1,239	2,365	32,000	8	19	55	82.5	271,939
Kiruka-Ngutugua private	1	1,239	2,160	32,000	7	20	10	15	280,000
Kiruka-Kiambajo private	1	1,239	15,820	32,000	8	20	20	30	265,000
Kiruka-Kithiringua private	1	1,239	6,500	32,000	8	20	10	15	390,000
Kiruka-Nchaau private	1	1,239	10,623	32,000	8	20	10	15	207,144
Kiruka-Nturutimi private	1	1,239	20,679	32,000	8	20	40	60	19,987.8
Kiruka-Mukangu private	1	1,239	19,501	32,000	8	20	20	30	221,867
Kiruka-Mbaabu private	1	1239	2,249	32,000	8	20	10	15	217,542
Kiruka-Mungatia private	1	1,239	3,866	32,000	8	20	20	30	217,500
Kiruka-Memeu private	1	1,239	20,092	32,000	8	20	10	15	217,500
Kiruka-Muthamia private	1	1,239	17,598	32,000	8	20	15	22.5	217,500

.../cont.

Efficiency Analysis of Health Systems in Africa

Appendix 19.1 (cont.)

Hospital name	Ownership	Preventive visits (y1)	Outpatient visits (y2)	Discharges (y3)	Doctors and clinical officers (x1)	Nurses (x2)	Allied personnel (x3)l	Admin (x4)	Medicines (x5)
Kiruka-Riungu private	1	1,239	7,754	32,000	8	20	20	30	217,500
Kiruka-Marangu private	1	1,239	4,636	32,000	8	20	20	30	204,176
Kiruka-Kaaria private	1	1,239	2,362	32,000	8	20	15	22.5	207,714.4
Kiruka-Nangithia private	1	1,239	24,410	32,000	8	20	35	52.5	199,867.8
Kiruka-Mungatia jwa kilo private	1	1,239	5,090	32,000	8	20	15	22.5	223,407
Kiruka-Ratanya private	1	1,239	16,676	32,000	8	20	20	30	201,867
Kiruka-Lubetaa private	1	1,239	9,788	32,000	8	20	45	67.5	199,867.8
Kiruka-Ithalii private	1	1,239	16,241	32,000	8	20	15	22.5	203,675.6
Kiruka-Guantaaru private	1	1,239	3,686	32,000	8	20	15	22.5	219,618
Lenity-Kainyu private 10	1	1,239	27,092	32,000	8	20	10	15	206,332
Rose-nabi private	1	1,239	56,000	32,000	8	20	10	15	918,000
Kirima private	1	1,239	6,600	32,000	8	20	10	15	682,600
Kibari private	1	1,239	4,356	32,000	7	20	20	30	682,600
Gaitune private	1	1,239	7,902	32,000	8	20	5	7.5	625,000
Mitungugu private	1	1,239	8,749	32,000	8	20	15	22.5	630,000
Miratina private	1	1,239	9,019	32,000	8	20	5	7.5	690,000
Mituntu private	1	1,239	9,674	32,000	8	20	10	15	683,000
Kierera private	1	1,239	20,394	32,000	8	20	15	22.5	683,000
Nkuene private	1	1,239	48,595	32,000	8	20	20	30	600,000
Gachiege private	1	1,239	58,696	32,000	8	20	10	15	610,000
Nchau private	0	1,239	27,363	32,000	8	20	15	22.5	547,000
Phineas-Nkanata private	0	1,239	16,253	32,000	8	20	25	37.5	567,000
Jessica Igoki private	0	1,239	17,398	32,000	8	20	5	7.5	538,000
Rose-Gakii private	0	1,239	19,400	32,000	8	20	20	30	460,000
Josphat-Kirigia private	0	1,239	19,049	32,000	7	20	5	7.5	560,000
Kaburi private	0	1,239	94,749	32,000	8	20	5	7.5	340,000
Karimi private	0	1,239	98,261	32,000	8	20	5	7.5	344,230
Kimathi private	0	1,239	49,487	32,000	8	20	15	22.5	271,939
Mugambi private	0	1,239	48,475	32,000	8	20	15	22.5	271,939

.../cont.

Appendix 19.1 (cont.)

Hospital name	Ownership	Preventive visits (y1)	Outpatient visits (y2)	Discharges (y3)	Doctors and clinical officers (x1)	Nurses (x2)	Allied personnel (x3)l	Admin (x4)	Medicines (x5)
Marimanti private	0	1,239	253,263	32,000	8	20	55	82.5	271,939
Muratina private	0	1,239	58,578	32,000	8	20	10	15	280,000
Muriati private	0	1,239	256,354	32,000	8	20	20	30	265,000
Muko-njira private	0	1,239	65,968	32,000	8	20	10	15	390,000
Ntiba-Ntangi public	0	25,790	46,452	49,681	10.5	20	10	15	207,144
Ntiba-Mbaine public	0	25,790	47,546	49,681	10.5	20	40	60	199,867.8
Ntiba-Thamburu public	0	25,790	111,332	49,681	10.5	20	20	30	221,867
Ntiba-Kibabu public	0	25,790	212,341	49,681	10.5	20	10	15	217,542
Ntiba-Kubai public	0	25,790	36,477	49,681	10.5	20	20	30	217,500
Ntiba-Kaburia public	0	25,790	43,521	49,681	10.5	20	10	15	217,500
Ntiba-Kiramana public	0	25,790	26,353	49,681	10.5	20	15	22.5	217,500
Ntiba-Murungi public	0	25,790	37,476	49,681	10.5	20	20	30	217,500
Ntiba-Kiruja public	0	25,790	25,353	49,681	10.5	20	20	30	204,176
Ntiba-Guantai public	0	25,790	28,393	49,681	10.5	20	15	22.5	207,714.4
Ntiba-Gichunge public	0	25,790	64,746	49,681	10.5	20	35	52.5	199,867.8
Ntiba-Miriti public	0	25,790	47,657	49,681	10.5	20	15	22.5	223,407
Ntiba-Mbarata public	0	25,790	24,353	49,681	10.5	20	20	30	201,867
Ntiba-Kiruka public	0	25,790	23,138	49,681	10.5	20	45	67.5	199,867.8
Ntiba-Rima public	0	25,790	74,664	49,681	10.5	20	15	22.5	203,675.6
Ntiba-Michubu public	0	25,790	56,475	49,681	10.5	20	15	22.5	219,618
Ntiba-Gitangiira public	0	25,790	14,242	49,681	10.5	20	10	15	206,332
Ntiba-Mbaringo public	0	25,790	125,436	49,681	10.5	20	10	15	918,000
Ntiba-Meeme public	0	25,790	26,364	49,681	10.5	20	15	22.5	682,600
Ntiba-Ngutugua public	0	25,790	46,454	49,681	10.5	20	20	30	682,600
Ntiba-Kiambajo public	0	25,790	253,536	49,681	10.5	20	20	30	625,000
Ntiba-Kithiringua public	0	25,790	353,464	49,681	10.5	20	15	22.5	630,000
Ntiba-Nchaau public	0	25,790	464,643	49,681	10.5	20	35	52.5	690,000
Ntiba-Nturutimi public	0	25,790	464,537	49,681	10.5	20	15	22.5	683,000
Ntiba-Mukangu public	0	25,790	123,256	49,681	10.5	20	20	30	683,000

.../cont.

Appendix 19.1 (cont.)

Hospital name	Ownership	Preventive visits (y1)	Outpatient visits (y2)	Discharges (y3)	Doctors and clinical officers (x1)	Nurses (x2)	Allied personnel (x3)	Admin (x4)	Medicines (x5)
Ntiba-Mbaabu public	0	25,790	253,438	49,681	10.5	20	45	67.5	600,000
Ntiba-Mungatia public	0	25,790	342,521	49,681	10.5	20	15	22.5	610,000
Ntiba-Memeu public	0	25,790	231,429	49,681	10.5	20	15	22.5	547,000
Ntiba-Muthamia public	0	25,790	253,636	49,681	10.5	20	10	15	567,000
Ntiba-Riungu public	0	25,790	364,647	49,681	10.5	20	10	15	538,000
Ntiba-Marangu public	0	25,790	586,960	49,681	10.5	20	15	22.5	460,000
Ntiba-Kaaria public	0	25,790	846,463	49,681	10.5	20	20	30	560,000
Ntiba-Nangithia public	0	25,790	234,262	49,681	10.5	20	20	30	340,000
Ntiba-Jwa kilo public	0	25,790	585,747	49,681	10.5	20	15	22.5	344,230
Ntiba-Ratanya public	0	25,790	352,542	49,681	10.5	20	35	52.5	271,939
Ntiba-Lubetaa public	0	25,790	364,641	49,681	10.5	20	15	22.5	271,939
Ntiba-Ithalii public	0	25,790	326,373	49,681	10.5	20	20	30	271,939
Ntiba-Guantaaru public	0	25,790	253,536	49,681	10.5	20	45	67.5	280,000

.../cont.

Appendix 19.1 (cont.)

Hospital name	Supplies (x6)	Beds (x7)	Price (w1)	Price (w2)	Price (w3)	Price (w4)	Price (w5)	Price (w6)	Price (w7)
Njuri-Ncheke private	650,000	150	100,000	50,000	30,000	25,000	120	30	5,500
Kiruka-Ntangi private	640,253	150	100,000	50,000	30,000	25,000	120	30	5,500
Kiruka-Mbaine private	640,253	150	100,000	50,000	30,000	25,000	120	30	5,500
Kiruka-Thamburu private	530,000	150	100,000	50,000	30,000	25,000	120	30	5,500
Kiruka-Kibabu private	510,000	150	100,000	50,000	30,000	25,000	120	30	5,500
Kiruka-Kubai private	480,000	150	100,000	50,000	30,000	25,000	120	30	5,500
Kiruka-Kaburia private	440,000	150	100,000	50,000	30,000	25,000	120	30	5,500
Kiruka-Kiramana private	440,000	150	100,000	50,000	30,000	25,000	120	30	5,500
Kiruka-Murungi private	430,000	150	100,000	50,000	30,000	25,000	120	30	5,500
Kiruka-Kiruja private	410,000	150	100,000	50,000	30,000	25,000	120	30	5,500
Kiruka-Guantai private	390,000	150	100,000	50,000	30,000	25,000	120	30	5,500
Kiruka-Gichunge private	380,000	150	100,000	50,000	30,000	25,000	120	30	5,500
Kiruka-Miriti private	340,000	150	100,000	50,000	30,000	25,000	120	30	5,500
Kiruka-Mbarata private	330,000	150	100,000	50,000	30,000	25,000	120	30	5,500
Kiruka-Mathiita private	314,000	150	100,000	50,000	30,000	25,000	120	30	5,500
Kiruka-Rima private	290,000	150	100,000	50,000	30,000	25,000	120	30	5,500
Kiruka-Michubu private	270,000	150	100,000	50,000	30,000	25,000	120	30	5,500
Kiruka-Gitangiira private	265,294	150	100,000	50,000	30,000	25,000	120	30	5,500
Kiruka-Mbaringo private	256,394	150	100,000	50,000	30,000	25,000	120	30	5,500
Kiruka-Meeme private	256,394	150	100,000	50,000	30,000	25,000	120	30	5,500
Kiruka-Ngutugua private	255,000	150	100,000	50,000	30,000	25,000	120	30	5,500
Kiruka-Kiambajo private	251,000	150	100,000	50,000	30,000	25,000	120	30	5,500
Kiruka-Kithiringua private	245,000	150	100,000	50,000	30,000	25,000	120	30	5,500
Kiruka-Nchaau private	204,000	150	100,000	50,000	30,000	25,000	120	30	5,500
Kiruka-Nturutimi private	199,867.8	150	100,000	50,000	30,000	25,000	120	30	5,500
Kiruka-Mukangu private	199,500	150	100,000	50,000	30,000	25,000	120	30	5,500
Kiruka-Mbaabu private	198,638	150	100,000	50,000	30,000	25,000	120	30	5,500
Kiruka-Mungatia private	189,000	150	100,000	50,000	30,000	25,000	120	30	5,500
Kiruka-Memeu private	189,000	150	100,000	50,000	30,000	25,000	120	30	5,500

.../cont.

Efficiency Analysis of Health Systems in Africa

Appendix 19.1 (cont.)

Hospital name	Supplies (x6)	Beds (x7)	Price (w1)	Price (w2)	Price (w3)	Price (w4)	Price (w5)	Price (w6)	Price (w7)
Kiruka-Muthamia private	189,000	150	100,000	50,000	30,000	25,000	120	30	5,500
Kiruka-Riungu private	189,000	150	100,000	50,000	30,000	25,000	120	30	5,500
Kiruka-Marangu private	186,500	150	100,000	50,000	30,000	25,000	120	30	5,500
Kiruka-Kaaria private	184,000	150	100,000	50,000	30,000	25,000	120	30	5,500
Kiruka-Nangithia private	179,809.8	150	100,000	50,000	30,000	25,000	120	30	5,500
Kiruka-Mungatia jwa kilo private	204,320	150	100,000	50,000	30,000	25,000	120	30	5,500
Kiruka-Ratanya private	199,867.8	150	100,000	50,000	30,000	25,000	120	30	5,500
Kiruka-Lubetaa private	141,913.1	150	100,000	50,000	30,000	25,000	120	30	5,500
Kiruka-Ithalii private	199,867.8	150	100,000	50,000	30,000	25,000	120	30	5,500
Kiruka-Guantaaru private	200,000	150	100,000	50,000	30,000	25,000	120	30	5,500
Lenity-Kainyu private	141,913	150	100,000	50,000	30,000	25,000	120	30	5,500
Rose-nabi private	650,000	150	100,000	50,000	30,000	25,000	120	30	5,500
Kirima private	640,253	150	100,000	50,000	30,000	25,000	120	30	5,500
Kibari private	640,253	150	100,000	50,000	30,000	25,000	120	30	5,500
Gaitune private	530,000	150	100,000	50,000	30,000	25,000	120	30	5,500
Mitungugu private	510,000	150	100,000	50,000	30,000	25,000	120	30	5,500
Miratina private	480,000	150	100,000	50,000	30,000	25,000	120	30	5,500
Mituntu private	440,000	150	100,000	50,000	30,000	25,000	120	30	5,500
Kierera private	440,000	150	100,000	50,000	30,000	25,000	120	30	5,500
Nkuene private	430,000	150	100,000	50,000	30,000	25,000	120	30	5,500
Gachiege private	410,000	150	100,000	50,000	30,000	25,000	120	30	5,500
Nchau private	390,000	150	100,000	50,000	30,000	25,000	120	30	5,500
Phineas-Nkanata private	380,000	150	100,000	50,000	30,000	25,000	120	30	5,500
Jessica Igoki private	340,000	150	100,000	50,000	30,000	25,000	120	30	5,500
Rose-Gakii private	330,000	150	100,000	50,000	30,000	25,000	120	30	5,500
Josphat-Kirigia private	314,000	150	100,000	50,000	30,000	25,000	120	30	5,500
Kaburi private	290,000	150	100,000	50,000	30,000	25,000	120	30	5,500
Karimi private	270,000	150	100,000	50,000	30,000	25,000	120	30	5,500
Kimathi private	265,294	150	100,000	50,000	30,000	25,000	120	30	5,500
Mugambi private	256,394	150	100,000	50,000	30,000	25,000	120	30	5,500

.../cont.

Appendix 19.1 (cont.)

Hospital name	Supplies (x6)	Beds (x7)	Price (w1)	Price (w2)	Price (w3)	Price (w4)	Price (w5)	Price (w6)	Price (w7)
Marimanti private	256,394	150	100,000	50,000	30,000	25,000	120	30	5,500
Muratina private	255,000	150	100,000	50,000	30,000	25,000	120	30	5,500
Muriati private	251,000	150	100,000	50,000	30,000	25,000	120	30	5,500
Muko-njira private	245,000	150	100,000	50,000	30,000	25,000	120	30	5,500
Ntiba-Ntangi public	204,000	200	100,000	50,000	30,000	25,000	60	30	5,500
Ntiba-Mbaine public	199,867.8	200	100,000	50,000	30,000	25,000	60	30	5,500
Ntiba-Thamburu public	199,500	200	100,000	50,000	30,000	25,000	60	30	5,500
Ntiba-Kibabu public	198,638	200	100,000	50,000	30,000	25,000	60	30	5,500
Ntiba-Kubai public	189,000	200	100,000	50,000	30,000	25,000	60	30	5,500
Ntiba-Kaburia public	189,000	200	100,000	50,000	30,000	25,000	60	30	5,500
Ntiba-Kiramana public	189,000	200	100,000	50,000	30,000	25,000	60	30	5,500
Ntiba-Murungi public	189,000	200	100,000	50,000	30,000	25,000	60	30	5,500
Ntiba-Kiruja public	186,500	200	100,000	50,000	30,000	25,000	60	30	5,500
Ntiba-Guantai public	184,000	200	100,000	50,000	30,000	25,000	60	30	5,500
Ntiba-Gichunge public	179,809.8	200	100,000	50,000	30,000	25,000	60	30	5,500
Ntiba-Miriti public	204,320	200	100,000	50,000	30,000	25,000	60	30	5,500
Ntiba-Mbarata public	199,867.8	200	100,000	50,000	30,000	25,000	60	30	5,500
Ntiba-Kiruka public	141,913.1	200	100,000	50,000	30,000	25,000	60	30	5,500
Ntiba-Rima public	199,867.8	200	100,000	50,000	30,000	25,000	60	30	5,500
Ntiba-Michubu public	200,000	200	100,000	50,000	30,000	25,000	60	30	5,500
Ntiba-Gitangiira public	141,913	200	100,000	50,000	30,000	25,000	60	30	5,500
Ntiba-Mbaringo public	650,000	200	100,000	50,000	30,000	25,000	60	30	5,500
Ntiba-Meeme public	640,253	200	100,000	50,000	30,000	25,000	60	30	5,500
Ntiba-Ngutugua public	640,253	200	100,000	50,000	30,000	25,000	60	30	5,500
Ntiba-Kiambajo public	530,000	200	100,000	50,000	30,000	25,000	60	30	5,500
Ntiba-Kithiringua public	510,000	200	100,000	50,000	30,000	25,000	60	30	5,500
Ntiba-Nchaau public	480,000	200	100,000	50,000	30,000	25,000	60	30	5,500
Ntiba-Nturutimi public	440,000	200	100,000	50,000	30,000	25,000	60	30	5,500
Ntiba-Mukangu public	440,000	200	100,000	50,000	30,000	25,000	60	30	5,500
Ntiba-Mbaabu public	430,000	200	100,000	50,000	30,000	25,000	60	30	5,500

.../cont.

Appendix 19.1 (cont.)

Hospital name	Supplies (x6)	Beds (x7)	Price (w1)	Price (w2)	Price (w3)	Price (w4)	Price (w5)	Price (w6)	Price (w7)
Ntiba-Mungatia public	410,000	200	100,000	50,000	30,000	25,000	60	30	5,500
Ntiba-Memeu public	390,000	200	100,000	50,000	30,000	25,000	60	30	5,500
Ntiba-Muthamia public	380,000	200	100,000	50,000	30,000	25,000	60	30	5,500
Ntiba-Riungu public	340,000	200	100,000	50,000	30,000	25,000	60	30	5,500
Ntiba-Marangu public	330,000	200	100,000	50,000	30,000	25,000	60	30	5,500
Ntiba-Kaaria public	314,000	200	100,000	50,000	30,000	25,000	60	30	5,500
Ntiba-Nangithia public	290,000	200	100,000	50,000	30,000	25,000	60	30	5,500
Ntiba-Jwa kilo public	270,000	200	100,000	50,000	30,000	25,000	60	30	5,500
Ntiba-Ratanya public	265,294	200	100,000	50,000	30,000	25,000	60	30	5,500
Ntiba-Lubetaa public	256,394	200	100,000	50,000	30,000	25,000	60	30	5,500
Ntiba-Ithalii public	256,394	200	100,000	50,000	30,000	25,000	60	30	5,500
Ntiba-Guantaaru public	255,000	200	100,000	50,000	30,000	25,000	60	30	5,500

Appendix 19.2   DEAP Data file called "eg4.dta"

1239	6000	32000	8	19	10	15	918000	650000	150	100000	50000	30000	25000	120	30	5500
1239	13525	32000	8	19	10	15	682600	640253	150	100000	50000	30000	25000	120	30	5500
1239	6008	32000	8	19	20	30	682600	640253	150	100000	50000	30000	25000	120	30	5500
1239	55800	32000	8	19	5	7.5	625000	530000	150	100000	50000	30000	25000	120	30	5500
1239	6480	32000	8	19	15	23	630000	510000	150	100000	50000	30000	25000	120	30	5500
1239	1680	32000	8	19	5	5	690000	480000	150	100000	50000	30000	25000	120	30	5500
1239	10000	32000	8	19	10	15	683000	440000	150	100000	50000	30000	25000	120	30	5500
1239	3509	32000	8	19	15	23	683000	440000	150	100000	50000	30000	25000	120	30	5500
1239	3348	32000	8	19	20	30	600000	430000	150	100000	50000	30000	25000	120	30	5500
1239	4200	32000	8	19	10	15	610000	410000	150	100000	50000	30000	25000	120	30	5500
1239	3700	32000	8	19	15	23	547000	390000	150	100000	50000	30000	25000	120	30	5500
1239	24000	32000	8	19	25	38	567000	380000	150	100000	50000	30000	25000	120	30	5500
1239	4548	32000	8	19	5	7.5	538000	340000	150	100000	50000	30000	25000	120	30	5500
1239	12600	32000	8	19	20	30	460000	330000	150	100000	50000	30000	25000	120	30	5500
1239	1480	32000	8	19	5	7.5	560000	314000	150	100000	50000	30000	25000	120	30	5500
1239	2241	32000	8	19	5	7.5	340000	290000	150	100000	50000	30000	25000	120	30	5500
1239	3600	32000	8	19	5	7.5	344230	270000	150	100000	50000	30000	25000	120	30	5500
1239	4682	32000	8	19	15	23	271939	265294	150	100000	50000	30000	25000	120	30	5500
1239	9334	32000	8	19	15	23	271939	256394	150	100000	50000	30000	25000	120	30	5500
1239	2365	32000	8	19	55	83	271939	256394	150	100000	50000	30000	25000	120	30	5500
1239	2160	32000	7	20	10	15	280000	255000	150	100000	50000	30000	25000	120	30	5500
1239	15820	32000	8	20	20	30	265000	251000	150	100000	50000	30000	25000	120	30	5500
1239	6500	32000	8	20	10	15	390000	245000	150	100000	50000	30000	25000	120	30	5500
1239	10623	32000	8	20	10	15	207144	204000	150	100000	50000	30000	25000	120	30	5500
1239	20679	32000	8	20	40	60	199868	199867.8	150	100000	50000	30000	25000	120	30	5500
1239	19501	32000	8	20	20	30	221867	199500	150	100000	50000	30000	25000	120	30	5500
1239	2249	32000	8	20	10	15	217542	198638	150	100000	50000	30000	25000	120	30	5500
1239	3866	32000	8	20	20	30	217500	189000	150	100000	50000	30000	25000	120	30	5500
1239	20092	32000	8	20	10	15	217500	189000	150	100000	50000	30000	25000	120	30	5500
1239	17598	32000	8	20	15	23	217500	189000	150	100000	50000	30000	25000	120	30	5500
1239	7754	32000	8	20	20	30	217500	189000	150	100000	50000	30000	25000	120	30	5500
1239	4636	32000	8	20	20	30	204176	186500	150	100000	50000	30000	25000	120	30	5500

.../cont.

Efficiency Analysis of Health Systems in Africa

Appendix 19.2 (cont.)

1239	2362	32000	8	20	15	23	207714	184000	150	100000	50000	30000	25000	120	30	5500
1239	24410	32000	8	20	35	53	199868	179809.8	150	100000	50000	30000	25000	120	30	5500
1239	5090	32000	8	20	15	23	223407	204320	150	100000	50000	30000	25000	120	30	5500
1239	16676	32000	8	20	20	30	201867	199867.8	150	100000	50000	30000	25000	120	30	5500
1239	9788	32000	8	20	45	68	199868	141913.1	150	100000	50000	30000	25000	120	30	5500
1239	16241	32000	8	20	15	23	203676	199867.8	150	100000	50000	30000	25000	120	30	5500
1239	3686	32000	8	20	15	23	219618	200000	150	100000	50000	30000	25000	120	30	5500
1239	27092	32000	8	20	10	15	206332	141913	150	100000	50000	30000	25000	120	30	5500
1239	56000	32000	8	20	10	15	918000	650000	150	100000	50000	30000	25000	120	30	5500
1239	6600	32000	8	20	10	15	682600	640253	150	100000	50000	30000	25000	120	30	5500
1239	4356	32000	7	20	20	30	682600	640253	150	100000	50000	30000	25000	120	30	5500
1239	7902	32000	8	20	5	7.5	625000	530000	150	100000	50000	30000	25000	120	30	5500
1239	8749	32000	8	20	15	23	630000	510000	150	100000	50000	30000	25000	120	30	5500
1239	9019	32000	8	20	5	7.5	690000	480000	150	100000	50000	30000	25000	120	30	5500
1239	9674	32000	8	20	10	15	683000	440000	150	100000	50000	30000	25000	120	30	5500
1239	20394	32000	8	20	15	23	683000	440000	150	100000	50000	30000	25000	120	30	5500
1239	48595	32000	8	20	20	30	600000	430000	150	100000	50000	30000	25000	120	30	5500
1239	58696	32000	8	20	10	15	610000	410000	150	100000	50000	30000	25000	120	30	5500
1239	27363	32000	8	20	15	23	547000	390000	150	100000	50000	30000	25000	120	30	5500
1239	16253	32000	8	20	25	38	567000	380000	150	100000	50000	30000	25000	120	30	5500
1239	17398	32000	8	20	5	7.5	538000	340000	150	100000	50000	30000	25000	120	30	5500
1239	19400	32000	8	20	20	30	460000	330000	150	100000	50000	30000	25000	120	30	5500
1239	19049	32000	7	20	5	7.5	560000	314000	150	100000	50000	30000	25000	120	30	5500
1239	94749	32000	8	20	5	7.5	340000	290000	150	100000	50000	30000	25000	120	30	5500
1239	98261	32000	8	20	5	7.5	344230	270000	150	100000	50000	30000	25000	120	30	5500
1239	49487	32000	8	20	15	23	271939	265294	150	100000	50000	30000	25000	120	30	5500
1239	48475	32000	8	20	15	23	271939	256394	150	100000	50000	30000	25000	120	30	5500
1239	253263	32000	8	20	55	83	271939	256394	150	100000	50000	30000	25000	120	30	5500
1239	58578	32000	8	20	10	15	280000	255000	150	100000	50000	30000	25000	120	30	5500
1239	256354	32000	8	20	20	30	265000	251000	150	100000	50000	30000	25000	120	30	5500
1239	65968	32000	8	20	10	15	390000	245000	150	100000	50000	30000	25000	120	30	5500

.../cont.

Appendix 19.2 (cont.)

25790	46452	49681	11	20	10	15	207144	204000	200	100000	50000	30000	25000	60	30	5500
25790	47546	49681	11	20	40	60	199868	199867.8	200	100000	50000	30000	25000	60	30	5500
25790	111332	49681	11	20	20	30	221867	199500	200	100000	50000	30000	25000	60	30	5500
25790	212341	49681	11	20	10	15	217542	198638	200	100000	50000	30000	25000	60	30	5500
25790	36477	49681	11	20	20	30	217500	189000	200	100000	50000	30000	25000	60	30	5500
25790	43521	49681	11	20	10	15	217500	189000	200	100000	50000	30000	25000	60	30	5500
25790	26353	49681	11	20	15	23	217500	189000	200	100000	50000	30000	25000	60	30	5500
25790	37476	49681	11	20	20	30	217500	189000	200	100000	50000	30000	25000	60	30	5500
25790	25353	49681	11	20	20	30	204176	186500	200	100000	50000	30000	25000	60	30	5500
25790	28393	49681	11	20	15	23	207714	184000	200	100000	50000	30000	25000	60	30	5500
25790	64746	49681	11	20	35	53	199868	179809.8	200	100000	50000	30000	25000	60	30	5500
25790	47657	49681	11	20	15	23	223407	204320	200	100000	50000	30000	25000	60	30	5500
25790	24353	49681	11	20	20	30	201867	199867.8	200	100000	50000	30000	25000	60	30	5500
25790	23138	49681	11	20	45	68	199868	141913.1	200	100000	50000	30000	25000	60	30	5500
25790	74664	49681	11	20	15	23	203676	199867.8	200	100000	50000	30000	25000	60	30	5500
25790	56475	49681	11	20	15	23	219618	200000	200	100000	50000	30000	25000	60	30	5500
25790	14242	49681	11	20	10	15	206332	141913	200	100000	50000	30000	25000	60	30	5500
25790	125436	49681	11	20	10	15	918000	650000	200	100000	50000	30000	25000	60	30	5500
25790	26364	49681	11	20	15	23	682600	640253	200	100000	50000	30000	25000	60	30	5500
25790	46454	49681	11	20	20	30	682600	640253	200	100000	50000	30000	25000	60	30	5500
25790	253536	49681	11	20	20	30	625000	530000	200	100000	50000	30000	25000	60	30	5500
25790	353464	49681	11	20	15	23	630000	510000	200	100000	50000	30000	25000	60	30	5500
25790	464643	49681	11	20	35	53	690000	480000	200	100000	50000	30000	25000	60	30	5500
25790	464537	49681	11	20	15	23	683000	440000	200	100000	50000	30000	25000	60	30	5500
25790	123256	49681	11	20	20	30	683000	440000	200	100000	50000	30000	25000	60	30	5500
25790	253438	49681	11	20	45	68	600000	430000	200	100000	50000	30000	25000	60	30	5500
25790	342521	49681	11	20	15	23	610000	410000	200	100000	50000	30000	25000	60	30	5500
25790	231429	49681	11	20	15	23	547000	390000	200	100000	50000	30000	25000	60	30	5500
25790	253636	49681	11	20	10	15	567000	380000	200	100000	50000	30000	25000	60	30	5500
25790	364647	49681	11	20	10	15	538000	340000	200	100000	50000	30000	25000	60	30	5500

.../cont.

Appendix 19.2 (cont.)

25790	586960	49681	11	20	15	23	460000	200	100000	50000	30000	25000	60	30	5500
25790	846463	49681	11	20	20	30	560000	200	100000	50000	30000	25000	60	30	5500
25790	234262	49681	11	20	20	30	340000	200	100000	50000	30000	25000	60	30	5500
25790	585747	49681	11	20	15	23	344230	200	100000	50000	30000	25000	60	30	5500
25790	352542	49681	11	20	35	53	271939	200	100000	50000	30000	25000	60	30	5500
25790	364641	49681	11	20	15	23	256394	200	100000	50000	30000	25000	60	30	5500
25790	326373	49681	11	20	20	30	256394	200	100000	50000	30000	25000	60	30	5500
25790	253536	49681	11	20	45	68	255000	200	100000	50000	30000	25000	60	30	5500

Appendix 19.3   Listing of instruction file EG4.INS

Eg4.dta	DATA FILE NAME
Eg4.out	OUTPUT FILE NAME
100	NUMBER OF FIRMS
1	NUMBER OF TIME PERIODS
3	NUMBER OF OUTPUTS
7	NUMBER OF INPUTS
0	0 = INPUT AND 1 = OUTPUT ORIENTATED
1	0 = CRS AND 1=VRS
1	0 = DEA (MULTI-STAGE), 1 = COST-DEA, 2 = MALMQUIST-DEA, 3 = DEA (1-STAGE), 4 = DEA (2-STAGE)

Appendix 19.4   Listing of output file EG4.OUT

Results from DEAP Version 2.1
Instruction file = eg4.ins
Data file = eg4.dta
Cost efficiency DEA
Scale assumption: VRS

Efficiency summary

Firm	TE	AE	CE	Firm	TE	AE	CE
1	1.000	0.243	0.243				
2	1.000	0.310	0.310	20	1.000	0.693	0.693
3	1.000	0.308	0.308	21	1.000	0.727	0.727
4	1.000	0.350	0.350	22	1.000	0.746	0.746
5	1.000	0.342	0.342	23	1.000	0.563	0.563
				24	1.000	0.943	0.943
6	1.000	0.323	0.323				
7	1.000	0.328	0.328	25	1.000	0.915	0.915
8	1.000	0.327	0.327	26	1.000	0.883	0.883
9	1.000	0.364	0.364	27	1.000	0.914	0.914
10	1.000	0.364	0.364	28	1.000	0.904	0.904
				29	1.000	0.922	0.922
11	1.000	0.399	0.399				
12	1.000	0.386	0.386	30	1.000	0.913	0.913
13	1.000	0.416	0.416	31	1.000	0.904	0.904
14	1.000	0.468	0.468	32	1.000	0.949	0.949
15	1.000	0.406	0.406	33	1.000	0.948	0.948
				34	1.000	0.940	0.940
16	1.000	0.617	0.617				
17	1.000	0.618	0.618	35	1.000	0.884	0.884
18	1.000	0.732	0.732	36	1.000	0.945	0.945
19	1.000	0.736	0.736	37	1.000	0.953	0.953
				38	1.000	0.948	0.948

.../cont.

Appendix 19.4 (cont)

Efficiency summary

Firm	TE	AE	CE	Firm	TE	AE	CE
39	1.000	0.898	0.898	71	1.000	0.893	0.893
40	1.000	1.000	1.000	72	1.000	0.922	0.922
41	1.000	0.247	0.247	73	1.000	0.932	0.932
42	1.000	0.309	0.309	74	1.000	0.920	0.920
43	1.000	0.308	0.308	75	1.000	0.880	0.880
44	1.000	0.344	0.344	76	1.000	0.910	0.910
45	1.000	0.342	0.342	77	1.000	0.917	0.917
46	1.000	0.323	0.323	78	1.000	0.947	0.947
47	1.000	0.328	0.328	79	1.000	0.898	0.898
48	1.000	0.327	0.327	80	1.000	1.000	1.000
49	1.000	0.368	0.368	81	1.000	0.278	0.278
50	1.000	0.371	0.371	82	1.000	0.320	0.320
51	1.000	0.399	0.399	83	1.000	0.322	0.322
52	1.000	0.386	0.386	84	1.000	0.414	0.414
53	1.000	0.416	0.416	85	1.000	0.465	0.465
54	1.000	0.468	0.468	86	1.000	0.484	0.484
55	1.000	0.407	0.407	87	1.000	0.508	0.508
56	1.000	0.641	0.641	88	1.000	0.371	0.371
57	1.000	0.643	0.643	89	1.000	0.435	0.435
58	1.000	0.740	0.740	90	1.000	0.497	0.497
59	1.000	0.744	0.744	91	1.000	0.480	0.480
60	1.000	0.811	0.811	92	1.000	0.486	0.486
61	1.000	0.739	0.739	93	1.000	0.582	0.582
62	1.000	0.877	0.877	94	1.000	0.792	0.792
63	1.000	0.576	0.576	95	1.000	1.000	1.000
64	1.000	0.932	0.932	96	1.000	0.697	0.697
65	1.000	0.875	0.875	97	1.000	1.000	1.000
66	1.000	0.909	0.909	98	1.000	0.894	0.894
67	1.000	1.000	1.000	99	1.000	0.957	0.957
68	1.000	0.893	0.893	100	1.000	0.909	0.909
69	1.000	0.923	0.923	**Mean**	**1.000**	**0.652**	
70	1.000	0.901	0.901			**0.652**	

Note: TE = Technical efficiency   AE = Allocative efficiency = CE/TE
    CE = Cost efficiency

Appendix 19.4 (cont)

Summary of cost-minimising input quantities

				Input quantities			
Firm	Input 1	Input 2	Input 3	Input 4	Input 5	Input 6	Input 7
1	8.000	20.000	10.000	15.000	206,332.000	141,913.000	150.000
2	8.000	20.000	10.000	15.000	206,332.000	141,913.000	150.000
3	8.000	20.000	10.000	15.000	206,332.000	141,913.000	150.000
4	8.387	20.000	10.000	15.000	208,069.211	150,703.662	157.748
5	8.000	20.000	10.000	15.000	206,332.000	141,913.000	150.000
6	8.000	20.000	10.000	15.000	206,332.000	141,913.000	150.000
7	8.000	20.000	10.000	15.000	206,332.000	141,913.000	150.000
8	8.000	20.000	10.000	15.000	206,332.000	141,913.000	150.000
9	8.000	20.000	10.000	15.000	206,332.000	141,913.000	150.000
10	8.000	20.000	10.000	15.000	206,332.000	141,913.000	150.000
11	8.000	20.000	10.000	15.000	206,332.000	141,913.000	150.000
12	8.000	20.000	10.000	15.000	206,332.000	141,913.000	150.000
13	8.000	20.000	10.000	15.000	206,332.000	141,913.000	150.000
14	8.000	20.000	10.000	15.000	206,332.000	141,913.000	150.000
15	8.000	20.000	10.000	15.000	206,332.000	141,913.000	150.000
16	8.000	20.000	10.000	15.000	206,332.000	141,913.000	150.000
17	8.000	20.000	10.000	15.000	206,332.000	141,913.000	150.000
18	8.000	20.000	10.000	15.000	206,332.000	141,913.000	150.000
19	8.000	20.000	10.000	15.000	206,332.000	141,913.000	150.000
20	8.000	20.000	10.000	15.000	206,332.000	141,913.000	150.000
21	8.000	20.000	10.000	15.000	206,332.000	141,913.000	150.000
22	8.000	20.000	10.000	15.000	206,332.000	141,913.000	150.000
23	8.000	20.000	10.000	15.000	206,332.000	141,913.000	150.000
24	8.000	20.000	10.000	15.000	206,332.000	141,913.000	150.000
25	8.000	20.000	10.000	15.000	206,332.000	141,913.000	150.000
26	8.000	20.000	10.000	15.000	206,332.000	141,913.000	150.000
27	8.000	20.000	10.000	15.000	206,332.000	141,913.000	150.000
28	8.000	20.000	10.000	15.000	206,332.000	141,913.000	150.000
29	8.000	20.000	10.000	15.000	206,332.000	141,913.000	150.000
30	8.000	20.000	10.000	15.000	206,332.000	141,913.000	150.000
31	8.000	20.000	10.000	15.000	206,332.000	141,913.000	150.000
32	8.000	20.000	10.000	15.000	206,332.000	141,913.000	150.000
33	8.000	20.000	10.000	15.000	206,332.000	141,913.000	150.000
34	8.000	20.000	10.000	15.000	206,332.000	141,913.000	150.000
35	8.000	20.000	10.000	15.000	206,332.000	141,913.000	150.000
36	8.000	20.000	10.000	15.000	206,332.000	141,913.000	150.000
37	8.000	20.000	10.000	15.000	206,332.000	141,913.000	150.000
38	8.000	20.000	10.000	15.000	206,332.000	141,913.000	150.000
39	8.000	20.000	10.000	15.000	206,332.000	141,913.000	150.000
40	8.000	20.000	10.000	15.000	206,332.000	141,913.000	150.000
41	8.390	20.000	10.000	15.000	208,081.314	150,764.904	157.802
42	8.000	20.000	10.000	15.000	206,332.000	141,913.000	150.000
43	8.000	20.000	10.000	15.000	206,332.000	141,913.000	150.000

…/cont.

Appendix 19.4 (cont.)

Firm	Input 1	Input 2	Input 3	Input 4	Input 5	Input 6	Input 7
				Input quantities			
44	8.000	20.000	10.000	15.000	206,332.000	141,913.000	150.000
45	8.000	20.000	10.000	15.000	206,332.000	141,913.000	150.000
46	8.000	20.000	10.000	15.000	206,332.000	141,913.000	150.000
47	8.000	20.000	10.000	15.000	206,332.000	141,913.000	150.000
48	8.000	20.000	10.000	15.000	206,332.000	141,913.000	150.000
49	8.290	20.000	10.000	15.000	207,633.214	148,497.422	155.804
50	8.427	20.000	10.000	15.000	208,244.458	151,590.444	158.530
51	8.004	20.000	10.000	15.000	206,348.399	141,995.983	150.073
52	8.000	20.000	10.000	15.000	206,332.000	141,913.000	150.000
53	8.000	20.000	10.000	15.000	206,332.000	141,913.000	150.000
54	8.000	20.000	10.000	15.000	206,332.000	141,913.000	150.000
55	8.000	20.000	10.000	15.000	206,332.000	141,913.000	150.000
56	8.913	20.000	10.000	15.000	210,426.138	162,630.215	168.261
57	8.960	20.000	10.000	15.000	210,638.660	163,705.622	169.209
58	8.302	20.000	10.000	15.000	207,687.192	148,770.561	156.045
59	8.289	20.000	10.000	15.000	207,625.953	148,460.677	155.771
60	10.500	20.000	10.548	15.822	231,425.886	206,458.645	200.000
61	8.425	20.000	10.000	15.000	208,237.317	151,554.312	158.498
62	10.500	20.000	10.589	15.884	232,474.591	207,049.369	200.000
63	8.525	20.000	10.000	15.000	208,684.509	153,817.200	160.493
64	10.500	20.000	10.000	15.000	208,154.695	151,136.228	200.000
65	10.500	20.000	10.000	15.000	208,216.602	151,449.491	200.000
66	10.500	20.000	10.000	15.000	211,826.116	169,714.404	200.000
67	10.500	20.000	10.000	15.000	217,542.000	198,638.000	200.000
68	10.500	20.000	10.000	15.000	207,590.231	148,279.919	200.000
69	10.500	20.000	10.000	15.000	207,988.836	150,296.946	200.000
70	10.500	20.000	10.000	15.000	207,017.336	145,380.945	200.000
71	10.500	20.000	10.000	15.000	207,646.763	148,565.980	200.000
72	10.500	20.000	10.000	15.000	206,960.748	145,094.598	200.000
73	10.500	20.000	10.000	15.000	207,132.775	145,965.093	200.000
74	10.500	20.000	10.000	15.000	209,189.914	156,374.655	200.000
75	10.500	20.000	10.000	15.000	208,222.884	151,481.276	200.000
76	10.500	20.000	10.000	15.000	206,904.160	144,808.252	200.000
77	10.500	20.000	10.000	15.000	206,835.406	144,460.340	200.000
78	10.500	20.000	10.000	15.000	209,751.152	159,214.642	200.000
79	10.500	20.000	10.000	15.000	208,721.875	154,006.281	200.000
80	10.500	20.000	10.000	15.000	206,332.000	141,913.000	200.000
81	10.500	20.000	10.000	15.000	212,624.231	173,753.038	200.000
82	10.500	20.000	10.000	15.000	207,017.958	145,384.095	200.000
83	10.500	20.000	10.000	15.000	208,154.808	151,136.801	200.000
84	10.500	20.000	10.552	15.827	231,518.509	206,510.818	200.000
85	10.500	20.000	11.890	17.835	265,421.763	225,608.160	200.000
86	10.500	20.000	13.378	20.068	303,142.220	246,855.692	200.000
87	10.500	20.000	13.377	20.065	303,106.257	246,835.434	200.000
88	10.500	20.000	10.000	15.000	212,500.870	173,128.802	200.000
89	10.500	20.000	10.550	15.825	231,485.259	206,492.089	200.000

.../cont.

Appendix 19.4 (cont.)

Firm	Input quantities						
	Input 1	Input 2	Input 3	Input 4	Input 5	Input 6	Input 7
90	10.500	20.000	11.743	17.615	261,709.056	223,516.832	200.000
91	10.500	20.000	10.256	15.383	224,018.116	202,285.927	200.000
92	10.500	20.000	10.553	15.829	231,552.436	206,529.929	200.000
93	10.500	20.000	12.039	18.059	269,215.895	227,745.354	200.000
94	10.500	20.000	15.023	22.535	345,233.885	270,204.713	200.000
95	10.500	20.000	20.000	30.000	560,000.000	314,000.000	200.000
96	10.500	20.000	10.294	15.440	224,979.287	202,827.345	200.000
97	10.500	20.000	15.000	22.500	344,230.000	270,000.000	200.000
98	10.500	20.000	11.877	17.816	265,108.949	225,431.956	200.000
99	10.500	20.000	12.039	18.059	269,213.860	227,744.208	200.000
100	10.500	20.000	11.527	17.290	256,230.414	220,430.771	200.000

-20-

Measurement of Efficiency Change and Productivity Growth:

A Case Study of National Health Systems in the African Union

Joses Kirigia

INTRODUCTION

A national health system (NHS) has been described as a body encompassing all the activities whose primary purpose is to promote, restore, or maintain health (i.e., quantity and health-related quality of life). A national health system performs the functions of *(a)* stewardship (oversight); *(b)* health financing including revenue collection, pooling of resources, sharing of financial risk, and purchasing of health services; *(c)* creation of resources or inputs for producing health, including human resources for health; and *(d)* provision of health services with a view to improving responsiveness to people's non-medical expectations, ensuring fair financial contribution to health systems, and ultimately improving health (these three being goals of a health system) [1]. The World Health Report for 2000 ranked the 191 Member States of the World Health Organization (WHO) on the basis of their overall health system goals performance [2]. A majority of the African Union (AU) countries' national health systems performed poorly.

In May 2006, the ministers of health at a special session of the AU decided to undertake a number of measures to strengthen the health financing function of their health systems [3] with a view to mobilising more domestic resources for massive expansion of the coverage of health interventions envisaged in the United Nations MDGs [4]. The health ministers undertook to institutionalise efficiency monitoring within the national health information management systems. To date, no other study has estimated the technical efficiency, scale efficiency, efficiency change, technical progress, and productivity growth for all the AU countries' national health systems (NHSs). The African Union identified the need for a study aimed at contributing to bridging that knowledge gap by establishing baseline efficiency and productivity growth scores for use to monitor changes in the performance of NHSs as countries strive to strengthen their health financing systems.

The chair of the AU established a steering committee consisting of departmental directors to develop the terms of reference for a regional expert to undertake a study aimed at bridging the above-mentioned knowledge gaps. The committee, through the Economic Commission for Africa (ECA), identified Professor Rosenabi Deborah Aburi, an internationally acclaimed professor of health economics from the University of Kibari (a continental centre of excellence) to design and undertake the study.

After extensive discussions involving Professor Aburi, the steering committee, and ECA it was agreed that the study should (*a*) assess the technical efficiency of national health systems of AU countries in producing male and female life expectancy, (*b*) assess changes in health productivity over time with a view to analysing changes in efficiency and changes in technology, (*c*) identify the best performing NHSs whose practice could be emulated by others, and (*d*) highlight to health sector policymakers the implications for policy.

METHODOLOGY

Professor Aburi downloaded numerous articles on efficiency and productivity measurement in health from the Internet. She undertook extensive critical literature review to gain deeper understanding of the actual knowledge gaps, output and input variables employed by other studies, and methods and software used for measurement of efficiency and productivity growth.

The literature review revealed two main approaches to the measurement of health services efficiency: parametric (econometric) methods that include estimation of production and cost functions with *a priori* well-defined functional form and construction of index numbers using non-parametric methods including data envelopment analysis (DEA). The DEA technique has the advantage of easily accommodating multiple input-multiple output production and does not make behavioural assumptions (such as profit maximisation) about the NHSS (decision-making units). For these reasons Professor Aburi opted for DEA to estimate technical efficiency and productivity of national health systems in the African continent.

Variables

In her extensive literature review, Professor Aburi found some parametric studies [5] that used health-adjusted life expectancy (HALE) as a measure of NHS outcomes and per capita total health expenditure as a composite input. After extensive discussions with the steering committee and the ECA, it was agreed that (*a*) the unit of analysis in the study should be a country's NHS; (*b*) the ultimate outputs for each individual country NHS are male and female life expectancies at birth (in years); (*c*) the inputs should include per capita total health expenditure (international dollars) and adult literacy rate; and (*d*) due to the dearth of research resources data gathering should be confined to WHO and UN secondary sources.

Data Sources

Professor Aburi obtained data for the period 1999 to 2003 on life expectancy and per capita total health expenditure from the tabular annexes of the World Health Reports 2001 to 2005 [6-11]. Data on adult literacy rate were obtained from the statistical annexes of the United Nations Development Programme Human Development Reports for 2001 to 2005 [12-16]. Data on inputs and outcomes are contained in Appendix 20.1.

Analysis

Professor Aburi used the free DEAP software developed by Professor Tim Coelli of the University of New Queensland, Australia. She followed the following steps:

1. Download the DEAP Version 2.1 software from http://www.uq.edu/economics/cepa/deap.htm into a folder on your computer. DEAP comprises five files [17] as follows:

   a) The executable file called DEAP.EXE, which is supplied with the program;

   b) The start-up file called DEAP.000, which stores key parameter values and comes with the program;

   c) The data file, e.g., EG2.DTA, which you have to create prior to execution;

   d) An instruction file, e.g., EG2.INS, which you have to create prior to execution;

   e) The output file, e.g., EG2.OUT, which is created by DEAP during execution.

2. Enter the data contained in Appendix 20.1 on an Excel spreadsheet. Data for each decision-making unit (firm) should occupy one row. There must be one column for each output and each input with all outputs listed first and then all inputs. In this Malmquist case study, you have panel data for 53 countries' national health systems, each observed for five years (i.e., 1999 to 2003). You must list all the data for 1999 and then for 2000 in the same order as the NHSs. All NHSs must be observed in all the time

periods (i.e., the panel must be "balanced"). For the purpose of this case study, listing of the data will be as follows:

a) Column 1: Names of countries (i.e., NHSs)

b) Column 2: Output1{O} = Male life expectancy (list the values for the five years starting with 1999 as the base year)

c) Column 3: Output2{O} = Female life expectancy (list the values for the five years starting with 1999 as the base year)

d) Column 4: Input1{I} = Per capita total health expenditure, PCTHE, (list the values for the five years starting with 1999 as the base year)

e) Column 5: Input2{I} = Adult literacy rate (list the values for the five years starting with 1999 as the base year)

3. Using the computer mouse, copy only the data values of outputs and inputs without the names of the health systems, outputs, or inputs.

4. Choose **Start**, **Program**, **Accessories,** and then finally **Notepad**. This will open the Notepad software.

5. In Notepad, choose **File** and then **Open**. Browse for the folder where you saved the DEAP software. Click on the data file, for example EG2.DTA, and open it. Delete the contents, paste your data on the Notepad, and click on **Save**. The data, once pasted on Notepad, will appear as indicated in Appendix 20.2.

6. Choose **File** and then **New**. Locate the DEAP instruction file called EG2.INS and open it. The contents of this file will appear as in Appendix 20.3. Modify the instruction file to reflect the data file name (Eg2.dta), output file name (Eg2.out), number of firms (53), number of time periods (5), number of outputs (2), number of inputs (2,) model orientation (1 for output oriented), type of model (0 for CRS) , and type of DEA analysis (2 for MALMQUIST-DEA). For Malmquist total factor productivity analysis, Professor Aburi used 2=MALMQUIST-DEA. Remember to save the file. Please read the DEA manual contained in the PDF file that comes with the software.

7. Close Notepad and go to the folder in which you saved the DEAP software. Locate and select the execution file named DEAP.EXE.

8. The DEAP programme will prompt you to enter the name of the instruction file. At the prompt, type EG2.INS. Within a few seconds the estimations will be completed and the results sent to your output file EG2.OUT. The EG2.OUT file will look like Appendix 20.4.

9. Choose EG2.OUT and when prompted to indicate the software in which it should be opened, make your selection. If you select Excel, the listing of your output will look like Appendix 20.4. It will contain summaries of

efficiency (firm efficiency, constant returns to scale technical efficiency, variable returns to scale technical efficiency, and scale efficiency); output and input slacks; peers, peer weights and peer count; output and input targets; and firm by firm results.

10. You can then proceed to do the exercise in the next section.

Exercise

1. Estimate the descriptive statistics (mean, median, standard deviation, maximum value, minimum value) of the outcomes and the two inputs for each of the five years (1999–2003). Tabulate and discuss the results.

2. Estimate the constant returns to scale technical efficiency, variable returns to scale technical efficiency, and scale efficiency for individual NHSs for each year during 1999–2003. Tabulate and discuss the results.

3. Prepare a table presenting the frequency (and percentage) distribution of technical and scale efficiency scores for the national health systems in the African Union during 1999–2003. Discuss the results.

4. Apply the Malmquist total factor productivity (TFP) index to analyse the temporal differences in productivity and to decompose the sources of productivity change, that is technological change and efficiency change (decomposed into pure efficiency change and scale change). Use the year 1999 as the technology reference. Tabulate and discuss the results.

REFERENCES

1. Murray CJL, Frenk J. A framework for assessing the performance of health systems. *Bulletin of the World Health Organization* 2000;78(6):717–731.

2. World Health Organization. *The world health report 2000 — improving performance of health systems*. Geneva: World Health Organization; 2000.

3. African Union. *Universal access to HIV/AIDS, tuberculosis and malaria services by a united Africa by 2010*. Resolution Sp/Assembly/ATM/5(I) Rev. 3 of the Ministers of Health on health financing in Africa. Addis Ababa: African Union; 2006.

4. United Nations: *Millennium Development Declaration. Resolution A/55/L.2*. New York: United Nations; 2000.

5. Evans DB, Tandon A, Murray CJL, Lauer JA. Comparative efficiency of national health systems: cross national econometric analysis. *British Medical Journal* 2001;323:307–310.

6. World Health Organization. *The world health report 2001: mental health: new understanding, new hope*. Geneva: World Health Organization; 2001.

7. World Health Organization. *The world Health report 2002: Reducing health risks, promoting healthy life*. Geneva: World Health Organization; 2002.

8. World Health Organization. *The world health report 2003: Shaping the future.* Geneva: World Health Organization; 2003.

9. World Health Organization. *The world health report 2004: Changing history.* Geneva: World Health Organization; 2004.

10. World Health Organization: *The world health report 2005: Make every mother and child count.* Geneva: World Health Organization; 2005.

11. World Health Organization: *The world health report 2006: Working together for health.* Geneva: World Health Organization; 2006.

12. United Nations Development Programme. *Human development report 2001.* New York: Oxford University Press; 2001.

13. United Nations Development Programme. *Human development report 2002.* New York: Oxford University Press; 2002.

14. United Nations Development Programme. *Human development report 2003.* New York: Oxford University Press; 2003.

15. United Nations Development Programme. *Human development report 2004.* New York: Oxford University Press; 2004.

16. United Nations Development Programme. *Human development report 2005.* New York: Oxford University Press; 2005.

17. Coelli TJ. *A guide to DEAP version 2.1: a data envelopment analysis [computer] program,* Centre for Efficiency and Productivity Analysis (CEPA) Working Paper 96/08. Department of Econometrics, University of New England, Armidale, NSW Australia; 1996.

Appendix 20.1   *Male life expectancy, female life expectancy, per capita total health expenditure, and adult literacy rates for African countries during 1999 to 2003*

Country	Code	Period	MLE[a]	FLE[b]	PCTHE[c]	Adult Literacy
				1999		
Algeria	1	1	68.2	68.8	137	66.6
Angola	2	1	46.3	49.1	43	42
Benin	3	1	51.3	53.3	34	39
Botswana	4	1	39.5	39.3	259	76.4
Burkina Faso	5	1	44.1	45.7	55	23
Burundi	6	1	43.2	43.8	14	46.9
Cameroon	7	1	49.9	52.0	62	74.8
Cape Verde	8	1	64.2	71.8	148	73.6
CAR	9	1	43.3	44.9	44	45.4
Chad	10	1	47.3	50.1	37	41
Comoros	11	1	56.0	58.1	30	59.2
Congo	12	1	53.6	55.2	25	79.5
Côte d'Ivoire	13	1	47.2	48.3	87	45.7
DRC	14	1	45.1	46.5	12	60.3
Djibouti	15	1	45.0	45.0	61	63.4
Egypt	16	1	64.2	65.8	173	54.6
Equatorial Guinea	17	1	51.4	55.4	125	82.2
Eritrea	18	1	46.6	46.5	47	52.7
Ethiopia	19	1	41.4	43.1	17	37.4
Gabon	20	1	54.6	57.5	250	63
Gambia	21	1	56.0	58.9	76	35.7
Ghana	22	1	54.2	55.6	100	70.3
Guinea	23	1	46.2	48.9	74	35
Guinea-Bissau	24	1	45.0	47.0	45	37.7
Kenya	25	1	47.3	48.1	60	81.5
Lesotho	26	1	44.1	45.1	91	82.9
Liberia	27	1	42.5	44.9	26	32
Libya	28	1	65.0	67.0	234	79.1
Madagascar	29	1	45.0	47.7	20	65.7
Malawi	30	1	37.3	38.4	47	59.2
Mali	31	1	41.3	44.0	27	39.8
Mauritania	32	1	49.5	53.0	32	41.6
Mauritius	33	1	66.7	74.1	281	84.2
Morocco	34	1	65.0	66.8	167	48
Mozambique	35	1	41.8	44.0	34	43.2
Namibia	36	1	43.3	43.0	328	81.4
Niger	37	1	37.2	40.6	27	15.3
Nigeria	38	1	46.8	48.2	48	62.6
Rwanda	39	1	41.2	42.3	33	65.8
STP	40	1	62.1	64.9	94	83.1
Senegal	41	1	53.5	56.2	44	36.4
Seychelles	42	1	64.9	70.5	548	88

.../cont.

Appendix 20.1 (cont)

Country	Code	Period	MLE[a]	FLE[b]	PCTHE[c]	Adult Literacy
Sierra Leone	43	1	33.2	35.4	19	32
Somalia	44	1	44.0	44.7	18	32
South Africa	45	1	47.3	49.7	595	84.9
Sudan	46	1	53.1	54.7	42	56.9
Swaziland	47	1	45.8	46.8	305	78.9
Togo	48	1	48.9	50.8	59	56.3
Tunisia	49	1	67.0	67.9	343	69.9
Uganda	50	1	41.9	42.4	55	66.1
Tanzania	51	1	44.4	45.6	23	74.7
Zambia	52	1	38.0	39.0	45	77.2
Zimbabwe	53	1	40.9	40.0	185	88
2000						
Algeria	1	2	68.1	71.2	132	66.7
Angola	2	2	44.3	48.3	34	42
Benin	3	2	51.7	53.8	34	37.4
Botswana	4	2	44.6	44.4	294	77.2
Burkina Faso	5	2	42.6	43.6	54	23.9
Burundi	6	2	40.6	41.3	14	48
Cameroon	7	2	49.0	50.4	58	75.8
Cape Verde	8	2	66.5	72.3	163	73.8
CAR	9	2	41.6	42.5	50	46.7
Chad	10	2	47.4	51.1	40	42.6
Comoros	11	2	55.3	58.1	25	55.9
Congo	12	2	50.1	52.9	20	80.7
Côte d'Ivoire	13	2	46.4	48.4	79	46.8
DRC	14	2	41.6	44.0	13	61.4
Djibouti	15	2	43.5	44.7	63	64.6
Egypt	16	2	65.4	69.1	190	55.3
Equatorial Guinea	17	2	53.5	56.2	106	83.2
Eritrea	18	2	49.1	51.0	48	55.7
Ethiopia	19	2	42.8	44.7	19	39.1
Gabon	20	2	54.6	56.9	229	71
Gambia	21	2	55.9	58.7	88	36.6
Ghana	22	2	55.0	57.9	102	71.5
Guinea	23	2	49.0	52.0	76	41
Guinea-Bissau	24	2	44.5	46.9	38	38.5
Kenya	25	2	48.2	49.6	61	82.4
Lesotho	26	2	42.0	42.2	100	83.4
Liberia	27	2	46.6	49.1	23	36
Libya	28	2	67.5	71.0	220	80
Madagascar	29	2	51.7	54.6	20	66.5
Malawi	30	2	37.1	37.8	41	60.1
Mali	31	2	42.7	44.6	32	41.5
Mauritania	32	2	51.7	53.5	32	40.2
Mauritius	33	2	67.6	74.6	331	84.5

.../cont.

Appendix 20.1 (cont.)

Country	Code	Period	MLE[a]	FLE[b]	PCTHE[c]	Adult Literacy
Morocco	34	2	66.1	70.4	175	48.9
Mozambique	35	2	37.9	39.5	40	44
Namibia	36	2	42.8	42.6	340	82
Niger	37	2	42.7	43.9	25	15.9
Nigeria	38	2	49.8	51.4	39	63.9
Rwanda	39	2	38.5	40.5	32	66.8
STP	40	2	60.3	61.9	84	83.1
Senegal	41	2	54.0	56.1	45	37.3
Seychelles	42	2	66.5	74.2	555	88
Sierra Leone	43	2	37.0	38.8	24	36
Somalia	44	2	43.8	45.9	18	36
South Africa	45	2	49.6	52.1	579	85.3
Sudan	46	2	55.4	57.8	40	57.8
Swaziland	47	2	44.7	45.6	302	79.6
Togo	48	2	50.5	53.0	49	57.1
Tunisia	49	2	69.2	73.4	367	71
Uganda	50	2	43.5	44.6	60	67.1
Tanzania	51	2	45.8	47.2	25	75.1
Zambia	52	2	39.2	39.5	46	78.1
Zimbabwe	53	2	45.4	46.0	168	88.7
2001						
Algeria	1	3	67.7	71.1	149	67.8
Angola	2	3	34.1	38.3	48	42
Benin	3	3	51.0	53.3	38	38.6
Botswana	4	3	39.3	38.6	284	78.1
Burkina Faso	5	3	42.2	43.5	55	24.8
Burundi	6	3	38.4	42.3	15	49.2
Cameroon	7	3	48.9	50.5	62	72.4
Cape Verde	8	3	65.7	72.0	186	74.9
CAR	9	3	42.0	43.3	49	48.2
Chad	10	3	47.0	50.2	43	44.2
Comoros	11	3	59.8	63.8	21	56
Congo	12	3	51.8	53.8	23	81.8
Côte d'Ivoire	13	3	45.0	47.0	65	49.7
DRC	14	3	42.1	45.5	10	62.7
Djibouti	15	3	47.9	50.4	64	65.5
Egypt	16	3	65.3	67.8	208	56.1
Equatorial Guinea	17	3	52.3	55.1	152	84.2
Eritrea	18	3	52.3	55.0	53	56.7
Ethiopia	19	3	46.8	49.2	21	40.3
Gabon	20	3	58.0	60.5	235	71
Gambia	21	3	56.2	61.0	92	37.8
Ghana	22	3	55.8	58.9	94	72.7
Guinea	23	3	50.1	53.8	81	41
Guinea-Bissau	24	3	45.9	48.7	38	39.6
Kenya	25	3	48.2	49.6	62	83.3

.../cont.

Appendix 20.1 (cont.)

Country	Code	Period	MLE[a]	FLE[b]	PCTHE[c]	Adult Literacy
Lesotho	26	3	40.1	39.8	103	83.9
Liberia	27	3	44.6	48.0	21	36
Libya	28	3	68.3	73.1	391	80.8
Madagascar	29	3	53.3	56.4	19	67.3
Malawi	30	3	35.7	36.9	48	61
Mali	31	3	44.2	46.2	32	26.4
Mauritania	32	3	50.9	53.1	38	40.7
Mauritius	33	3	67.5	74.9	373	84.8
Morocco	34	3	67.5	71.3	196	49.8
Mozambique	35	3	43.7	45.9	39	45.2
Namibia	36	3	48.4	49.0	323	82.7
Niger	37	3	41.9	43.2	26	16.5
Nigeria	38	3	50.6	52.6	50	65.4
Rwanda	39	3	38.9	42.8	31	68
STP	40	3	62.9	65.0	107	83.1
Senegal	41	3	54.4	57.2	51	38.3
Seychelles	42	3	66.7	76.5	535	91
Sierra Leone	43	3	32.7	35.9	25	36
Somalia	44	3	41.0	45.4	18	36
South Africa	45	3	47.7	50.3	626	85.6
Sudan	46	3	54.1	57.9	44	58.8
Swaziland	47	3	40.2	40.1	308	80.3
Togo	48	3	50.3	53.1	58	58.4
Tunisia	49	3	69.0	73.5	396	72.1
Uganda	50	3	45.3	47.7	70	68
Tanzania	51	3	45.8	47.2	27	76
Zambia	52	3	36.7	37.0	51	79
Zimbabwe	53	3	37.1	36.5	184	89.3
2002						
Algeria	1	4	67.5	71.2	174	68.9
Angola	2	4	37.9	42.0	41	42
Benin	3	4	50.1	52.4	37	39.8
Botswana	4	4	40.2	40.6	312	78.9
Burkina Faso	5	4	40.6	42.6	62	12.8
Burundi	6	4	38.7	43.0	15	50.4
Cameroon	7	4	47.2	49.0	66	67.9
Cape Verde	8	4	66.6	72.9	193	75.7
CAR	9	4	42.1	43.7	51	48.6
Chad	10	4	46.1	49.3	44	45.8
Comoros	11	4	61.6	64.9	27	56.2
Congo	12	4	51.6	54.5	22	82.8
Côte d'Ivoire	13	4	43.1	48.0	62	49.7
DRC	14	4	41.0	46.1	11	62.7
Djibouti	15	4	48.6	50.7	67	65.5

.../cont.

Appendix 20.1 (cont.)

Country	Code	Period	MLE[a]	FLE[b]	PCTHE[c]	Adult Literacy
Egypt	16	4	65.3	69.0	231	55.6
Equatorial Guinea	17	4	51.9	54.8	193	84.2
Eritrea	18	4	55.8	59.3	51	56.7
Ethiopia	19	4	46.8	49.4	21	41.5
Gabon	20	4	57.3	61.4	244	71
Gambia	21	4	55.4	58.9	84	37.8
Ghana	22	4	56.3	58.8	95	73.8
Guinea	23	4	50.9	53.7	90	41
Guinea-Bissau	24	4	45.7	48.7	49	39.6
Kenya	25	4	49.8	51.9	66	84.3
Lesotho	26	4	32.9	38.2	125	81.4
Liberia	27	4	40.1	43.7	20	36
Libya	28	4	70.4	75.5	360	81.7
Madagascar	29	4	54.4	58.4	24	67.3
Malawi	30	4	39.8	40.6	44	61.8
Mali	31	4	43.9	45.7	35	19
Mauritania	32	4	49.8	54.5	53	41.2
Mauritius	33	4	68.4	75.5	398	84.3
Morocco	34	4	68.8	72.8	205	50.7
Mozambique	35	4	41.2	43.9	45	46.5
Namibia	36	4	48.1	50.5	318	83.3
Niger	37	4	42.6	42.7	27	17.1
Nigeria	38	4	48.0	49.6	49	66.8
Rwanda	39	4	41.9	46.8	35	69.2
STP	40	4	61.7	63.6	95	83.1
Senegal	41	4	54.3	57.3	55	39.3
Seychelles	42	4	67.0	77.2	554	91.9
Sierra Leone	43	4	32.4	35.7	32	36
Somalia	44	4	43.0	45.7	45.7	36
South Africa	45	4	48.8	52.6	649	86
Sudan	46	4	54.9	59.3	47	59.9
Swaziland	47	4	36.9	40.4	315	80.9
Togo	48	4	50.0	53.3	54	59.6
Tunisia	49	4	69.5	73.9	396	73.2
Uganda	50	4	47.9	50.8	75	68.9
Tanzania	51	4	45.5	47.5	28	77.1
Zambia	52	4	39.1	40.2	53	79.9
Zimbabwe	53	4	37.7	38.0	161	90
2003						
Algeria	1	5	69	72	186	69.8
Angola	2	5	38	42	49	66.8
Benin	3	5	52	54	36	33.6
Botswana	4	5	37	36	375	78.9
Burkina Faso	5	5	44	46	68	12.8

.../cont.

Appendix 20.1 (cont.)

Country	Code	Period	MLE[a]	FLE[b]	PCTHE[c]	Adult Literacy
Burundi	6	5	40	45	15	58.9
Cameroon	7	5	47	48	64	67.9
Cape Verde	8	5	67	73	185	75.7
CAR	9	5	42	43	47	48.6
Chad	10	5	44	47	51	25.5
Comoros	11	5	62	66	25	56.2
Congo	12	5	53	55	23	82.8
Côte d'Ivoire	13	5	42	49	57	48.1
DRC	14	5	42	47	14	65.3
Djibouti	15	5	53	56	72	65.5
Egypt	16	5	65	69	235	55.6
Equatorial Guinea	17	5	50	52	179	84.2
Eritrea	18	5	58	61	50	56.7
Ethiopia	19	5	49	51	20	41.5
Gabon	20	5	55	60	255	71
Gambia	21	5	56	59	96	37.8
Ghana	22	5	57	60	98	54.1
Guinea	23	5	51	53	95	41
Guinea-Bissau	24	5	45	48	45	39.6
Kenya	25	5	50	49	65	73.6
Lesotho	26	5	35	40	106	81.4
Liberia	27	5	40	43	17	29.6
Libya	28	5	71	76	327	81.7
Madagascar	29	5	55	59	24	70.6
Malawi	30	5	41	42	46	64.1
Mali	31	5	44	46	39	19
Mauritania	32	5	48	53	59	51.2
Mauritius	33	5	69	76	430	84.3
Morocco	34	5	69	73	218	50.7
Mozambique	35	5	44	46	45	46.5
Namibia	36	5	50	53	359	85
Niger	37	5	42	41	30	14.4
Nigeria	38	5	45	46	51	66.8
Rwanda	39	5	43	46	32	64
STP	40	5	58	60	93	83.1
Senegal	41	5	54	57	58	39.3
Seychelles	42	5	67	77	599	91.9
Sierra Leone	43	5	37	39	34	29.6
Somalia	44	5	43	45	45	29.6
South Africa	45	5	48	50	669	82.4
Sudan	46	5	57	62	54	59
Swaziland	47	5	33	36	324	79.2
Togo	48	5	50	54	62	53
Tunisia	49	5	70	74	409	74.3

…/cont.

Appendix 20.1 (cont.)

Country	Code	Period	MLE[a]	FLE[b]	PCTHE[c]	Adult Literacy
Uganda	50	5	47	50	75	68.9
Tanzania	51	5	44	46	29	69.4
Zambia	52	5	39	39	51	67.9
Zimbabwe	53	5	37	36	132	90

Note: [a]Male life expectancy

[b]Female life expectancy

[c]Per capita total health expenditure

Efficiency Analysis of Health Systems in Africa

Appendix 20.2   Listing of Malmquist Data File EG2.DTA

68.2	68.8	137	66.6	41.3	44.0	27	39.8	66.5	72.3	163	73.8	38.5	40.5	32	66.8
46.3	49.1	43	42	49.5	53.0	32	41.6	41.6	42.5	50	46.7	60.3	61.9	84	83.1
51.3	53.3	34	39	66.7	74.1	281	84.2	47.4	51.1	40	42.6	54.0	56.1	45	37.3
39.5	39.3	259	76.4	65.0	66.8	167	48	55.3	58.1	25	55.9	66.5	74.2	555	88
44.1	45.7	55	23	41.8	44.0	34	43.2	50.1	52.9	20	80.7	37.0	38.8	24	36
43.2	43.8	14	46.9	43.3	43.0	328	81.4	46.4	48.4	79	46.8	43.8	45.9	18	36
49.9	52.0	62	74.8	37.2	40.6	27	15.3	41.6	44.0	13	61.4	49.6	52.1	579	85.3
64.2	71.8	148	73.6	46.8	48.2	48	62.6	43.5	44.7	63	64.6	55.4	57.8	40	57.8
43.3	44.9	44	45.4	41.2	42.3	33	65.8	65.4	69.1	190	55.3	44.7	45.6	302	79.6
47.3	50.1	37	41	62.1	64.9	94	83.1	53.5	56.2	106	83.2	50.5	53.0	49	57.1
56.0	58.1	30	59.2	53.5	56.2	44	36.4	49.1	51.0	48	55.7	69.2	73.4	367	71
53.6	55.2	25	79.5	64.9	70.5	548	88	42.8	44.7	19	39.1	43.5	44.6	60	67.1
47.2	48.3	87	45.7	33.2	35.4	19	32	54.6	56.9	229	71	45.8	47.2	25	75.1
45.1	46.5	12	60.3	44.0	44.7	18	32	55.9	58.7	88	36.6	39.2	39.5	46	78.1
45.0	45.0	61	63.4	47.3	49.7	595	84.9	55.0	57.9	102	71.5	45.4	46.0	168	88.7
64.2	65.8	173	54.6	53.1	54.7	42	56.9	49.0	52.0	76	41	67.7	71.1	149	67.8
51.4	55.4	125	82.2	45.8	46.8	305	78.9	44.5	46.9	38	38.5	34.1	38.3	48	42
46.6	46.5	47	52.7	48.9	50.8	59	56.3	48.2	49.6	61	82.4	51.0	53.3	38	38.6
41.4	43.1	17	37.4	67.0	67.9	343	69.9	42.0	42.2	100	83.4	39.3	38.6	284	78.1
54.6	57.5	250	63	41.9	42.4	55	66.1	46.6	49.1	23	36	42.2	43.5	55	24.8
56.0	58.9	76	35.7	44.4	45.6	23	74.7	67.5	71.0	220	80	38.4	42.3	15	49.2
54.2	55.6	100	70.3	38.0	39.0	45	77.2	51.7	54.6	20	66.5	48.9	50.5	62	72.4
46.2	48.9	74	35	40.9	40.0	185	88	37.1	37.8	41	60.1	65.7	72.0	186	74.9
45.0	47.0	45	37.7	68.1	71.2	132	66.7	42.7	44.6	32	41.5	42.0	43.3	49	48.2
47.3	48.1	60	81.5	44.3	48.3	34	42	51.7	53.5	32	40.2	47.0	50.2	43	44.2
44.1	45.1	91	82.9	51.7	53.8	34	37.4	67.6	74.6	331	84.5	59.8	63.8	21	56
42.5	44.9	26	32	44.6	44.4	294	77.2	66.1	70.4	175	48.9	51.8	53.8	23	81.8
65.0	67.0	234	79.1	42.6	43.6	54	23.9	37.9	39.5	40	44	45.0	47.0	65	49.7
45.0	47.7	20	65.7	40.6	41.3	14	48	42.8	42.6	340	82	42.1	45.5	10	62.7
37.3	38.4	47	59.2	49.0	50.4	58	75.8	42.7	43.9	25	15.9	47.9	50.4	64	65.5
								49.8	51.4	39	63.9	65.3	67.8	208	56.1

…/cont.

Appendix 20.2 (cont.)

52.3	55.1	152	84.2	40.2	40.1	308	80.3	45.7	48.7	49	39.6	69	72	186	69.8
52.3	55.0	53	56.7	50.3	53.1	58	58.4	49.8	51.9	66	84.3	38	42	49	66.8
46.8	49.2	21	40.3	69.0	73.5	396	72.1	32.9	38.2	125	81.4	52	54	36	33.6
58.0	60.5	235	71	45.3	47.7	70	68	40.1	43.7	20	36	37	36	375	78.9
56.2	61.0	92	37.8	45.8	47.2	27	76	70.4	75.5	360	81.7	44	46	68	12.8
55.8	58.9	94	72.7	36.7	37.0	51	79	54.4	58.4	24	67.3	40	45	15	58.9
50.1	53.8	81	41	37.1	36.5	184	89.3	39.8	40.6	44	61.8	47	48	64	67.9
45.9	48.7	38	39.6	67.5	71.2	174	68.9	43.9	45.7	35	19	67	73	185	75.7
48.2	49.6	62	83.3	37.9	42.0	41	42	49.8	54.5	53	41.2	42	43	47	48.6
40.1	39.8	103	83.9	50.1	52.4	37	39.8	68.4	75.5	398	84.3	44	47	51	25.5
44.6	48.0	21	36	40.2	40.6	312	78.9	68.8	72.8	205	50.7	62	66	25	56.2
68.3	73.1	391	80.8	40.6	42.6	62	12.8	41.2	43.9	45	46.5	53	55	23	82.8
53.3	56.4	19	67.3	38.7	43.0	15	50.4	48.1	50.5	318	83.3	42	49	57	48.1
35.7	36.9	48	61	47.2	49.0	66	67.9	42.6	42.7	27	17.1	42	47	14	65.3
44.2	46.2	32	26.4	66.6	72.9	193	75.7	48.0	49.6	49	66.8	53	56	72	65.5
50.9	53.1	38	40.7	42.1	43.7	51	48.6	41.9	46.8	35	69.2	65	69	235	55.6
67.5	74.9	373	84.8	46.1	49.3	44	45.8	61.7	63.6	95	83.1	50	52	179	84.2
67.5	71.3	196	49.8	61.6	64.9	27	56.2	54.3	57.3	55	39.3	58	61	50	56.7
43.7	45.9	39	45.2	51.6	54.5	22	82.8	67.0	77.2	554	91.9	49	51	20	41.5
48.4	49.0	323	82.7	43.1	48.0	62	49.7	32.4	35.7	32	36	55	60	255	71
41.9	43.2	26	16.5	41.0	46.1	11	62.7	43.0	45.7	45.7	36	56	59	96	37.8
50.6	52.6	50	65.4	48.6	50.7	67	65.5	48.8	52.6	649	86	57	60	98	54.1
38.9	42.8	31	68	65.3	69.0	231	55.6	54.9	59.3	47	59.9	51	53	95	41
62.9	65.0	107	83.1	51.9	54.8	193	84.2	36.9	40.4	315	80.9	45	48	45	39.6
54.4	57.2	51	38.3	55.8	59.3	51	56.7	50.0	53.3	54	59.6	50	49	65	73.6
66.7	76.5	535	91	46.8	49.4	21	41.5	69.5	73.9	396	73.2	35	40	106	81.4
32.7	35.9	25	36	57.3	61.4	244	71	47.9	50.8	75	68.9	40	43	17	29.6
41.0	45.4	18	36	55.4	58.9	84	37.8	45.5	47.5	28	77.1	71	76	327	81.7
47.7	50.3	626	85.6	56.3	58.8	95	73.8	39.1	40.2	53	79.9	55	59	24	70.6
54.1	57.9	44	58.8	50.9	53.7	90	41	37.7	38.0	161	90	41	42	46	64.1

.../cont.

Appendix 20.2 (cont.)

44	46	39	19	42	41	30	14.4	37	39	34	29.6	70	74	409	74.3
48	53	59	51.2	45	46	51	66.8	43	45	45	29.6	47	50	75	68.9
69	76	430	84.3	43	46	32	64	48	50	669	82.4	44	46	29	69.4
69	73	218	50.7	58	60	93	83.1	57	62	54	59	39	39	51	67.9
44	46	45	46.5	54	57	58	39.3	33	36	324	79.2	37	36	132	90
50	53	359	85	67	77	599	91.9	50	54	62	53				

Appendix 20.3   Listing of Malmquist instruction file EG2.INS

```
Eg1.dta DATA FILE NAME
Eg1.out OUTPUT FILE NAME
53 NUMBER OF FIRMS
5 NUMBER OF TIME PERIODS
2 NUMBER OF OUTPUTS
2 NUMBER OF INPUTS
0 0=INPUT AND 1=OUTPUT ORIENTATED
0 0=CRS AND 1=VRS
2 0=DEA(MULTI-STAGE), 1=COST-DEA, 2=MALMQUIST-DEA, 3=DEA(1-STAGE), 4=DEA(2-STAGE)
```

Appendix 20.4 Listing of Malmquist output file EG2.OUT

Results from DEAP Version 2.1

Instruction file = EG2.INS

Data file = eg2.dta

Output orientated Malmquist DEA

Distances summary

Year = 1

firm crs te rel to tech in yr vrs

no. ********************** te

t-1 t t+1

1	0.000	0.421	0.381	1.000	28	0.000	0.338	0.307	0.958
2	0.000	0.622	0.584	0.863	29	0.000	0.762	0.810	0.922
3	0.000	0.799	0.763	1.000	30	0.000	0.399	0.389	0.646
4	0.000	0.213	0.193	0.579	31	0.000	0.728	0.726	0.867
5	0.000	0.789	0.720	0.996	32	0.000	0.790	0.773	0.994
					33	0.000	0.332	0.319	1.000
6	0.000	1.000	1.074	1.000					
7	0.000	0.415	0.402	0.845	34	0.000	0.557	0.504	1.000
8	0.000	0.368	0.353	1.000	35	0.000	0.624	0.609	0.806
9	0.000	0.551	0.514	0.787	36	0.000	0.219	0.198	0.635
10	0.000	0.697	0.667	0.910	37	0.000	1.000	0.961	1.000
					38	0.000	0.481	0.473	0.806
11	0.000	0.754	0.772	1.000					
12	0.000	0.716	0.764	1.000	39	0.000	0.498	0.514	0.731
13	0.000	0.425	0.385	0.797	40	0.000	0.399	0.363	1.000
14	0.000	1.000	1.174	1.000	41	0.000	0.756	0.684	1.000
15	0.000	0.411	0.384	0.756	42	0.000	0.303	0.290	0.968
					43	0.000	0.774	0.787	0.785
16	0.000	0.484	0.438	0.973					
17	0.000	0.282	0.251	0.806	44	0.000	1.000	1.056	1.000
18	0.000	0.531	0.504	0.823	45	0.000	0.229	0.212	0.700
19	0.000	0.952	0.975	0.955	46	0.000	0.610	0.605	0.934
20	0.000	0.356	0.331	0.827	47	0.000	0.239	0.216	0.673
					48	0.000	0.482	0.444	0.841
21	0.000	0.645	0.598	1.000					
22	0.000	0.362	0.311	0.852	49	0.000	0.394	0.357	0.983
23	0.000	0.543	0.506	0.840	50	0.000	0.393	0.379	0.712
24	0.000	0.619	0.557	0.836	51	0.000	0.637	0.682	0.850
25	0.000	0.380	0.377	0.796	52	0.000	0.356	0.370	0.658
					53	0.000	0.191	0.173	0.600
26	0.000	0.288	0.261	0.702					
27	0.000	0.846	0.821	0.943	Mean	0.000	0.546	0.533	0.86

.../cont.

Appendix 20.4 (cont.)

Year = 2

firm crs te rel to tech in yr vrs

no. *********** te

t-1 t t+1

firm no.	t-1	t	t+1	te	firm no.	t-1	t	t+1	te
1	0.420	0.387	0.408	1.000	28	0.347	0.321	0.339	0.986
2	0.695	0.675	0.687	0.873	29	0.868	0.924	0.835	1.000
3	0.823	0.781	0.803	1.000	30	0.417	0.421	0.427	0.648
4	0.238	0.215	0.228	0.648	31	0.665	0.651	0.662	0.815
5	0.733	0.664	0.702	0.887	32	0.814	0.793	0.812	0.993
6	0.931	1.000	0.925	1.000	33	0.333	0.320	0.337	1.000
7	0.416	0.409	0.418	0.827	34	0.556	0.521	0.550	1.000
8	0.371	0.355	0.374	1.000	35	0.513	0.487	0.500	0.693
9	0.489	0.446	0.464	0.740	36	0.215	0.194	0.206	0.620
10	0.670	0.637	0.654	0.901	37	1.187	1.000	1.059	1.000
11	0.867	0.886	0.855	1.000	38	0.556	0.570	0.575	0.874
12	0.767	0.833	0.744	0.969	39	0.484	0.491	0.482	0.687
13	0.419	0.375	0.395	0.787	40	0.410	0.379	0.393	0.967
14	0.904	1.000	0.883	1.000	41	0.746	0.667	0.695	1.000
15	0.388	0.361	0.373	0.727	42	0.318	0.305	0.322	0.995
16	0.486	0.453	0.477	0.978	43	0.716	0.716	0.721	0.771
17	0.321	0.288	0.301	0.826	44	0.989	1.000	0.996	1.000
18	0.538	0.515	0.530	0.852	45	0.239	0.221	0.233	0.717
19	0.904	0.919	0.909	0.941	46	0.653	0.649	0.658	0.970
20	0.316	0.290	0.306	0.796	47	0.231	0.209	0.221	0.649
21	0.628	0.581	0.613	1.000	48	0.544	0.524	0.535	0.872
22	0.360	0.316	0.333	0.857	49	0.401	0.374	0.395	1.000
23	0.492	0.459	0.484	0.870	50	0.389	0.369	0.380	0.731
24	0.662	0.625	0.643	0.852	51	0.627	0.666	0.616	0.828
25	0.382	0.378	0.386	0.809	52	0.359	0.375	0.377	0.678
					53	0.211	0.191	0.202	0.665
26	0.260	0.232	0.242	0.653	**Mean**	**0.551**	**0.535**	**0.540**	**0.867**
27	0.924	0.929	0.931	0.991					

.../cont.

Appendix 20.4 (cont.)

Year = 3

firm crs te rel to tech in yr vrs

no. **************** te

t-1 t t+1

1	0.380	0.401	0.395	1.000	28	0.328	0.346	0.272	0.993
2	0.421	0.437	0.464	0.650	29	0.982	0.883	0.979	0.942
3	0.709	0.731	0.779	0.957	30	0.364	0.372	0.395	0.581
4	0.187	0.198	0.172	0.574	31	0.774	0.806	0.854	0.942
5	0.635	0.670	0.659	0.886	32	0.695	0.714	0.762	0.938
6	0.958	0.856	0.941	0.892	33	0.320	0.337	0.275	1.000
7	0.396	0.407	0.431	0.785	34	0.519	0.547	0.462	1.000
8	0.348	0.367	0.352	1.000	35	0.571	0.584	0.625	0.774
9	0.453	0.470	0.496	0.721	36	0.218	0.230	0.197	0.705
10	0.588	0.606	0.646	0.842	37	0.948	1.000	1.050	1.000
11	1.103	1.000	1.132	1.000	38	0.490	0.501	0.534	0.822
12	0.777	0.707	0.785	0.864	39	0.529	0.508	0.561	0.665
13	0.395	0.413	0.436	0.752	40	0.331	0.346	0.365	0.966
14	1.344	1.000	1.130	1.000	41	0.615	0.644	0.680	1.000
15	0.397	0.409	0.436	0.767	42	0.304	0.321	0.253	1.000
16	0.438	0.462	0.398	0.964	43	0.646	0.651	0.702	0.671
17	0.237	0.250	0.256	0.774	44	0.989	0.975	1.067	1.000
18	0.517	0.530	0.566	0.851	45	0.213	0.224	0.177	0.691
19	0.936	0.931	1.012	0.951	46	0.608	0.616	0.663	0.889
20	0.309	0.325	0.290	0.851	47	0.186	0.197	0.169	0.587
21	0.584	0.616	0.594	1.000	48	0.464	0.478	0.510	0.812
22	0.341	0.357	0.377	0.868	49	0.369	0.389	0.306	1.000
23	0.475	0.501	0.505	0.879	50	0.349	0.361	0.384	0.721
24	0.643	0.661	0.706	0.859	51	0.629	0.584	0.659	0.761
25	0.373	0.381	0.404	0.773	52	0.328	0.332	0.356	0.595
26	0.216	0.226	0.234	0.618	53	0.155	0.164	0.160	0.547
27	0.959	0.955	1.038	0.965	Mean	**0.529**	**0.528**	**0.548**	**0.842**

...*/cont.*

Appendix 20.4 (cont.)

Year = 4

firm crs te rel to tech in yr vrs

no. *********************** te

t-1 t t+1

no.	t-1	t	t+1	te	no.	t-1	t	t+1	te
1	0.395	0.377	0.350	0.999	28	0.353	0.287	0.273	1.000
2	0.532	0.567	0.548	0.721	29	0.786	0.882	0.871	0.952
3	0.722	0.772	0.739	0.925	30	0.435	0.463	0.431	0.639
4	0.201	0.171	0.158	0.575	31	0.919	0.938	0.917	1.000
5	1.271	1.000	0.955	1.000	32	0.585	0.618	0.627	0.929
6	0.861	0.944	0.959	1.000	33	0.342	0.272	0.259	0.996
7	0.386	0.411	0.396	0.747	34	0.548	0.460	0.435	1.000
8	0.368	0.351	0.326	1.000	35	0.505	0.539	0.520	0.720
9	0.457	0.485	0.475	0.711	36	0.232	0.198	0.187	0.687
10	0.579	0.617	0.595	0.815	37	0.981	1.000	1.049	1.000
11	0.916	1.000	0.933	1.000	38	0.477	0.507	0.474	0.768
12	0.719	0.794	0.835	0.935	39	0.520	0.568	0.515	0.717
13	0.436	0.461	0.465	0.754	40	0.370	0.389	0.387	0.959
14	0.972	1.000	1.248	1.000	41	0.607	0.640	0.658	0.992
15	0.400	0.425	0.415	0.769	42	0.321	0.252	0.234	1.000
16	0.474	0.394	0.373	0.946	43	0.560	0.599	0.569	0.655
17	0.249	0.243	0.225	0.760	44	0.566	0.599	0.606	0.825
18	0.586	0.626	0.597	0.899	45	0.234	0.184	0.170	0.696
19	0.918	1.000	0.921	1.000	46	0.602	0.647	0.601	0.900
20	0.330	0.291	0.274	0.835	47	0.191	0.162	0.153	0.540
21	0.595	0.586	0.541	1.000	48	0.499	0.533	0.508	0.805
22	0.352	0.372	0.377	0.875	49	0.386	0.303	0.281	0.993
23	0.500	0.494	0.456	0.884	50	0.365	0.388	0.382	0.757
24	0.559	0.591	0.595	0.846	51	0.564	0.637	0.626	0.738
25	0.377	0.403	0.377	0.788					
					52	0.344	0.368	0.339	0.624
26	0.183	0.192	0.200	0.549	53	0.165	0.166	0.164	0.563
27	0.891	0.971	0.858	1.000	Mean	0.522	0.531	0.518	0.845

.../cont.

Appendix 20.4 (cont.)

Year = 5

firm crs te rel to tech in yr vrs

no. *********************** te

t-1 t t+1

1	0.372	0.346	0.000	1.000	28	0.299	0.283	0.000	1.000
2	0.428	0.393	0.000	0.626	29	0.873	0.870	0.000	0.918
3	0.855	0.841	0.000	1.000	30	0.458	0.426	0.000	0.652
4	0.149	0.140	0.000	0.522	31	0.925	0.859	0.000	1.000
5	1.084	1.000	0.000	1.000	32	0.523	0.521	0.000	0.813
6	0.905	0.953	0.000	0.954	33	0.271	0.254	0.000	0.997
7	0.411	0.399	0.000	0.738	34	0.451	0.429	0.000	1.000
8	0.355	0.329	0.000	1.000	35	0.564	0.545	0.000	0.752
9	0.505	0.491	0.000	0.705	36	0.197	0.187	0.000	0.704
10	0.708	0.665	0.000	0.916	37	1.123	1.000	0.000	1.000
11	1.062	1.000	0.000	1.000	38	0.463	0.435	0.000	0.713
12	0.798	0.831	0.000	0.908	39	0.608	0.556	0.000	0.694
13	0.505	0.505	0.000	0.772	40	0.373	0.369	0.000	0.893
14	0.912	1.000	0.000	1.000	41	0.612	0.635	0.000	0.968
15	0.447	0.441	0.000	0.828	42	0.252	0.233	0.000	1.000
16	0.391	0.371	0.000	0.939	43	0.668	0.664	0.000	0.758
17	0.234	0.216	0.000	0.728	44	0.627	0.653	0.000	0.851
18	0.653	0.619	0.000	0.921	45	0.184	0.169	0.000	0.676
19	1.075	1.000	0.000	1.000	46	0.622	0.594	0.000	0.922
20	0.281	0.264	0.000	0.808	47	0.145	0.137	0.000	0.475
21	0.569	0.529	0.000	0.983	48	0.510	0.509	0.000	0.815
22	0.434	0.427	0.000	0.882	49	0.299	0.277	0.000	0.993
23	0.481	0.446	0.000	0.873	50	0.382	0.376	0.000	0.735
24	0.619	0.615	0.000	0.820	51	0.631	0.603	0.000	0.708
25	0.423	0.406	0.000	0.784					
					52	0.399	0.374	0.000	0.618
26	0.227	0.231	0.000	0.575	53	0.175	0.181	0.000	0.555
27	1.141	1.000	0.000	1.000	Mean	0.541	0.521	0.000	0.839

Note that t-1 in year 1 and t+1 in the final year are not defined

Malmquist index summary
Year = 2

Firm	Effch	Techch	Pech	Sech	Tfpch	Firm	Effch	Techch	Pech	Sech	Tfpch
1	0.918	1.095	1.000	0.918	1.005	28	0.951	1.091	1.029	0.924	1.037
2	1.085	1.047	1.011	1.073	1.136	29	1.212	0.940	1.085	1.117	1.139
3	0.978	1.050	1.000	0.978	1.027	30	1.055	1.008	1.004	1.051	1.063
4	1.012	1.105	1.118	0.905	1.117	31	0.894	1.012	0.940	0.951	0.905
5	0.842	1.100	0.891	0.945	0.926	32	1.004	1.024	0.999	1.005	1.028
6	1.000	0.931	1.000	1.000	0.931	33	0.964	1.040	1.000	0.964	1.003
7	0.986	1.025	0.978	1.008	1.011	34	0.936	1.085	1.000	0.936	1.016
8	0.965	1.042	1.000	0.965	1.006	35	0.781	1.039	0.860	0.908	0.811
9	0.810	1.084	0.941	0.860	0.878	36	0.888	1.105	0.976	0.910	0.981
10	0.913	1.049	0.989	0.923	0.958	37	1.000	1.111	1.000	1.000	1.111
11	1.175	0.978	1.000	1.175	1.149	38	1.185	0.997	1.084	1.093	1.181
12	1.164	0.928	0.969	1.201	1.080	39	0.987	0.977	0.939	1.051	0.964
13	0.882	1.112	0.988	0.893	0.981	40	0.950	1.090	0.967	0.982	1.036
14	1.000	0.877	1.000	1.000	0.877	41	0.882	1.112	1.000	0.882	0.981
15	0.877	1.073	0.962	0.912	0.941	42	1.007	1.043	1.028	0.980	1.050
16	0.936	1.090	1.005	0.931	1.020	43	0.925	0.991	0.982	0.942	0.917
17	1.020	1.121	1.025	0.995	1.144	44	1.000	0.968	1.000	1.000	0.968
18	0.970	1.049	1.036	0.937	1.018	45	0.965	1.081	1.024	0.943	1.044
19	0.965	0.980	0.985	0.980	0.946	46	1.063	1.007	1.038	1.024	1.071
20	0.814	1.084	0.964	0.845	0.883	47	0.876	1.105	0.963	0.909	0.967
21	0.900	1.081	1.000	0.900	0.973	48	1.087	1.062	1.036	1.049	1.155
22	0.875	1.151	1.006	0.869	1.007	49	0.950	1.087	1.017	0.934	1.033
23	0.846	1.071	1.037	0.816	0.907	50	0.938	1.046	1.027	0.914	0.981
24	1.010	1.084	1.020	0.990	1.095	51	1.045	0.938	0.974	1.073	0.980
25	0.996	1.009	1.016	0.980	1.005	52	1.053	0.960	1.030	1.022	1.011
						53	0.997	1.105	1.109	0.899	1.101
26	0.803	1.113	0.931	0.863	0.895						
27	1.098	1.012	1.051	1.045	1.111	Mean	0.966	1.043	1.000	0.966	1.007

.../cont.

Appendix 20.4 (cont.)

Year = 3

Firm	Effch	Techch	Pech	Sech	Tfpch	Firm	Effch	Techch	Pech	Sech	Tfpch
1	1.036	0.948	1.000	1.036	0.982	28	1.075	0.948	1.007	1.067	1.019
2	0.648	0.973	0.744	0.871	0.630	29	0.956	1.110	0.942	1.014	1.060
3	0.936	0.972	0.957	0.978	0.909	30	0.884	0.981	0.896	0.987	0.867
4	0.921	0.946	0.887	1.039	0.871	31	1.238	0.971	1.156	1.071	1.203
5	1.010	0.947	0.999	1.011	0.956	32	0.901	0.975	0.945	0.953	0.878
6	0.856	1.100	0.892	0.959	0.942	33	1.055	0.948	1.000	1.055	1.000
7	0.996	0.975	0.949	1.050	0.971	34	1.049	0.948	1.000	1.049	0.994
8	1.035	0.948	1.000	1.035	0.981	35	1.197	0.977	1.117	1.072	1.169
9	1.054	0.962	0.973	1.083	1.014	36	1.186	0.946	1.138	1.042	1.121
10	0.951	0.973	0.935	1.017	0.925	37	1.000	0.946	1.000	1.000	0.946
11	1.128	1.069	1.000	1.128	1.206	38	0.879	0.985	0.940	0.935	0.866
12	0.849	1.109	0.892	0.951	0.941	39	1.034	1.030	0.968	1.069	1.065
13	1.103	0.952	0.956	1.154	1.050	40	0.914	0.959	0.999	0.915	0.877
14	1.000	1.234	1.000	1.000	1.234	41	0.966	0.957	1.000	0.966	0.924
15	1.135	0.969	1.055	1.075	1.099	42	1.051	0.948	1.005	1.046	0.997
16	1.020	0.948	0.986	1.034	0.967	43	0.909	0.992	0.870	1.045	0.902
17	0.869	0.953	0.937	0.927	0.828	44	0.975	1.009	1.000	0.975	0.984
18	1.029	0.974	0.998	1.031	1.002	45	1.015	0.948	0.964	1.052	0.962
19	1.014	1.008	1.011	1.003	1.022	46	0.949	0.987	0.916	1.036	0.936
20	1.121	0.948	1.069	1.049	1.063	47	0.943	0.946	0.904	1.043	0.891
21	1.061	0.948	1.000	1.061	1.006	48	0.913	0.975	0.931	0.980	0.890
22	1.128	0.954	1.012	1.115	1.076	49	1.040	0.948	1.000	1.040	0.986
23	1.091	0.948	1.010	1.080	1.035	50	0.977	0.969	0.986	0.991	0.947
24	1.059	0.972	1.008	1.051	1.029	51	0.878	1.079	0.919	0.955	0.947
25	1.006	0.980	0.956	1.052	0.986	52	0.885	0.991	0.878	1.008	0.877
						53	0.858	0.946	0.822	1.045	0.812
26	0.977	0.955	0.946	1.032	0.933						
27	1.028	1.001	0.975	1.055	1.029	**Mean**	**0.990**	**0.981**	**0.968**	**1.023**	**0.972**

.../cont.

Appendix 20.4 (cont.)

Year = 4

Firm	Effch	Techch	Pech	Sech	Tfpch	Firm	Effch	Techch	Pech	Sech	Tfpch
1	0.942	1.030	0.999	0.943	0.970	28	0.831	1.249	1.007	0.825	1.039
2	1.297	0.940	1.109	1.169	1.220	29	0.999	0.896	1.010	0.989	0.896
3	1.056	0.937	0.967	1.092	0.990	30	1.245	0.941	1.100	1.132	1.171
4	0.861	1.163	1.001	0.860	1.001	31	1.163	0.962	1.062	1.095	1.119
5	1.492	1.136	1.129	1.322	1.696	32	0.865	0.941	0.991	0.873	0.815
6	1.104	0.911	1.120	0.985	1.005	33	0.805	1.243	0.996	0.809	1.001
7	1.008	0.943	0.952	1.058	0.950	34	0.840	1.188	1.000	0.840	0.999
8	0.956	1.045	1.000	0.956	0.999	35	0.923	0.936	0.931	0.991	0.864
9	1.033	0.945	0.986	1.047	0.976	36	0.858	1.172	0.975	0.880	1.005
10	1.019	0.938	0.968	1.053	0.956	37	1.000	0.967	1.000	1.000	0.967
11	1.000	0.899	1.000	1.000	0.899	38	1.012	0.939	0.935	1.083	0.950
12	1.123	0.903	1.082	1.037	1.014	39	1.119	0.910	1.078	1.038	1.018
13	1.116	0.946	1.002	1.114	1.056	40	1.124	0.949	0.992	1.133	1.067
14	1.000	0.928	1.000	1.000	0.928	41	0.993	0.948	0.992	1.001	0.942
15	1.040	0.939	1.002	1.037	0.976	42	0.786	1.271	1.000	0.786	0.999
16	0.853	1.182	0.981	0.870	1.008	43	0.920	0.931	0.976	0.943	0.856
17	0.972	0.999	0.981	0.991	0.971	44	0.614	0.930	0.825	0.745	0.571
18	1.181	0.936	1.056	1.118	1.105	45	0.819	1.271	1.006	0.814	1.041
19	1.074	0.919	1.051	1.022	0.987	46	1.051	0.930	1.012	1.038	0.977
20	0.895	1.128	0.981	0.912	1.009	47	0.821	1.173	0.921	0.891	0.962
21	0.950	1.027	1.000	0.950	0.975	48	1.114	0.937	0.991	1.124	1.044
22	1.042	0.947	1.008	1.034	0.987	49	0.779	1.271	0.993	0.784	0.990
23	0.985	1.003	1.006	0.979	0.988	50	1.076	0.940	1.050	1.025	1.012
24	0.893	0.941	0.985	0.907	0.841	51	1.091	0.886	0.970	1.125	0.966
25	1.059	0.938	1.019	1.039	0.993	52	1.110	0.934	1.048	1.059	1.036
						53	1.012	1.008	1.029	0.983	1.020
26	0.849	0.960	0.887	0.956	0.815						
27	1.016	0.919	1.036	0.981	0.934	Mean	0.985	0.998	1.002	0.983	0.984

.../cont.

Appendix 20.4 (cont.)

Year = 5

Firm	Effch	Techch	Pech	Sech	Tfpch	Firm	Effch	Techch	Pech	Sech	Tfpch
1	0.917	1.076	1.001	0.916	0.986	28	0.984	1.054	1.000	0.984	1.038
2	0.693	1.062	0.869	0.797	0.736	29	0.987	1.008	0.965	1.023	0.994
3	1.089	1.031	1.081	1.008	1.123	30	0.920	1.074	1.020	0.902	0.989
4	0.821	1.070	0.909	0.904	0.878	31	0.916	1.050	1.000	0.916	0.961
5	1.000	1.065	1.000	1.000	1.065	32	0.843	0.995	0.875	0.963	0.839
6	1.009	0.967	0.954	1.058	0.976	33	0.936	1.057	1.001	0.935	0.989
7	0.973	1.033	0.988	0.985	1.005	34	0.933	1.055	1.000	0.933	0.984
8	0.938	1.078	1.000	0.938	1.011	35	1.011	1.036	1.044	0.968	1.048
9	1.012	1.025	0.992	1.020	1.037	36	0.944	1.057	1.024	0.921	0.997
10	1.078	1.051	1.124	0.959	1.133	37	1.000	1.035	1.000	1.000	1.035
11	1.000	1.067	1.000	1.000	1.067	38	0.859	1.067	0.928	0.925	0.916
12	1.046	0.956	0.971	1.078	1.000	39	0.978	1.099	0.968	1.011	1.075
13	1.095	0.995	1.024	1.069	1.090	40	0.948	1.008	0.931	1.018	0.956
14	1.000	0.855	1.000	1.000	0.855	41	0.992	0.968	0.976	1.016	0.960
15	1.037	1.020	1.076	0.964	1.058	42	0.924	1.080	1.000	0.924	0.997
16	0.943	1.055	0.993	0.950	0.995	43	1.110	1.029	1.157	0.959	1.141
17	0.890	1.082	0.958	0.929	0.963	44	1.091	0.974	1.032	1.057	1.062
18	0.989	1.052	1.025	0.965	1.040	45	0.922	1.082	0.972	0.949	0.998
19	1.000	1.080	1.000	1.000	1.080	46	0.919	1.062	1.024	0.897	0.975
20	0.908	1.063	0.968	0.938	0.965	47	0.848	1.057	0.880	0.964	0.897
21	0.903	1.080	0.983	0.918	0.974	48	0.954	1.025	1.012	0.942	0.978
22	1.148	1.001	1.008	1.139	1.149	49	0.914	1.080	0.999	0.914	0.987
23	0.903	1.082	0.988	0.914	0.976	50	0.970	1.015	0.972	0.998	0.984
24	1.040	1.000	0.969	1.073	1.040	51	0.946	1.032	0.959	0.986	0.976
25	1.008	1.055	0.995	1.013	1.063	52	1.016	1.076	0.990	1.026	1.093
						53	1.091	0.989	0.987	1.105	1.079
26	1.204	0.971	1.048	1.149	1.169						
27	1.030	1.136	1.000	1.030	1.170	**Mean**	**0.970**	**1.038**	**0.992**	**0.978**	**1.007**

Malmquist index summary of annual means

Year	Effch	Techch	Pech	Sech	Tfpch
2	0.966	1.043	1.000	0.966	1.007
3	0.990	0.981	0.968	1.023	0.972
4	0.985	0.998	1.002	0.983	0.984
5	0.970	1.038	0.992	0.978	1.007
Mean	**0.978**	**1.015**	**0.990**	**0.987**	**0.992**

.../cont.

Appendix 20.4 (cont.)

Malmquist index summary of firm means

Firm	Effch	Techch	Pech	Sech	Tfpch	Firm	Effch	Techch	Pech	Sech	Tfpch
1	0.952	1.036	1.000	0.952	0.986	28	0.956	1.080	1.011	0.946	1.033
2	0.892	1.004	0.923	0.966	0.895	29	1.034	0.985	0.999	1.035	1.018
3	1.013	0.996	1.000	1.013	1.009	30	1.017	1.000	1.002	1.014	1.016
4	0.901	1.068	0.975	0.924	0.962	31	1.042	0.998	1.036	1.006	1.040
5	1.061	1.060	1.001	1.060	1.125	32	0.901	0.984	0.951	0.948	0.886
6	0.988	0.975	0.988	1.000	0.963	33	0.936	1.067	0.999	0.937	0.999
7	0.990	0.993	0.967	1.025	0.984	34	0.937	1.066	1.000	0.937	0.998
8	0.973	1.027	1.000	0.973	0.999	35	0.966	0.996	0.983	0.983	0.963
9	0.972	1.003	0.973	0.999	0.974	36	0.961	1.066	1.026	0.936	1.025
10	0.988	1.001	1.002	0.987	0.990	37	1.000	1.013	1.000	1.000	1.013
11	1.073	1.001	1.000	1.073	1.074	38	0.975	0.996	0.970	1.006	0.971
12	1.038	0.971	0.976	1.063	1.008	39	1.028	1.001	0.987	1.042	1.030
13	1.044	0.999	0.992	1.053	1.043	40	0.981	1.000	0.972	1.009	0.981
14	1.000	0.963	1.000	1.000	0.963	41	0.957	0.994	0.992	0.965	0.951
15	1.018	0.999	1.023	0.995	1.016	42	0.936	1.079	1.008	0.929	1.011
						43	0.963	0.985	0.991	0.971	0.948
16	0.936	1.065	0.991	0.944	0.997						
17	0.936	1.037	0.975	0.960	0.970	44	0.899	0.970	0.960	0.936	0.872
18	1.039	1.001	1.028	1.010	1.040	45	0.927	1.090	0.991	0.935	1.010
19	1.012	0.995	1.012	1.001	1.008	46	0.993	0.995	0.997	0.997	0.989
20	0.928	1.054	0.994	0.933	0.978	47	0.871	1.067	0.917	0.950	0.929
						48	1.013	0.999	0.992	1.022	1.012
21	0.951	1.032	0.996	0.956	0.982						
22	1.042	1.010	1.009	1.034	1.053	49	0.916	1.091	1.002	0.914	0.999
23	0.952	1.025	1.010	0.943	0.975	50	0.989	0.992	1.008	0.981	0.981
24	0.998	0.998	0.995	1.003	0.996	51	0.986	0.981	0.955	1.033	0.967
25	1.017	0.995	0.996	1.021	1.011	52	1.012	0.989	0.984	1.029	1.001
						53	0.986	1.010	0.981	1.005	0.996
26	0.946	0.998	0.951	0.995	0.944						
27	1.043	1.014	1.015	1.027	1.057	Mean	0.978	1.015	0.990	0.987	0.992

Note that all Malmquist index averages are geometric means

Part IV

Advancing Knowledge and Skills
in Efficiency Analysis using
Data Envelopment Analysis

Learning Objectives

By the end of Part 4 you should have a good understanding of:

1. Web sites containing information on DEA.

2. Existing productivity analysis journals.

3. Some of the internationally available DEA textbooks.

4. International courses offered in DEA.

5. How to access DEA software.

6. How to access information on the Operational Research Society.

7. How to undertake DEA analyses using either secondary or primary data.

-21-

Advancing Knowledge and Skills in Data Envelopment Analysis

Joses M. Kirigia

INTRODUCTION

> There are only two qualities in the world: efficiency and inefficiency, and only two sorts of people: the efficient and the inefficient.

George Bernard Shaw 1907, *John Bull's Other Island*, Act IV.

I hope that this book has stimulated in you the enthusiasm for the application of DEA in performance measurement for all types of DMUs. Although the book has focused on health-related circumstances, DEA is a very versatile tool and can be used in many other areas. The literature attests to the application of DEA in agriculture, commerce, the courts, education, industry, market research, prisons, sports, transport, and tourism among other areas. Even though DEA has not received widespread application in those other sectors in Africa, I believe that the time is ripe for such pioneering use.

I envision that over the next two decades Africa shall witness a revolutionary growth in studies involving the application of tools such as DEA in productivity and efficiency monitoring. If you are reading this chapter, I presume that you intend to become an active participant, and not just a passive observer, in that revolution. Should the former be the case, you will need to advance your knowledge and hone your skills in efficiency measurement and DEA application. The various complementary ways of mustering knowledge about DEA and becoming accustomed to the application of this important technique of efficiency measurement are described in this chapter and include the following:

1.   Browsing DEA websites
2.   Reading productivity analysis journals

3. Reading textbooks on DEA
4. Taking courses in DEA
5. Browsing through the relevant software and manuals
6. Joining the Operational Research Society
7. Undertaking DEA analyses using secondary and primary data

Browsing DEA Websites

It is recommended that you browse the following DEA websites:

1. Ali Emrouznejad's DEA homepage at http://www.deazone.com. This is the most comprehensive and resourceful DEA web page globally. It features a DEA glossary, bibliography, list of books, tutorials, datasets, links, models, people and their contacts, courses, software, and discussion lists [1].

2. The Website of Centre for Management of Technology and Entrepreneurship (CMTE) at the University of Toronto at http://www.cmte.utoronto.ca/ and at http://cmte.chem-eng.utoronto.ca/ research/dea.shtml. It has an online library that features lecture notes, thesis abstracts, papers, and presentations. It reports significant CMTE applications of DEA in the service sector. Its programme covers [2]:

    i)   Performance in the financial services and impact of IT investments.

    ii) Incorporating quality into the performance measurement of service organisations.

    iii) Design of benchmarking and continuous improvement programmes.

    iv) Development of visual interactive DEA and managerial tools for benchmarking.

    v)   Transfer of technology to the financial services industry.

3. World Wide Web for operations research and management science (WORMS) housed at the University of Melbourne, Australia [3]: http://www.worms.ms.unimelb.edu.au.

4. Holger Scheel's DEA Website [4] at http://www.wiso.uni-dortmund.de/ lsfg/or/doordea.htm. The site features links, Scheel's research work, text data, and lists of commercial and free software.

Reading Productivity Analysis Journals

Some of the journals that publish articles in DEA include:

1. *Journal of Medical Systems* published by Springer Netherlands. ISSN: 0148-5598 (print version) and 1573-689X (online version). The journal can be accessed at http://www.springer.com/journal/10916. Online submission of manuscripts for consideration can be made at: http://joms.edmgr.com.

2. *Socio-Economic Planning Sciences* journal (ISSN 0038-0121) published by Elsevier.

3. *Journal of Productivity Analysis* published by Springer Netherlands. ISSN: 0895-562X (print version) and ISSN: 1573-0441 (electronic version) The journal publishes theoretical and applied research covering the measurement, explanation, and improvement of productivity..

4. *European Journal of Operational Research* (ISSN: 0377-2217) published by Elsevier Science. The journal publishes original papers that contribute to the methodology of operational research (OR) and to the practice of decision making. It consists of the following sections: continuous optimisation; discrete optimisation; production, manufacturing and logistics; stochastics and statistics; decision support; computing, artificial intelligence and information management; operational research applications; and interfaces with other disciplines. More details about the journal can be found at http://www.elsevier.com/ wps/find/journaldescription.cws_home/505543/description.

5. *International Journal of Production Economics* (ISSN: 0925-5273) published by Elsevier. It focuses on topics covering the interface between engineering, economics, and management. This interdisciplinary journal considers whole cycles of activities such as the product life cycle (research, design, development, test, launch and disposal) and the material flow cycle (supply, production, and distribution). You can find more information about the journal at http://www.elsevier.com/wps/find/journaleditorialboard.cws_home/5056 47/.

6. *Journal of Operational Research Society* (ISSN: 0160-5682) published by Palgrave Macmillan. The web page for the journal is http://www.palgrave-journals.com/jors/index.html.

7. *Annals of Operations Research Journal* (Print version ISSN 0254-5330; online version 1572-9338) published by Springer Netherlands. Website: http://www.springerlink.com/content/1572-9338/.

8. *Journal of Management Studies* (Print version ISSN: 0022-2380; online version ISSN: 1467-6486) published by Blackwell. This is a multidisciplinary journal that publishes theoretical and empirical articles on organisation theory and behavior and strategic and human resource management. More information about the journal can be accessed at http://www.blackwellpublishing.com/.

9.   *Health Care Management Science* journal (Print version ISSN: 1386-9620; online version 1572-9389) published by Springer Netherlands. This interdisciplinary journal covers areas such as productivity analysis and operations analysis in health care, health information systems, health care financial management, strategic management in health care, managed care, and systems dynamics. More information about the journal and how to subscribe can be found at http://www.springer.com/.

Reading DEA Textbooks

1.   Ali Emrouznejad and Victor Podinovski (Editors). *Data envelopment analysis and performance management*. Birmingham: University of Aston; 2004. ISBN: 090268373X. The book covers articles on Olympic games, banking services, teacher qualifications, telecommunications, water and sewerage services, electric services, health, wine production, insurance companies, agriculture, environment, tourism, research, and railroads. The book can be downloaded for free from: http://www.deazone.com/books/index.htm or through email from DEAbook@DEAzone.com.

2.   Ali Emrouznejad, Rodney Green, and Vladimir Krivonozhko (editors). *Efficiency and Productivity Analysis in the 21st Century: International DEA Symposium 2002.* Moscow: Institute for Systems Analysis of Russian Academy of Sciences and Global S. Consulting Company; 2002. The book features articles on theory and methodology, financial institutions, production systems, applications in the public sector, applications in agriculture, and novel applications of DEA.

3.   Emmanuel Thanassoulis. *Introduction to the Theory and Application of Data Envelopment Analysis: A Foundation Text with Integrated Software.* Boston: Kluwer Academic Publisher; 2001. This book is specifically aimed at readers with no prior exposure to DEA and who wish to learn the essentials, how DEA works, its key uses, and the mechanics of using it.

4.   Jati K. Sengupta: *Dynamic and Stochastic Efficiency Analysis: Economics of Data Envelopment Analysis.* London: World Scientific Publishing; 2000. This book extends the dynamic and stochastic analysis of economic efficiency by using the techniques of data envelopment analysis. It provides information on finance and management, treatment of private sector industries, portfolio models in finance, quality control techniques in managerial performance, and the role of market competition and more.

5.   William W. Cooper, Lawrence M. Seiford, Kaoru Tone: *Data Envelopment Analysis: A Comprehensive Text with Models, Applications, References and DEA-Solver Software.* Boston: Kluwer Academic Publisher; 2006.

6.   Tim Coelli, D.S. Prasada Rao, Christopher J. O'Donnell, George E. Battese: *An Introduction to Efficiency and Productivity Analysis*. New York: Springer; 2005. The book is an authoritative introduction to efficiency and productivity analysis that discusses, in an accessible manner, the least-squares econometric production models, total factor productivity (TFP) indices, data envelopment analysis (DEA), and stochastic frontiers.

7.   Rolf Färe, Shawna Grosskopf, R. Robert Russell (eds.): *Index Numbers Essays in Honour of Sten Malmquist*. Boston: Kluwer Academic Publishers; 1997. This is an important book for those who wish to get a good grasp of the work of Malmquist and its subsequent applications.

8.   Abraham Charnes, William W. Cooper, Arie Y. Lewin, Lawrence M. Seiford: *Data Envelopment Analysis: Theory, Methodology and Applications*. Boston: Kluwer Academic Publishers; 1995.

Other references for additional books on efficiency measurement can be accessed by selecting the "Books" icon at http://www.deazone.com/software/index.htm.

Taking Courses in DEA

(a)   The Centre for Efficiency and Productivity Analysis (CEPA of the University of New Queensland offers doctorate and masters degree programmes on productivity and efficiency analysis. In addition, CEPA provides short courses and workshops on productivity and efficiency analysis. These courses are very relevant for economists who wish to hone their knowledge and skills on efficiency measurement within a short period. Refer to the CEPA website at http://www.uq.edu/economics/cepa/teaching.htm to view the forthcoming and past workshops. At the CEPA website you will also find several theoretical and applied discussion papers on productivity and efficiency measurements. The papers employ parametric (econometric) and non-parametric (mathematical programming) approaches. I highly recommend that you make this website one of your favourite sites.

(b)   Aston University offers a course on performance management. This is the University where Dr Ali Emrouznejad and other DEA gurus are based. You can get more information on the courses offered at Aston from http://www.deazone.com/course/index.htm.

Browsing Through DEA Software and Manuals

Free software

1.   *DEAP (Version 2.1):* This software can be used to construct DEA frontiers for calculation of technical, allocative, and cost efficiencies and Malmquist total factor productivity (TFP) indices. The software [6] and

its manual [7] can be downloaded for free at http://www.uq.edu/economics/cepa/deap.htm. The manual explains and demonstrates how to set up your data and execute DEA estimations. The software was developed by Professor Tim Coelli, School of Economics, University of New Queensland.

2. *Efficiency Measurement System (EMS):* This software [8] and manual [9] can be downloaded for free at http://www.wiso.uni-dortmund.de/lsfg/or/scheel/ems/. The manual explains how to prepare the input-output data; how to prepare weights restricts; how to start EMS and load data; how to run a DEA model; and how results are displayed in a table. The software was developed by Dr. Holger Scheel, Operations Research, Und Wirtschaftsinformatik, Universitat Dortmund, D-44221 Dortmund, Germany. Dr. Scheel welcomes questions and suggestions for further development of the software.

Commercial software

1. *Banxia Frontier Analyst:* This commercial software is good for estimating technical efficiency of DMUs. The software is user friendly and has a graphic facility for presenting DEA results. Currently, it does not have a facility for estimating allocative and cost efficiencies and the Malmquist TFP indices. It is available at www.banxia.com.

2. *OnFront2:* I have not used this software, but I understand it is good for measuring economic productivity and quality.

3. *PIM-DEAsoft V1:* The software was developed by Professor Thanssoulis and Dr. Ali Emrouznejad. It can be used to assess DMUs under constant or variable returns to scale, non-increasing or non-decreasing returns to scale, restrictions on the input/output weights, and restrictions (applying either to the unit assessed only or to all units) on the product of input/output weights and corresponding input/output level; the restriction. In addition, the software can be used to estimate performance targets with varying priorities over the improvement of inputs/outputs; assess the super efficiency of units; identify whether increasing, constant, or decreasing returns to scale hold locally for units efficient under variable returns to scale; and compute Malmquist productivity indices and their decomposition into boundary shift and efficiency catch-up among other applications. You can get more information on the software at: http://deasoftware.co.uk/AboutDevelopers.asp.

Joining the Operational Research Society

The Operational Research Society (OR) was founded over 50 years ago to succeed the Operational Research Club, which was set up in 1948. The OR Society is the world's oldest learned society catering to the Operational Research (OR) profession. It is also one of the largest professional societies in the world with 3,000 members in 53 countries. Some of the key activities of the OR society include [10]:

1. Providing extensive training programme in OR.

2. Publishing journals to disseminate the latest developments in OR.

3. Maintaining a library of International Abstracts in OR.

4. Facilitating free exchange of conference presentations, case studies, lecture notes, and many other types of documents.

5. Production of publications such as *Issue Explorer* and a downloadable multimedia presentation package designed for use in schools.

6. Sponsoring summer schools for researchers and research projects on OR.

7. Establishing and supporting OR archive and sponsoring the official history of OR.

8. Supporting conferences to further OR knowledge.

Undertaking DEA analyses using secondary and primary data

An effective way of acquiring skills for DEA analysis is to immerse yourself in an actual analysis using secondary or primary data. Irrespective of the kind of data you might be using, you will need to go through a number of sequential steps as follows:

1. *Define the research problem:* These are the knowledge or information gaps that you intend to bridge with your analysis.

2. *Determine/select the input and output variables:* The choice of variables should be guided by (*a*) research questions you are intent on answering, for example, if the question relates to allocative efficiency, you will need both quantities of outputs and quantities and prices of inputs; (*b*) published literature; and (*c*) availability of data.

3. *Determine the type of model:* This entails choosing between input-oriented and output-oriented model. The minimisation of input usage, cost, or expenditure implies the use of the input-oriented model. On the other hand, the maximisation of outcomes, outputs, revenues, or profits entails the use of the output-oriented model.

4. *Obtain data:* It is cost-effective to first explore the availability of suitable/appropriate secondary data from national and/or international sources. National statistical reports from the national central bureau of statistics, sectoral management information systems, and national research institutions may be a good starting point. On the other hand,

international organisations (e.g., the World Bank, IMF, WHO, UNDP human development reports, and other United Nations Agencies) usually publish statistical tables in their databases or annual technical reports. These reports are usually available online for free downloading at the various organisational websites. If there is no appropriate data available from secondary sources to address your research problem, you will have to design and implement a primary study to gather the data directly from the DMUs, for example, hospitals, university departments, schools, business firms, and farms, among other sources. It is beyond the scope of this book to delve into the research methodologies, but you are encouraged to consult any research methodology textbook in your library.

5. ***Choice of DEA software:*** The choice of the software to use will depend on a number of considerations including (*a*) size of your dataset vis-à-vis the size that can be handled by various software; (*b*) operating capacity of your computer; (*c*) cost of the software vis-à-vis your resources; (*d*) capacity of the software to handle your problem (e.g., some software are only capable of estimating technical efficiency).

6. ***Analysis of factual data about DMUs' performance:*** Here, I suggest that you follow the instructions contained in the manual of the software you have chosen to use.

7. ***Report writing:*** The report may have the following sections:

   (a) *Abstract:* Aim at having one or two sentences on background, purpose/objective, method, results, and conclusion in this section.

   (b) *Introduction:* This section should contain a paragraph on the background/context, a paragraph on pertinent literature highlighting knowledge/information gaps, a paragraph on objectives of the study, and a paragraph on the rationale of the study.

   (c) *Methods:* This section should cover the conceptual framework; model, inputs and outputs; population/sample size, location, sampling technique, materials (description of data collection instruments), data sources and collection procedures; and data analysis process (including mention of software used).

   (d) *Results:* This section usually includes three elements [11]: (i) a statement that locates the table(s) or figure(s) where results can be found; (ii) statements that present the most important findings; and (iii) statements that comment on the results. I suggest that you refer to the preceding chapters and other published literature on how DEA results are usually presented in tabular and graphic forms.

   (e) *Discussion:* Ideally, the section contains six informational elements as follows:

(i) a reference to the main purpose or hypothesis of the study; (ii) a review of the most important findings, whether or not they support the original hypothesis, and whether they agree with the findings of other researchers; (iii) possible explanations for or speculations about the findings; (iv) limitations of the study that restrict the extent to which the findings can be generalised; (v) implications of the study (generalisations from the results); and (vi) recommendations for future research and practical applications. [11, p.162]

(f) Conclusion.

8. ***Working out the plan of productivity improvement:*** In light of the results, your client might request you, in conjunction with his/her management team(s), to prepare a plan for productivity improvement taking the best practice into account. Software like DEAP will have provided you with target inputs and outputs. In the light of that you will need to discuss with the managers feasible ways of alleviating the inefficiencies obserbved in the use of various inputs; what it would cost (if anything); timeframe; and responsible persons. There may be need for a detailed study of the operations of the "best practice" DMUs that can be emulated by the inefficient ones.

REFERENCES

1 http://www.DEAzone.com.

2. http://cmte.chem-eng.utoronto.ca/research/dea.shtml.

3. http://www.worms.ms.unimelb.edu.au.

4. http://www.wiso.uni-dortmund.de/lsfg/or/doordea.htm.

5. http://www.uq.edu/economics/cepa/teaching.htm.

6. http://www.uq.edu/economics/cepa/deap.htm.

7. Coelli TJ. *A guide to DEAP version 2.1: a data envelopment analysis [computer] program.* Centre for Efficiency and Productivity Analysis (CEPA) Working Paper 96/08. University of New England, Armidale, NSW Australia; 1996.

8. http://www.wiso.uni-dortmund.de/lsfg/or/scheel/ems/.

9. Scheel H. EMS. *Efficiency measurement system user's manual*, version 1.3. Dortmund: University of Dortmund. http://www.wiso.uni-dortmund.de/lsfg/or/scheel/ems/.

10. http://www.theorsociety.com/.

11. Weissberg R, Buker S. *Writing up research.* London: Prentice-Hall; 1987.

Glossary

Allocative efficiency: A situation where for any level of health service production of a decision-making unit (DMU), inputs are used in the proportion that minimises the cost of production, given input prices. Estimation of allocative efficiency requires data on quantities of health service outputs, health system inputs, and input prices.

Benchmarking: The process of comparing the performance of an individual health system DMU against a benchmark or ideal level of performance. Benchmarks can be set on the basis of performance over time across a sample of similar DMUs or against some externally set standard.

Best practice: The set of management and work practices which results in the highest potential or optimal quantity and combination of health service outputs for a given quantity and combination of inputs (*productivity*) for a group of similar DMUs (e.g., health programme, health post, health centre, district hospital, provincial hospital, tertiary hospital, district health system, national and international health system). Thus, best practice can be identified at any of those levels of health systems.

Cost efficiency: A scenario where a health system DMU is *technically efficient* and *allocatively efficient* and hence produces a given quantity, quality, and mix of health outputs at minimum possible cost given existing knowledge of technologies and people's preferences.

Data envelopment analysis (DEA): A *linear programming* technique which identifies *best practice* within a sample or population of health system DMUs. DEA measures *efficiency* based on differences between observed and best practice DMUs.

Decision-making units (DMUs): The production units (e.g., health programmes, health posts, health centres, hospitals, hospital departments, and national health systems) being examined in a DEA study.

Dynamic efficiency: Success with which health entrepreneurs alter technology and products following changes in consumer preferences and productive opportunities.

Effectiveness: Degree to which the outputs of a health DMU achieve its stated objectives (e.g., the objective of a health centre might be to optimise provision of antenatal, delivery, and postnatal services; immunisation and growth monitoring services; health education; protection of water sources; and promotion of ventilated improved pit latrines).

Efficiency: Degree to which the observed use of health resources (inputs) to produce health-related outputs of a given quality matches the optimal use of resources to produce outputs of a given quality. This can be assessed in terms of *technical efficiency* and *allocative efficiency*.

External operating environment: Factors which affect the productivity of DMUs that are not in the direct control of health managers (e.g., weather, epidemics, natural disasters, cultural beliefs and practices).

Health: WHO defines health as a state of complete physical, mental and social well-being and not merely absence of disease or infirmity. Social scientists define health as the ability to perform one's societal expected functions (or roles).

Health system: All actors, institutions, and resources that undertake health actions and where the primary intent of a health action is to improve health.

Health system building blocks: WHO health system framework consists of the six building blocks of service delivery; health workforce; information; medical products, vaccines and technologies; financing; and leadership/governance.

Health system goals: The WHO recognises the four health system goals/outcomes of improved health (level and equity); responsiveness; social and financial risk protection; and improved efficiency.

Input: A factor or resource used in the production of a good or service (e.g., human resources for health, medicines, non-pharmaceutical supplies, buildings, medical equipment, vehicles, computers and software, and utilities such as water, electricity, telephone, fax, Internet, and email).

Linear programme: A set of linear mathematical equations for which a solution can be obtained subject to an upper bound (maximisation) or a lower bound (minimisation).

Outputs: Goods and services provided to entities or persons outside the production unit. For example: (i) outputs of pharmaceutical companies are quantities of quality drugs produced; (ii) outputs of Expanded Programme for Immunisation are the numbers of children who are fully immunised with specific antigens; (iii) outputs of health education programme are the number of persons educated; (iv) outputs of health centres are the number of curative outpatient visits, number of people reached by the preventive services; (v) outputs of hospitals are numbers of outpatient visits, preventive services provided, admissions/discharges, students trained, and research outputs.

Peers: In DEA studies, the group of *best practice* health system DMUs with which a relatively inefficient DMU is compared.

Production frontier: The curve plotting the minimum amount of a health input(s) necessary to produce a given quantity of health-related output(s).

Production technology: Know-how incorporated in health service production processes that determine the manner in which health system inputs can be converted to health system outputs.

Productivity: A measure of the physical health system output produced from the use of a given quantity of health system inputs. This may include all health system inputs and all health system outputs (*total factor productivity*) or a subset of health system inputs and health system outputs (*partial productivity*). DMU productivity varies as a result of differences in *production technology*, differences in the *technical efficiency* of the health system or its component, and the *external environment* in which production occurs.

Pure technical efficiency (PTE): Proportion of health system DMU *technical efficiency* that cannot be attributed to deviations from optimal scale (*scale efficiency*).

Returns to scale: Relationship between health system DMU output and inputs. Returns to scale can be constant, increasing, or decreasing depending on whether output increases in proportion to, more than or less than inputs, respectively. In the case of multiple inputs and outputs, it refers to how outputs change when all inputs are varied by an equal proportion.

Scale efficiency: The extent to which a health system DMU can take advantage of returns to scale by altering its size towards optimal scale (which is defined as the region in which there are constant *returns to scale* in the relationship between outputs and inputs).

Slacks: The extra amount by which a health system input (output) can be reduced (increased) to attain *technical efficiency* after all inputs (outputs) have been reduced (increased) in equal proportions to reach the *production frontier*. This is a feature of the piece-wise linear production frontier derived when using DEA.

Technical efficiency: A scenario in which a health-related DMU produces optimal/maximum outputs from the available health service inputs. Alternatively, it can be viewed as a situation in which a DMU produces a given level of outputs with the least quantities of inputs.

Total factor productivity (TFP): Ratio of the quantity of all health system DMU outputs to the quantity of all inputs. TFP can be measured by an index of the ratio of all outputs (weighted by revenue shares) to all inputs (weighted by cost shares).

Index

Abuja Declaration, 247
Adolescent fertility rate. *see* maternal health
Africa, 37
 disease burden, 37
 health challenges, 38
 health status, 3
 Regional Child Survival Strategy, 6
African Union, 53, 479
Algiers Declaration, 39, *see also* Ouagadougou Declaration
Allocative efficiency, 53, 108, 118, 219, 272, 373, 516
Antenatal care. *see* maternal health
Antiretroviral therapy, 9
Average product, 73
Average total cost, 99
Average variable cost, 98
Banxia Frontier Analyst software, 512, *See also* DEA software
Benchmarking, 516
Best practice, 516
Best practice frontier, 205, 249
Botswana, 367
Centre for Efficiency and Productivity Analysis (CEPA), 511
Child mortality, 4
Cobb-Douglas production, 82, 83
Coelli, Tim. *See* DEAP Version 2.1 software
Constant returns to scale, 145, 250, 294, *See also* increasing returns to scale, decreasing returns to scale
Constant returns to scale efficiency change, 128
Convex isoquant, 79
Cost efficiency, 516, *See also* total economic efficiency
 calculating, 118
Cost function, 94
Data envelope. *See* best practice frontier
Data envelopment analysis, 58, 133, 516, *See also* efficiency, methods of
 advantages, 63, 219
 application, 143, 161, 171, 204, 217, 239
 disadvantages, 64
 strengths and weaknesses, 148, 403
DEA resources, 507–15
DEA software, 346, 511
DEAP Version 2.1 software, 116, 129, 251, 454, 455, *See also* Efficiency Measurement System software
Decision-making units (DMUs), 516

Declaration on Primary Health Care and Health Systems, 39
Decreasing returns to scale, 145, 250, 294, *See also* increasing returns to scale, constant returns to scale
Diarrhoeal diseases, 14
Disability-adjusted life expectancy, 62
Disability-adjusted life years, 62
Diseconomies of scale. *See* decreasing returns to scale
DOTS. *see* tuberculosis
Dynamic efficiency, 516
Economic efficiency, 53, 106, 273, 340, 373
Economies of scale. *See* increasing returns to scale
Edgeworth box, 89
Effectiveness, 516
Efficiency, 52, 53, 85, 205, 219, 255, 300, 516
 measurement challenges, 105
 measurement concepts, 106
 measurement methods, 111
 measurement of, 55, 317
 strategies for improvement, 300
Efficiency analysis, 52
 methods of, 219
Efficiency frontier, 58, 115
Efficiency Measurement System software (EMS), 454, *See also* DEA software
Efficiency monitoring, 351
Elasticity of substitution, 83
EMS. *See* Efficiency Measurement System software
External operating environment, 517
Factor intensity, 84
Family planning. *see* maternal health
Fifty-Sixth WHO Regional Committee for Africa, 351
Fisher index, 343
Free Disposal Hall, 317, 399
Ghana, 139, 141
Health, 517
Health financing, 16–19, 48
Health information, 47
Health infrastructure, 16
Health promotion, 155, 255
Health services
 cost, 93
Health system, 15, 43, 267, 517
 factors of production, 69
 leadership and governance, 48
 outputs, 71

production technology, 71
WHO framework, 44
Health system building blocks, 517
Health system goals, 517
Health technologies, 47
Health workforce, 15, 45
HIV/AIDS, 8
mother-to-child transmission, 9
Hotelling's T-squared generalised means test, 222
Immunisation, 5
Increasing returns to scale, 145, 250, *See also* decreasing returns to scale, constant returns to scale
Infant mortality. *see* child mortality
Input, 517
Integrated Management of Childhood Illness, 6
Isocost, 272
Isoquant, 272
Isoquant map, 80
Kenya, 161
Kinked isoquant. *See* linear programming isoquant
Law of diminishing marginal returns, 75
Leontief isoquant, 76
Linear isoquant, 77
Linear programme, 517
Linear programming isoquant, 79
Luenberger indicators, 371
Malaria, 8
mortality rate, 10
Malmquist productivity index, 343
advantages, 375
Malmquist Total Factor Productivity Index, 126
Marginal cost, 99
Marginal physical product, 73
Marginal product, 81
Marginal rate of technical substitution, 78, 83
Marginal rate of transformation, 92
MDG 2, 13
MDG 4. *See* child mortality
MDG 6, 8
MDG 7, 13
Millenium Development Goals, 3, 26
health-related, 3
Neonatal mortality. *See* child mortality
New Partnership for Africa's Development (NEPAD), 269
Non-communicable diseases, 11
OnFront2. See DEA software
Oral rehydration therapy, 6
Ouagadougou Declaration, 19, 39, 256

framework for implementation, 39
Outputs, 517
Overall efficiency. *See* total economic efficiency
Pareto-Koopman efficiency, 400
Paris Declaration, 40
Peers, 517
PIM-DEAsoft V1. See DEAsoftware
Product transformation curve. *See* production possibilities frontier
Production contract curve, 91
Production frontier, 517
Production function, 71, 272
multiple output, 89
Production possibilities frontier, 91, *see* also technical efficiency
Production technology, 517
Productivity, 343, 375, 518
Property of free disposal, 76
Pure technical efficiency, 518
Quality-adjusted life years, 62
Returns to scale, 144, 250, 294, 518
Roll Back Malaria Partnership, 11
Sanitation, 14
Scale efficiency, 518
Scale efficiency change, 324
Service delivery, 44
Seychelles, 312
Slacks, 518
STATA software, 222
Stochastic Frontier Analysis, 270
Stochastic frontier regression analysis. *See* efficiency analysis, methods of
sub-Saharan Africa
health challenges, 218
Technical efficiency, 85, 121, 219, 249, 272, 315, 373, 518
meaning and types of, 53
measuring, 112
Tornqvist index, 343
Total economic cost, 95
Total economic efficiency, 108
Total factor productivity, 518
Total fixed costs, 95
Total variable costs, 96
Vaccine-preventable diseases, 5, *See also* child mortality
Variable returns to scale technical efficiency, 116
WHO, 53
WHO Commission on Macroeconomics and Health, 21, 247, 269, 338
World Bank, 53
World Health Assembly Resolutions on NCDs, 12